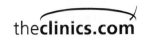

MEDICAL CLINICS

OF NORTH AMERICA

Atrial Fibrillation

GUEST EDITORS
Ranjan K. Thakur, MD
Andrea Natale, MD, FACC, FHRS

January 2008 • Volume 92 • Number 1

SAUNDERS

An Imprint of Elsevier, Inc.
PHILADELPHIA LONDON TORONTO MONTREAL SYDNEY TOKYO

W.B. SAUNDERS COMPANY
A Division of Elsevier Inc.

1600 John F. Kennedy Boulevard • Suite 1800 • Philadelphia, Pennsylvania 19103-2899

http://www.theclinics.com

MEDICAL CLINICS OF NORTH AMERICA
January 2008
Editor: Rachel Glover

Volume 92, Number 1
ISSN 0025-7125
ISBN-13: 978-1-4160-5860-1
ISBN-10: 1-4160-5860-5

The ideas and opinions expressed in *Medical Clinics of North America* do not necessarily reflect those of the Publisher. The Publisher does not assume any responsibility for any injury and/or damage to persons or property arising out of or related to any use of the material contained in this periodical. The reader is advised to check the appropriate medical literature and the product information currently provided by the manufacturer of each drug to be administered to verify the dosage, the method and duration of administration, or contraindications. It is the responsibility of the treating physician or other health care professional, relying on independent experience and knowledge of the patient, to determine drug dosages and the best treatment for the patient. Mention of any product in this issue should not be construed as endorsement by the contributors, editors, or the Publisher of the product or manufacturers' claims.

Medical Clinics of North America (ISSN 0025-7125) is published bimonthly by W.B. Saunders, 360 Park Avenue South, New York, NY 10010-1710. Business and editorial offices: 1600 John F. Kennedy Boulevard, Suite 1800, Philadelphia, PA 19103-2899. Accounting and circulation offices: 6277 Sea Harbor Drive, Orlando, FL 32887-4800. Periodicals postage paid at New York, NY, and additional mailing offices. Subscription prices are USD 173 per year for US individuals, USD 306 per year for US institutions, USD 89 per year for US students, USD 220 per year for Canadian individuals, USD 389 per year for Canadian institutions, USD 131 per year for Canadian students, USD 250 per year for international individuals, USD 389 per year for international institutions and USD 131 per year for international students. To receive student/resident rate, orders must be accompanied by name of affiliated institution, date of term, and the *signature* of program/residency coordinator on institution letterhead. Orders will be billed at individual rate until proof of status is received. Foreign air speed delivery is included in all *Clinics* subscription prices. All prices are subject to change without notice. POSTMASTER: Send address changes to *Medical Clinics of North America*, Elsevier Periodicals Customer Service, 6277 Sea Harbor Drive, Orlando, FL 32887-4800. **Customer Service: 1-800-654-2452 (US). From outside of the USA, call (+1) 407-345-1000. E-mail: hhspcs@harcourt.com.**

Reprints. For copies of 100 or more, of articles in this publication, please contact the Commercial Reprints Department, Elsevier Inc., 360 Park Avenue South, New York, New York 10010-1710. Tel.: (+1) (212) 633-3813; Fax: (+1) (212) 462-1935; E-mail: reprints@elsevier.com.

Medical Clinics of North America is also published in Spanish by McGraw-Hill Interamericana Editores S. A., P.O. Box 5-237, 06500 Mexico, D.F., Mexico.

Medical Clinics of North America is covered in *Index Medicus, Current Contents, ASCA, Excerpta Medica, Science Citation Index,* and *ISI/BIOMED.*

Printed in the United States of America.

GOAL STATEMENT

The goal of *Medical Clinics of North America* is to keep practicing physicians up to date with current clinical practice by providing timely articles reviewing the state of the art in patient care.

ACCREDITATION

The *Medical Clinics of North America* is planned and implemented in accordance with the Essential Areas and Policies of the Accreditation Council for Continuing Medical Education (ACCME) through the joint sponsorship of the University of Virginia School of Medicine and Elsevier. The University of Virginia School of Medicine is accredited by the ACCME to provide continuing medical education for physicians.

The University of Virginia School of Medicine designates this educational activity for a maximum of 90 *AMA PRA Category 1 Credits*™. Physicians should only claim credit commensurate with the extent of their participation in the activity.

The American Medical Association has determined that physicians not licensed in the US who participate in this CME activity are eligible for *AMA PRA Category 1 Credits*™.

Credit can be earned by reading the text material, taking the CME examination online at http://www.theclinics.com/home/cme, and completing the evaluation. After taking the test, you will be required to review any and all incorrect answers. Following completion of the test and evaluation, your credit will be awarded and you may print your certificate.

FACULTY DISCLOSURE/CONFLICT OF INTEREST

The University of Virginia School of Medicine, as an ACCME accredited provider, endorses and strives to comply with the Accreditation Council for Continuing Medical Education (ACCME) Standards of Commercial Support, Commonwealth of Virginia statutes, University of Virginia policies and procedures, and associated federal and private regulations and guidelines on the need for disclosure and monitoring of proprietary and financial interests that may affect the scientific integrity and balance of content delivered in continuing medical education activities under our auspices.

The University of Virginia School of Medicine requires that all CME activities accredited through this institution be developed independently and be scientifically rigorous, balanced and objective in the presentation/discussion of its content, theories and practices.

All authors/editors participating in an accredited CME activity are expected to disclose to the readers relevant financial relationships with commercial entities occurring within the past 12 months (such as grants or research support, employee, consultant, stock holder, member of speakers bureau, etc.). The University of Virginia School of Medicine will employ appropriate mechanisms to resolve potential conflicts of interest to maintain the standards of fair and balanced education to the reader. Questions about specific strategies can be directed to the Office of Continuing Medical Education, University of Virginia School of Medicine, Charlottesville, Virginia.

The authors/editors listed below have identified no professional or financial affiliations for themselves or their spouse/partner:
Emelia J. Benjamin, MD, ScM; Thomas D. Callahan, IV, MD; Chung-Chuan Chou, MD; Emily Laine Conway, MD; Patrick T. Ellinor, MD, PhD; Rachel Glover (Acquisitions Editor); Krit Jongnarangsin, MD; Gautham Kalahasty, MD; William B. Kannel, MD, MPH, FACC; Atul Khasnis, MD; Susan S. Kim, MD; Bradley P. Knight, MD; Calum A. MacRae, MD, PhD; Simone Musco, MD; Andrea Natale, MD (Guest Editor); Navinder S. Sawhney, MD; Ranjan K. Thakur, MD, FRCP, FACC, FHRS (Guest Editor); and, B. Alexander Yi, MD, PhD.

The authors/editors listed below identified the following professional or financial affiliations for themselves or their spouse/partner:
Peng-Sheng Chen, MD is a consultant for Medtronic Inc., and has received research equipment from Medtronic Inc. and Cryocarth.
Kenneth Ellenbogen, MD is an independent contractor for Medtronic, Boston Scientific, and St. Jude Medical, is a consultant for Boston Scientific and Sun Biomedical, and serves on the Speaker's Bureau for Medtronic, Boston Scientific, St. Jude, and Sun.
Gregory K. Feld, MD is a consultant, on the advisory committee, and a stockowner in CryoCor; and is a consultant, on the advisory committee, a stockholder, and a patent holder for Medwaves.
A. Marc Gillinov, MD is a consultant for Edwards Lifesciences, AtriCure, and Medtronic; and is on the speaker's bureau for Guidant.
Peter Kowey, MD is a consultant for Sanofi-Aventis, Proctor and Gamble, Solvay, and Astella.
Hakan Oral, MD is a consultant, owns stock in, and is a patent holder for Ablation Frontiers, Inc. and has received research grants from St. Jude Medical, Boston Scientific, and Reliant Pharmaceuticals.
Benzy J. Padanilam, MD is a consultant for Boston Scientific.
Eric N. Prystowsky, MD is a consultant for BARD and Sanofi-Aventis and serves on the Board of Directors for Sterotaxis and Cardio Net.
Vivek Y. Reddy, MD is a consultant for Biosense-Webster, St. Jude Medical, and Boston Scientific.
Adam E. Saltman, MD, PhD is a consultant for Cardima Corp, Boston Scientific Corp, and Medtronic Corp.
Albert L. Waldo, MD is an independent contractor for Boehringer Ingelheim; is a consultant for CryoCor and GSK; and is a consultant and on the speaker's bureau for Reliant.

Disclosure of Discussion of non-FDA approved uses for pharmaceutical products and/or medical devices:
The University of Virginia School of Medicine, as an ACCME provider, requires that all faculty presenters identify and disclose any "off label" uses for pharmaceutical and medical device products. The University of Virginia School of Medicine recommends that each physician fully review all the available data on new products or procedures prior to instituting them with patients.

TO ENROLL

To enroll in the Medical Clinics of North America Continuing Medical Education program, call customer service at 1-800-654-2452 or visit us online at http://www.theclinics.com/home/cme. The CME program is available to subscribers for an additional fee of USD 205.

FORTHCOMING ISSUES

March 2008

Hospital Medicine
Scott A. Flanders, MD, Vikas I. Parekh, MD,
and Lakshmi Halasyamani, MD, *Guest Editors*

May 2008

Common Gastroenterologic and Hepatobiliary Complications
Mitchell S. Cappell, MD, PhD, *Guest Editor*

July 2008

Women's Health
Tony Ogburn, MD, and Carolyn Voss, MD,
Guest Editors

RECENT ISSUES

November 2007

Metabolic Syndrome
Robert T. Yanagisawa, MD and
Derek LeRoith, MD, PhD, *Guest Editors*

September 2007

Nanomedicine
Chiming Wei, MD, PhD, *Guest Editor*

July 2007

Acute Myocardial Infarction
Mandeep Singh, MD and
David R. Holmes, Jr., MD, *Guest Editors*

May 2007

Bariatric Surgery Primer for the Internist
Nilesh A. Patel, MD and Lisa S. Koche, MD,
Guest Editors

March 2007

Pain Management, Part II
Howard S. Smith, MD, *Guest Editor*

THE CLINICS ARE NOW AVAILABLE ONLINE!

Access your subscription at:
http://www.theclinics.com

GUEST EDITORS

RANJAN K. THAKUR, MD, Michigan State University, Thoracic and Cardiovascular Institute, Sparrow Health System, Lansing, Michigan

ANDREA NATALE, MD, FACC, FHRS, Consulting Professor of Medicine, Stanford University, Palo Alto, California

CONTRIBUTORS

EMELIA J. BENJAMIN, MD, ScM, Professor of Medicine and Epidemiology, Boston University School of Medicine and School of Public Health, Boston; The Framingham Heart Study, Framingham, Massachusetts

THOMAS D. CALLAHAN IV, MD, Fellow, Cardiac Pacing and Electrophysiology, Cleveland Clinic, Cleveland, Ohio

PENG-SHENG CHEN, MD, Professor of Medicine and Director, Krannert Institute of Cardiology and the Division of Cardiology, Department of Medicine, Indiana University School of Medicine, Indianapolis, Indiana

CHUNG-CHUAN CHOU, MD, Assistant Professor of Medicine, The Second Section of Cardiology, Chang Gung Memorial Hospital and Chang Gung University College of Medicine, Taipei, Taiwan

EMILY L. CONWAY, MD, Fellow, Division of Cardiovascular Diseases, Main Line Heart Center, Wynnewood, Pennsylvania

KENNETH ELLENBOGEN, MD, Kontos Professor of Medicine; Vice Chair, Division of Cardiology; Director, Cardiac Electrophysiology, Department of Internal Medicine, Virginia Commonwealth University, Richmond, Virginia

PATRICK T. ELLINOR, MD, PhD, Assistant Professor, Cardiac Arrhythmia Service and Cardiovascular Research Center, Massachusetts General Hospital and Harvard Medical School, Boston, Massachusetts

GREGORY K. FELD, MD, Professor of Medicine; Director, Clinical Cardiac Electrophysiology Program, Division of Cardiology, University of California Medical Center, San Diego, California

A. MARC GILLINOV, MD, Surgical Director, the Center for Atrial Fibrillation, The Judith Dion Pyle Endowed Chair in Heart Valve Research, Department of Thoracic and Cardiovascular Surgery, The Cleveland Clinic Foundation, Cleveland, Ohio

KRIT JONGNARANGSIN, MD, Assistant Professor, Division of Cardiovascular Medicine, University of Michigan, Veterans Affairs Ann Arbor Healthcare System, Ann Arbor, Michigan

GAUTHAM KALAHASTY, MD, Assistant Professor of Medicine, Division of Cardiology, Department of Internal Medicine, Virginia Commonwealth University, Richmond, Virginia

WILLIAM B. KANNEL, MD, MPH, FACC, Professor of Medicine and Epidemiology, Boston University School of Medicine, Boston; The Framingham Heart Study, Framingham, Massachusetts

ATUL KHASNIS, MD, Michigan State University, Thoracic and Cardiovascular Institute, Sparrow Health System, Lansing, Michigan

SUSAN S. KIM, MD, Assistant Professor of Medicine, Clinical Cardiac Electrophysiology, Section of Cardiology, Department of Medicine, University of Chicago Hospitals, University of Chicago, Chicago, Illinois

BRADLEY P. KNIGHT, MD, Professor of Medicine, Clinical Cardiac Electrophysiology, Section of Cardiology, Department of Medicine, University of Chicago Hospitals, University of Chicago; Director, Clinical Cardiac Electrophysiology Laboratory, University of Chicago Hospitals, Chicago, Illinois

PETER R. KOWEY, MD, Chief, Division of Cardiovascular Diseases, Main Line Heart Center, Wynnewood; Professor of Medicine and Clinical Pharmacology, Thomas Jefferson University, Philadelphia, Pennsylvania

CALUM A. MACRAE, MB, ChB, PhD, Assistant Professor, Cardiology Division and Cardiovascular Research Center, Massachusetts General Hospital and Harvard Medical School, Boston, Massachusetts

SIMONE MUSCO, MD, Fellow, Division of Cardiovascular Diseases, Main Line Heart Center, Wynnewood, Pennsylvania

ANDREA NATALE, MD, FACC, FHRS, Consulting Professor of Medicine, Stanford University, Palo Alto, California

HAKAN ORAL, MD, Associate Professor, Division of Cardiovascular Medicine, University of Michigan, Cardiovascular Center, Ann Arbor, Michigan

BENZY J. PADANILAM, MD, The Care Group, LLC, Indianapolis, Indiana

ERIC N. PRYSTOWSKY, MD, The Care Group, LLC, Indianapolis, Indiana

VIVEK Y. REDDY, MD, Endowed Faculty; Dean, Institute for Integrative Research in AF and Stroke, Cardiac Arrhythmia Service and Heart Center, Massachusetts General Hospital; Harvard Medical School, Boston, Massachusetts

ADAM E. SALTMAN, MD, PhD, Director, Cardiothoracic Surgery Research; Co-Director, Atrial Fibrillation Center, Maimonides Medical Center, Brooklyn, New York

NAVINDER S. SAWHNEY, MD, Clinical Fellow, Clinical Cardiac Electrophysiology Program, Division of Cardiology, University of California Medical Center, San Diego, California

RANJAN K. THAKUR, MD, Michigan State University, Thoracic and Cardiovascular Institute, Sparrow Health System, Lansing, Michigan

ALBERT L. WALDO, MD, Walter H. Pritchard Professor of Cardiology; Professor of Medicine; Professor of Biomedical Engineering, Department of Medicine, Division of Cardiovascular Medicine, Case Western Reserve University/University Hospitals of Cleveland Case Medical Center, Cleveland, Ohio

B. ALEXANDER YI, MD, PhD, Clinical and Research Fellow, Cardiology Division, Massachusetts General Hospital and Harvard Medical School, Boston, Massachusetts

CONTENTS

Atrial fibrillation (AF) undoubtedly has become one of the most
well studied arrhythmias today in terms of pathophysiology and
diagnostic and therapeutic (interventional) electrophysiology.
Although it lends itself to an apparently easy diagnosis on a
surface ECG, myriad electromechanical mechanisms underlie its
origin. An era of technology has been reached that makes AF not
only "treatable" but also potentially "curable." This article aims at
walking through the historical corridors and maze that have led to
the present-day understanding of this most common yet complex
arrhythmia.

Atrial fibrillation (AF), an increasingly common dysrhythmia, is
responsible for substantial morbidity and mortality. Currently in
the United States, approximately 2.3 million people are diagnosed
with AF and, based on the census, this number may rise to 5.6
million by 2050. Risk factors for AF include advancing age and
cardiovascular disease and its risk factors. The chief hazard of AF is
embolic stroke, which is increased four- to fivefold, assuming great
importance in advanced age when it becomes a dominant factor.
AF is associated with about a doubling of mortality.

fibrillation usually resolves spontaneously after heart rate is controlled; however, if patients are highly symptomatic or hemodynamically unstable, sinus rhythm should be restored by electrical or pharmacologic cardioversion. Patients with atrial fibrillation of more than 48 hours should receive antithrombotic therapy for thromboembolism prevention.

Pacemakers are used to facilitate medical management of atrial fibrillation with rate control agents and anti-arrhythmic drugs. Atrioventricular junction ablation in conjunction with pacemaker implantation can be an effective therapy for controlling a rapid ventricular rate during atrial fibrillation. The minimization of right ventricular apical pacing in patients with paroxysmal atrial fibrillation is an important objective. Cardiac resynchronization therapy devices are likely to be beneficial in select patients with chronic atrial fibrillation.

Atrial fibrillation is a common arrhythmia associated with significant morbidity including angina, heart failure and stroke. Medical therapy remains suboptimal with significant side effects and toxicities, as well as a high recurrence rate. Catheter ablation or modification of the atrio-ventricular node with pacemaker implantation provides rate control but subjects the patient to the risks of an implantable device and does nothing to reduce the risk of stroke. Pulmonary vein antrum isolation offers a nonpharmacologic means of restoring sinus rhythm, thereby eliminating the morbidity of atrial fibrillation and the need for anti-arrhythmic drugs.

For cardiac surgery patients presenting with atrial fibrillation (AF), surgeons offer an operation that corrects the structural heart disease and the AF. With this approach, it is estimated that surgeons will perform more than 10,000 ablation procedures in 2007. Surgeons are developing minimally invasive techniques for stand-alone, epicardial ablation of AF. This article (1) reviews the rationale for surgical ablation of AF, (2) describes the classic maze procedure and its results, (3) details new approaches to surgical ablation of AF, (4) emphasizes the importance of management of the left atrial appendage, and (5) considers challenges and future directions in the ablation of AF.

The primary goals in the management of patients who have atrial fibrillation are prevention of stroke and cardiomyopathy and amelioration of symptoms. Each patient presents to a physician with a specific constellation of symptoms and signs, but, fortunately, most patients can be assigned to broad categories of therapy. For some, anticoagulation and rate control suffice, whereas others require more aggressive attempts to restore and maintain sinus rhythm. Physicians and patients need to be willing to alter therapeutic plans if an initial strategy of rate or rhythm control is unsuccessful.

Atrial Fibrillation: Unanswered Questions and Future Directions

Vivek Y. Reddy

Just more than a decade ago, Haissaguerre and colleagues provided the seminal demonstration of the role of pulmonary vein triggers in the pathogenesis of atrial fibrillation (AF) and the potential therapeutic role of catheter ablation to treat patients who have paroxysmal AF. This initial observation ushered in the modern era of catheter ablation to treat patients who have AF, and tremendous progress has been made in understanding its pathogenesis and the catheter approaches to treating this rhythm. Although the current state of AF catheter ablation is well described earlier in this issue, this article reflects on some of the major unanswered questions about AF management, and the future technological and investigational directions being explored in the nonpharmacologic management of AF.

Index

ELSEVIER
SAUNDERS

THE MEDICAL
CLINICS
OF NORTH AMERICA

Med Clin N Am 92 (2008) xv–xvi

Preface

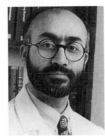 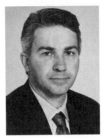

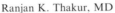

Ranjan K. Thakur, MD   Andrea Natale, MD, FACC, FHRS
Guest Editors

Atrial fibrillation is the most common sustained arrhythmia in man. Until recently, atrial fibrillation did not receive deserved attention, in part because we did not have much of a therapeutic armamentarium that could be brought to bear. A new wave of enthusiasm appeared about a decade ago after Haissaguerre and colleagues showed that atrial fibrillation could be initiated by ectopic beats originating in the pulmonary veins and that ablation of these sites can be curative.

Aeschylus, a sixth-century Greek dramatist wrote that a physician's goal should be "to cure, sometimes; to alleviate, often; to comfort, always." An incredible worldwide effort from physicians, scientists, and the entire industry over the last decade has brought forth new insights and therapeutic tools. We are fortunate to have achieved a level of understanding about this complex disease that we can, indeed, cure some patients. While we proceed at full speed ahead in the ongoing search for cures for other diseases, we have taken the opportunity in this issue of *Medical Clinics of North America* to reflect on how much we have learned and the task that still lies ahead.

This issue opens with a historical perspective, then discusses many of the clinical issues in the management of atrial fibrillation, such as cardioversion, anticoagulation, and ablation, and finally concludes with the current guidelines for treatment and a view of the future.

0025-7125/08/$ - see front matter © 2008 Elsevier Inc. All rights reserved.
doi:10.1016/j.mcna.2007.09.007   *medical.theclinics.com*

We are grateful to our colleagues who have contributed their time and energy in writing these reviews. All of the contributors are busy investigators and well-known experts in the field. We have enjoyed reading their perspectives, and we hope that the reader will also find these reviews helpful in obtaining an up-to-date understanding.

Ranjan K. Thakur, MD
Thoracic and Cardiovascular Institute
Sparrow Health System
Michigan State University
Lansing, MI 48910, USA

Andrea Natale, MD, FACC, FHRS
Stanford University
Palo Alto, CA

ELSEVIER
SAUNDERS

THE MEDICAL
CLINICS
OF NORTH AMERICA

Med Clin N Am 92 (2008) xvii

Dedication

To Jay, friend, colleague, sounding board, teacher, and son.
And to my wife, Niti, and my mother.
Ranjan K. Thakur

To my wife, Marina, and our daughters, Veronica and Eleonora.
Andrea Natale

doi:10.1016/j.mcna.2007.09.006   *medical.theclinics.com*

ELSEVIER
SAUNDERS

THE MEDICAL
CLINICS
OF NORTH AMERICA

Med Clin N Am 92 (2008) 1–15

Atrial Fibrillation: A Historical Perspective

Atul Khasnis, MD, Ranjan K. Thakur, MD*

*Michigan State University, Thoracic and Cardiovascular Institute, Sparrow Health System,
405 West Greenlawn, Suite 400, Lansing, MI 48910, USA*

If I have seen further, it is by standing on the shoulders of giants.
—Isaac Newton

Atrial fibrillation (AF) undoubtedly has become one of the most well studied arrhythmias in terms of pathophysiology and diagnostic and therapeutic (interventional) electrophysiology. Although it lends itself to an apparently easy diagnosis on a surface ECG, myriad electromechanical mechanisms underlie its origin. An era of technology has been reached that makes AF not only treatable but also potentially curable. This article aims at walking through the historical corridors and maze that have led to the present-day understanding of this most common yet complex arrhythmia.

Earliest clinical sightings

The earliest record of AF seems to be in the *Yellow Emperor's Classic of Internal Medicine* in the 17th century [1]. William Harvey, however, is credited with the first description of "auricular fibrillation" in animals in 1628. After Harvey's description, the misunderstanding that the pulse was independent of the heartbeat continued to prevail, likely because of the dissociation that frequently exists between the irregular heart contractions and the palpable radial pulse in AF. This is now well recognized as the "pulse deficit," which can be a valuable clue to bedside diagnosis of AF. In 1863, Chauveau and Marey [2] conducted various studies on cardiac physiology using the sphygmograph, an instrument that recorded the pulse graphically and, therein, described pulse tracings from patients who had

---

* Corresponding author.
E-mail address: thakur@msu.edu (R.K. Thakur).

0025-7125/08/$ - see front matter © 2008 Elsevier Inc. All rights reserved.
doi:10.1016/j.mcna.2007.08.001   *medical.theclinics.com*

AF [1]. Various descriptions of the irregular pulse as "intermission of the pulsation of the heart" (Laennec), "ataxia of the pulse" (Bouilland), "delirium cordis" (Nothnagel), and, finally, "pulsus irregularis perpetuus" (Hering) later ensued [3]. In 1907, Cushny and Edmunds [4], at University College of London, published the first case report of AF in their patient after surgery on an "ovarian fibroid" recorded with a "Jacques sphygmochronograph." This was the first correlative clinical report on the electrical record and palpated irregularity of the pulse in AF. The development of the string galvanometer in 1909 opened the door to the electrical nature of AF, allowing further correlation with the physical examination.

AF is associated most commonly with mitral valve disease. Jean Baptiste Senac connected AF (which he called "rebellious palpitation") and mitral stenosis (MS) in 1783 [5]. Adams [6] reported irregular pulses associated with MS in 1827. In 1897, Mackenzie [7] first described the loss of jugular "A wave" during AF in a patient who had MS and disappearance of the presystolic murmur when the patient developed an irregular rhythm. In more recent literature, AF is reported to occur in 29% of patients who have isolated MS and in 16% who have isolated mitral regurgitation [8]. The incidence increases to 52% in MS combined with regurgitation of rheumatic etiology [8].

In the years that followed, the pure clinical face of AF was accompanied by further electromechanical insight facilitated by ECG and, over the years, newer recording and imaging modalities.

Electrocardiography: revealing the electrical face of atrial fibrillation

The development of ECG by Einthoven [9] in 1902 allowed a simple means to record the electrical events that represent AF. His device consisted of a string galvanometer (with various complex attachments) and required transmission of electrical signals over telephone wires to his laboratory. He recorded 26 single-lead ECG strips of various cardiac rhythm disturbances, one of which depicted AF (he called this electrical pattern "pulsus inequalis and irregularis"). Lewis [10], in 1909, described the classic "absence of P waves" and "irregularity of the f waves" that define AF. In 1928, technical advances were made to amplify ECG recording [11]. Frank Sanborn developed the first portable ECG machine the same year [12]. This was a significant development in the miniaturization of ECG recording. Further research started focusing on finer points of the ECG to elucidate more useful and corroborative information regarding mechanisms and cardiac activity during AF. The atrial cycle length has been studied as a predictor of paroxysmal AF and a predictor of recurrence after cardioversion. This is done using frequency analysis of fibrillatory ECG [13]. Further studies have led to elucidation of initiating mechanisms for AF. In 1998, the pulmonary veins (PV) assumed an important role as the triggers driving paroxysmal AF. Ablation in the region of the PV also rewardingly treated AF, leading to an exciting chase to better identify anatomic and electrical characteristics of these veins. Certain ECG morphologies of the P waves can predict paroxysmal AF and identify the "culprit" pulmonary vein [14,15]. Newer technologies, such as the 65-lead ECG mapping system (Resolution Medical, Pleasanton, California), can facilitate noninvasive localization of AF trigger sites by matching the P-wave integral map morphology of a premature atrial contraction with the reference database of 34 mean paced P-wave integral map patterns [16]. AF also was appreciated later on intracardiac ECG (ICE) [17,18]. Algorithms have been developed that can help localize pulmonary vein activity using intracardiac recordings during spontaneous and paced pulmonary vein activity [19]. Time-frequency analysis of the surface ECG is reported to aid noninvasive monitoring effects of antiarrhythmic drugs on fibrillatory rate and waveform [20]. The role of ECG technology has come a long way since Einthoven but still uses the same basic principles of ECG diagnosis of AF. Many more advances will occur in understanding AF, but the ECG will remain a trusted, economic, and noninvasive source of invaluable information that assists in clinical decision-making.

Pathophysiology: what causes atrial fibrillation?

The understanding of mechanisms underlying the initiation and maintenance of AF has evolved over the past many decades. The question of reentry versus the earliest concept of reentry proposed by Winterberg [21] in 1906 and Lewis and Schleiter [22] in 1912 advocated that rapid focal activity from one or more centers accounted for AF. Mines [23] in 1913 showed that the mechanism of reentry was an impulse circling a large anatomic obstacle. Scherf [24], in 1947, revived the theory of focal trigger in AF. Moe, in the 1960s, supported the theory of randomly propagating multiple wavelets as the main mechanism underlying AF [25]. The reentrant wavelet hypothesis required the concept of "wavelength" of the arrhythmia circuit to be introduced. In the 1970s, Allessie and colleagues [26] introduced the concept of "leading circle reentry." In a goat model of AF, they demonstrated that the average circuit diameter was 20 to 30 mm and that a minimum of 5 to 8 random wavelets was required to sustain AF, but a solid theory of how AF is initiated was also required. Several alternative explanations were offered: a "stable background circuit" capable of initiating new AF when the earlier episode dies out, abnormal focal trigger sites in the atria, and the possibility of an echo beat from the AV node or from an accessory pathway. The current understanding is that AF requires a critical atrial mass needed to maintain the arrhythmia and that there is a critical rate above which organized atrial activity cannot continue. Thus, at a certain rate, organized atrial activity can disintegrate into AF provided the critical tissue mass is available to sustain it. Recent studies in isolated human atrial preparations show that a single meandering functional reentrant wavefront produces AF [27]. Recent work by Jalife and coworkers [28] questions the randomness of atrial activity in AF. Their study suggests the presence of a possible "mother circuit" that serves as a periodic background focus; the presence of anatomic obstacles (scar or orifices) serves to break up the wavefront from the mother circuit into multiple wavelets that spread in various directions. Wu and colleagues [29] have proposed the role of pectinate muscles as obstacles that break the activation wave, thus promoting reentry. They also may serve as an anchoring site for the wave leading to rotor like activity. The likelihood that focal activation plays some role in AF now is well accepted. In 1966, Nathan and Eliakim [30] reported that the proximal portion of the PV has a sleeve of myocardium that is a direct extension from the adjacent atrial tissue and that is coupled electrically to the atrium in an anatomic study of the left atrium-pulmonary vein junction in human hearts. Haissaguerre and coworkers [31] reported arrhythmogenicity of the PV as possible focal triggers in some cases of AF. The myocardial sleeves that extend from the left atrium onto the PV seem the pathologic correlate of the arrhythmogenic focus. Since then, many other foci of AF have been discovered in the thoracic venous structures connected to the atria, including the superior vena cava [32], coronary sinus [33], and the vein of Marshall [34]. The autonomic basis of AF also was explored by Coumel [35], who classified AF as adrenergic or vagally mediated. There also is research implicating genes that predispose to AF.

Genetics of atrial fibrillation: born with it?

Genetics, excitingly, has permeated every domain of medicine, and cardiac electrophysiology is no exception. Interest in the genetic basis of AF was driven by the occurrence of AF in families and its association with other arrhythmic conditions with genetic bases, such as Wolff-Parkinson-White syndrome [36] and hypertrophic cardiomyopathy [37]. Familial AF first was reported in 1943 [38]. Recent studies show that routinely encountered AF may have a genetic basis more commonly than considered previously [39]. In 1997, Brugada and colleagues [40] reported the first monogenic cause for familial AF, implicating a gene on chromosome 10. Ellinor and colleagues [41] mapped a gene for familial AF to chromosome 6. Genes coding for potassium channels have been discovered that are held responsible for AF [42]. More genes will continue to be discovered and, although remote at this time, someday genetic therapy may be a means to cure or prevent AF in those predisposed.

Mapping atrial fibrillation: localizing the origin of atrial fibrillation

The development of mapping techniques [43] is central to appreciating current success in treating AF with ablation. Mapping AF has helped clarify its mechanism and localize possible anatomic sites for effective radiofrequency (RF) ablation. Conventionally, this has been done by correlation of 12-lead surface ECG with intracardiac data. 3-D imaging of the triggering foci and correlation with the activation sequence can localize therapy better. Electroanatomic or CARTO mapping is a nonfluoroscopic mapping system that uses magnetic technology to determine the location and orientation of the mapping and ablation catheter accurately while simultaneously recording local electrograms from the catheter tip. Noncontact mapping using the EnSite 3000 (Endocardial Solutions, St. Paul, Minnesota) mapping system consists of a balloon or multielectrode array that detects endocardial activation recorded by noncontact intracavitary electrodes. The activation points are displayed as computed electrograms or isopotential maps [44]. Other techniques used include a basket catheter (Boston Scientific, Natick, Massachusetts) and amplification technique. The electrodes are coupled to achieve bipolar recordings and each electrode couple then is amplified and filtered separately for every channel (CardioLab System, Prucka Engineering, Houston). ICE can be a valuable tool in localizing anatomic areas for ablation. It allows for assessment of wall contact of ablation catheters for creation of long linear lesions for catheter ablative treatment of AF [45]. Inverse ECG images the activation time map on the entire surface of the heart from ECG mapping data, enabling reconstruction of unifocal, multifocal, and more distributed activation patterns [46,47]. MRI also shows promise in demonstrating pulmonary venous anatomy, which is central to the technique of RF ablation of focal AF [48]. Because of the focus on PV as triggers for AF, there is an increasing need to identify their anatomy and electrical functionality correctly. Ablation in the region of PV is fraught with risks [49], mandating that this procedure be made as successful yet as safe as possible. Newer technology aims precisely at doing this. One of the most logically developed technologies seems to be superimposition of a 3-D anatomic image (CT or MRI) on the image of the ablating catheter while correlating it with the electrical activation maps. This has been achieved successfully using a multislice multidetector CT combined with 3-D electroanatomic mapping [50]. The PV anatomy also has been studied using high-frequency intravascular ultrasound [51]. Other recent advances are the use of remote navigation combined with electroanatomic mapping [52] and the use of robotic surgery [53]. Mapping technology will continue to evolve, making ablation techniques safer and more successful. These hopefully will become more noninvasive, allowing ablations to become technically easier and analytically simpler, reducing procedure times.

Drugs for atrial fibrillation: from digitalis to dronedarone

Medical therapy for AF still is the primary modality of treatment, although ablation may become a first-line therapy for well-chosen patients in the future. Digitalis probably was the first drug available to treat AF. Digitalis was discovered in 1785 by Withering [54], who described its various qualities and uses. Quinidine likely was the next antiarrhythmic medication, used in 1950 to treat AF [55]. Amiodarone and disopyramide were explored in the 1970s to treat AF. Many studies regarding the efficacy of amiodarone in AF showed that is was useful and effective [56,57]. Disopyramide was reported as effective as quinidine in double-blind trials conducted in 1980 [58]. Vaughan-Williams [59] first classified antiarrhythmic drugs into four classes based on their pharmacologic actions in 1984. The class IC agent, encainide, was tried for treatment of AF in 1988 and had a 27% incidence of proarrhythmia [60]. After data from the Cardiac Arrhythmia Suppression Trial (CAST) [61] were reported, the class IA and IC agents have been relegated to treatment of AF in patients who do not have structural heart disease. Flecainide and propafenone recently made a comeback as effective medications for a "pill-in-the-pocket" approach to treating AF [62]. Sotalol was a class III drug that has received much approval for use in AF. Sotalol had electrophysiologic properties in addition to beta-receptor blockade [63]. Intravenous infusion of sotalol initially was reported as ineffective in restoration of sinus rhythm but effective in rate control in AF [64]; later, its antiarrhythmic efficacy also was proved. Dofetilide and ibutilide are the newer class III agents, studied in 1992 and 1993 as options in treating AF [65,66]. The toxicity of long-term amiodarone use has led to the discovery of a congener drug, dronedarone. Dronedarone, azimilide, tedisamal, and trecetilide (class III agents) are awaiting FDA approval pending long-term safety data regarding their clinical use. Future drug development and use are likely to be guided by a better molecular understanding of the electrical basis of AF. The long-standing battle of rate versus rhythm control strategy has been subdued, although not put to rest, after the recent Atrial Fibrillation Follow-up Investigation of Rhythm Management (AFFIRM) [67] and Rate Control Versus Electrical Cardioversion (RACE) [68] trials were published. These trials showed the noninferiority of rate control to rhythm control but this division is not as clear when it involves patients who have heart failure or symptomatic AF. AF portends a considerable risk for thromboembolism; this was reported as early as 1958 in a patient who had paroxysmal AF and normal heart [69]. Fisher [70] reported using anticoagulants for cerebral thrombosis in the same year. Today, it is considered standard of care to treat high-risk patients with anticoagulants and low-risk patients with antiplatelet therapy. This is facilitated by the CHADS$_2$ (Congetive heart failure, Hypertension, Age > 75, Diabetes mellitus, and prior Stroke or tansient ischemic attack) score [71]. The inflammatory nature of AF (as evinced by elevated C-reactive protein levels) is another pathophysiologic aspect of AF being explored, as it may have significant clinical and therapeutic implications.

Cardioversion: beating electricity with electricity

Cardioversion is the process of restoration of normal sinus rhythm by application of a synchronized external or internal current to the heart. It can be considered an interim measure in the management of AF, as it is more likely to be successful early in the course of AF and may ward off the need for more invasive therapy in some patients if normal sinus rhythm can be maintained on or off pharmacotherapy. In 1962, Lown and colleagues [72] described the first known device for application of electrical energy to the heart for correction of rhythm disturbances. The term, "cardioversion," first was used in the coming year (1963) for electrical correction of AF [73]. In 1963, Lown and colleagues showed that cardioversion was safer and more effective than quinidine. In 1968, diazepam was the first agent reported as an effective sedative for cardioversion [74]. It also was realized that cardioversion did not obviate anticoagulation if AF was present for more than a week [75]. The next step was to evaluate the long-term success of cardioversion in the management of AF. Within the next few years, longer duration of AF [76], increased left atrial size [77,78], and presence of congestive heart failure [79] came to be predictors of lower success rates with cardioversion. Cardioversion also was recognized as dangerous in the setting of digitalis toxicity [80]. The recognition of atrial stunning for 3 weeks after cardioversion next was recognized by pulsed Doppler studies [81]. These studies underscore the need for optimal anticoagulation that is recommended today in the pericardioversion period. The exact positioning of the external electrodes for successful cardioversion initially was considered unimportant as long as the current traveled along the long axis of the heart [82]; this also has been shown in recent studies [83]. If external cardioversion works, so should internal. This was the logic behind developing the atrial cardioverter (atrioverter) [84], the atrial rhythm control device counterpart of the implantable defibrillator that works well for ventricular arrhythmias. The atrial cardioverter still is being evaluated as useful therapy for AF because of problems with patient discomfort associated with the delivery of the shock. Studies show that it is accurate in targeting AF for cardioversion and not associated with ventricular proarrhythmias. Cardioversion currently is used widely and works for selected patients especially when used in combination with antiarrhythmic medications for conversion to and maintenance of normal sinus rhythm.

Ablating atrial fibrillation: learning while burning

In 1982, Scheinman and colleagues [85] used direct current energy to treat supraventricular tachycardia. RF energy has replaced direct current energy as a source of energy for catheter ablation of arrhythmias. Once again, the PV assumed center stage as the target for ablation therapy in AF. Other sites of ablation include the left atrium and the thoracic veins that now are identified as sustaining AF after PV ablation. In 1994, Haissaguerre and colleagues [86] reported successful treatment of AF by ablation of the PV. Since then, several techniques have been developed at various leading centers globally with varying success in curing AF ablation. The use of RF energy has been concerning as it can be thrombogenic and cause complications from damage to underlying structures depending on the site of ablation. Other sources of energy used successfully include cryoenergy (using a freeze-thaw cycle), microwave energy (by generation of frictional heat), ultrasound energy (using oscillation for heat generation), and laser (generates heat by harmonic oscillation in water molecules) [87]. These energy modalities have been used intraoperatively during the maze procedure for successful creation of endocardial lesions, thus interrupting AF. RF energy still is the most commonly used energy source and the other sources are used only at specific centers that are experienced in their use. Although ablation is not first-line therapy for paroxysmal AF at this time, trials are underway to evaluate this further [88]. RF ablation does not have pristine outcomes at this time; improved success rates, however, are reported. Like any other condition, optimal success rates likely are achieved only by correct patient selection; the criteria for selection only can be borne out of large randomized controlled trials. Until then, physicians treating patients with AF have to be content with attempting drug therapy first and considering ablation for failed drug therapy. Surgical intervention likely is used only in patients undergoing cardiac valve repair or other intracardiac procedures. Catheter technology continues to advance, permitting better energy delivery systems that ensure interruption of the AF circuits. When the only available ablation technology was RF energy applied through tip deflectable ablation catheters with a single electrode, long linear atrial lesions could be made only by a "drag" technique [89]. Multielectrode catheters were developed to surmount this problem so that a linear atrial lesion could be produced by placing it against the atrial wall and delivering energy [90]. Lesh and colleagues [91] developed a catheter design integrating a cylindrical ultrasound transducer within a water-filled balloon to produce narrow circumferential zones of hyperthermic tissue death at the pulmonary vein ostia. Newer catheters have been developed that permit the delivery of other energy modalities leading to better success rates of AF ablation.

Surgery for atrial fibrillation: down the corridor and inside the maze

The assumption that the electrophysiologic basis of AF is the multiple random circulating reentrant wavelets led to the development of the maze surgical procedure. In 1991, Cox and colleagues [92] reported success with the original maze procedure. Several surgical procedures were devised and tested in dogs, which finally led to a surgical approach that effectively creates an electrical maze in the atrium. The atrial incisions prevent reentry and allow sinus impulses to activate the entire atrial myocardium in a channeled manner, thereby preserving atrial transport function postoperatively. Thus, there is resolution of the electrical dysfunction and restoration of the atrial mechanical function. The procedure had been tried in seven patients since 1987 (five who had paroxysmal AF and two who had chronic AF) who had "cure" from AF and were free of postoperative antiarrhythmic medications. They went on to present further data on 75 patients in 1992 with a 98% cure rate for AF at average 3 months' follow-up [93]. By 1995, it was claimed that the procedure has been standardized to the extent that a good outcome likely was independent of the surgeon and without mapping guidance [94]. The same year, the maze procedure was modified twice culminating in the maze III procedure. This was intended to overcome the problems of chronotropic incompetence and left atrial dysfunction seen to result in some patients after the original maze procedure [95]. The maze III procedure then was combined with mitral valve surgery yielding a success rate of 79% for treatment of AF; fine fibrillatory waves and enlarged left atrium were predictive of failure [96]. Cox [97] emphasized that return of atrial mechanical function was key to the success of the maze procedure. In 1998, he reported return of right atrial contractile function in 99% cases and return of left atrial contractile function in 93% cases. These success rates were reported to persist 3 years later. In an attempt to restore left atrial function, modifications have been introduced to the maze III procedure [98]. The maze III procedure now can be performed through a minimally invasive approach, although there is skepticism about its success [99]. In 1997, Patwardhan and colleagues [100] reported success of the maze procedure using RF bipolar coagulation in patients who had rheumatic heart disease and AF to produce atrial lesions with a success rate of 80%. Pulsed wave Doppler evaluation at follow-up showed return of atrial transport function, presence of "a" wave in all these patients in tricuspid valve flow and in 75% patients in mitral valve flow. Calkins and colleagues [101] performed a maze-like procedure using the Guidant Heart Rhythm Technologies Linear Ablation System to create long transmural lesions. Bipolar RF ablation avoids the morbidity of cut-and-sew lesions, reduces procedural time, and increases the likelihood of transmurality and continuity of lesions created compared with unipolar devices [102]. A combination of energy sources also has been used successfully for the maze procedure [103]. The other surgical technique to treat AF is the corridor procedure. The procedure is a surgical open heart procedure designed to isolate a "corridor" from the right and the left atrium consisting of the sinus node area, the atrioventricular (AV) nodal junction, and the connecting right atrial mass. The principle of this surgery is to channel the electrical impulse from the sinus to the AV node through an atrial area small enough to prevent AF. Between 1987 and 1990, 20 patients who had severely disabling symptoms resulting from frequent paroxysmal AF underwent the corridor operation, with permanent success in 16 patients [104]. The corridor procedure has been used successfully in patients undergoing surgery for mitral valve disease with results comparable to the maze procedure (75% success rate) [105]. The surgical options for AF seem to be evolving and the focus seems to fluctuate from trying to isolate the trigger to trying to modify the substrate. The other area of focus to move to a minimally invasive mode for achieving successful interventional management of AF [106,107]. Surgical treatment of AF still is extremely rewarding when performed concomitant with surgery for associated surgically amenable cardiac disease.

Back to the future: looking through the crystal ball

Successful management (treatment for the most part and cure in some cases) of AF has come a long way. It is only when looking back that how much progress has been made can be appreciated. Although technology continues to advance, the efforts of those who have laid the foundation for clinical recognition, physical diagnosis, electrical documentation, drug therapy, and interventional and surgical management of this interesting disorder must be admired. The "grandfather arrhythmia" has come a long way; it continues to show newer mechanisms and presents newer challenges in its management. The future holds a lot in store regarding pharmacologic and nonpharmacologic therapies as more advanced molecular biology, imaging, and mapping techniques evolve. Which AF patients are treated best with which therapeutic modality needs to be ascertained, because not all AF is the same.

References

[1] Lip GYH, Beevers DG. ABC of atrial fibrillation: history, epidemiology and importance of atrial fibrillation. BMJ 1995;311:1361–7.
[2] Chauveau A, Marey EJ. Appareils et Expériences CardiographiquesDémonstration Nouvelle du Méchanisme des Mouvements du Coeur par l'Emploi des Instruments Enregistreurs à Indications Continuées. Paris: J.- B. Baillière; 1863.
[3] Flegel KM. From delirium cordis to atrial fibrillation: historical development of a disease concept. Ann Intern Med 1995;122:867–73.
[4] Cushny AR, Edmunds CW. Paroxysmal irregularity of the heart and auricular fibrillation. Am J Med Sci 1907;133:66–77.
[5] Schweitzer P, Keller S. A history of atrial fibrillation. Vnitr Lek 2002;48(1):24–6.
[6] Adams R. Cases of diseases of the heart, accompanied with pathological observations. Dublin Hospital Reports 1827;4:353–453.
[7] MacKenzie J. New methods of studying affections of the heart. V. The inception of the rhythm of the heart by the ventricle. Br Med J 1905;1:812–5.
[8] Diker E, Aydogdu S, Ozdemir M, et al. Prevalence and predictors of atrial fibrillation in rheumatic valvular heart disease. Am J Cardiol 1996;77:96–8.
[9] Einthoven W. Le telecardiogramme. Arch Int Physiol 1906;4:132–64.
[10] Lewis T. Auricular fibrillation: a common clinical condition. BMJ 1909;2:1528.
[11] Ernestene AC, Levine SA. A comparison of records taken with the Einthoven string galvanometer and the amplifier type electrocardiograph. Am Heart J 1928;4:725–31.
[12] ECG library. A (not so) brief history of electrocardiography. Available at: http://www.ecglibrary.com/ecghist.html. Accessed November 8, 2007.
[13] Holm M, Pehrson S, Ingemansson M, et al. Non-invasive assessment of the atrial cycle length during atrial fibrillation in man: introducing, validating and illustrating a new ECG method. Cardiovasc Res 1998;38(1):69–81.
[14] Dilaveris P, Gialafos E, Sideris S, et al. MD Simple electrocardiographic markers for the prediction of paroxysmal idiopathic atrial fibrillation. Am Heart J 1998;135(5):733–8.

[15] Rajawat YS, Gerstenfeld EP, Patel VV, et al. ECG criteria for localizing the pulmonary vein origin of spontaneous atrial premature complexes: validation using intracardiac recordings. Pacing Clin Electrophysiol 2004;27(2):182–8.

[16] Sippensgroenewegen A, Natale A, Marrouche NF, et al. Potential role of body surface ECG mapping for localization of atrial fibrillation trigger sites. J Electrocardiol 2004;37:47–52.

[17] Giraud G, Latour H, Levy A, et al. [Endocavitary electrocardiography and the mechanism of auricular fibrillation]. Montp Med 1952;41–42(7):625–39.

[18] Vitek B, Valenta J. [Auricular fibrillation in the intracardiac ECG]. Cesk Pediatr 1969; 24(5):401–7 [in Czech].

[19] O'Donnell D, Bourke JP, Furniss SS. P wave morphology during spontaneous and paced pulmonary vein activity: differences between patients with atrial fibrillation and normal controls. J Electrocardiol 2003;36(1):33–40.

[20] Husser D, Stridh M, Cannom DS, et al. Validation and clinical application of time-frequency analysis of atrial fibrillation electrocardiograms. J Cardiovasc Electrophysiol 2007;18(1):41–6.

[21] Winterberg H. Ueber Herzflimmern und seine Beeinflussung durch Kampher. Zeitschrift Experimental Pathologie Therapie 1906;3:182–208.

[22] Lewis T, Schleiter HG. The relation of regular tachycardias of auricular origin to auricular fibrillation. Heart 1912;3:173–93.

[23] Mines GR. On dynamic equilibrium in the heart. J Physiol 1913;46:349–82.

[24] Scherf D. Studies on auricular tachycardia caused by aconitine administration. Proc Soc Exp Biol Med 1947;64:233–9.

[25] Moe GK, Rheinboldt WC, Abildskov JA, et al. A computer model of atrial fibrillation. Am Heart J 1964;67:200–20.

[26] Allessie MA, Rensma PL, Brugada J, et al. Pathophysiology of atrial fibrillation. In: Zipes DP, Jalife J, editors. Cardiac electrophysiology: from cell to bedside. Philadelphia: WB Saunders; 1990. p. 548–59.

[27] Ikeda T, Czer L, Trento A, et al. Induction of meandering functional reentrant wavefront in isolated human atrial tissues. Circulation 1997;96:3013–20.

[28] Jalife J, Berenfeld O, Mansour M. Mother rotors and fibrillatory conduction: a mechanism of atrial fibrillation. Cardiovasc Res 2002;54:204–16.

[29] Wu TJ, Kim YH, Yashima M, et al. Progressive action potential duration shortening and the conversion from atrial flutter to atrial fibrillation in the isolated canine right atrium. J Am Coll Cardiol 2001;38:1757–65.

[30] Nathan H, Eliakim M. The junction between the left atrium and the pulmonary veins. An anatomic study of human hearts. Circulation 1966;34:412–22.

[31] Haissaguerre M, Jais P, Shah DC, et al. Spontaneous initiation of atrial fibrillation by ectopic beats originating in the pulmonary veins. N Engl J Med 1998;339:659–66.

[32] Li J, Wang L. Catheter ablation of atrial fibrillation originating from superior vena cava. Arch Med Res 2006;37(3):415–8.

[33] Haissaguerre M, Hocini M, Sanders P, et al. Localized sources maintaining atrial fibrillation organized by prior ablation. Circulation 2006;113(5):616–25.

[34] Chen PS, Chou CC, Tan AY, et al. The mechanisms of atrial fibrillation. J Cardiovasc Electrophysiol 2006;17(3):S2–7.

[35] Coumel P. Paroxysmal atrial fibrillation: a disorder of autonomic tone? Eur Heart J 1994; 15(Suppl A):9–16.

[36] Gollob MH, Seger JJ, Gollob TN, et al. Novel PRKAG2 mutation responsible for the genetic syndrome of ventricular preexcitation and conduction system disease with childhood onset and absence of cardiac hypertrophy. Circulation 2001;104(25):3030–3.

[37] Gruver EJ, Fatkin D, Dodds GA, et al. Familial hypertrophic cardiomyopathy and atrial fibrillation caused by Arg663His beta-cardiac myosin heavy chain mutation. Am J Cardiol 1999;83(12A):13H–8H.

[38] Wolff L. Familial auricular fibrillation. N Engl J Med 1943;229:396–8.

[39] Darbar D, Herron KJ, Ballew JD, et al. Familial atrial fibrillation is a genetically heterogeneous disorder. J Am Coll Cardiol 2003;41(12):2185–92.
[40] Brugada R, Tapscott T, Czernuszewicz GZ, et al. Identification of a genetic locus for familial atrial fibrillation. N Engl J Med 1997;336(13):905–11.
[41] Ellinor PT, Shin JT, Moore RK, et al. Locus for atrial fibrillation maps to chromosome 6q14-16. fCirculation 2003;107(23):2880–3.
[42] Chen YH, Xu SJ, Bendahhou S, et al. KCNQ1 gain-of-function mutation in familial atrial fibrillation. Science 2003;299(5604):251–4.
[43] Sra Jasbir, Thomas Joy M. New techniques for mapping cardiac arrhythmias. Indian Heart J 2001;53:423–44.
[44] Schneider MA, Schmitt C. Non-contact mapping: a simultaneous spatial detection in the diagnosis of arrhythmias. Z Kardiol 2000;89(3):177–85 [in German].
[45] Epstein LM, Mitchell MA, Smith TW, et al. Comparative study of fluoroscopy and intracardiac echocardiographic guidance for the creation of linear atrial lesions. Circulation 1998;98:1796–801.
[46] Tilg B, Fischer G, Modre R, et al. Electrocardiographic imaging of atrial and ventricular electrical activation. Med Image Anal 2003;7:391–8.
[47] Modre R, Tilg B, Fischer G, et al. Noninvasive myocardial activation time imaging: a novel inverse algorithm applied to clinical ECG mapping data. IEEE Trans Biomed Eng 2002;49:1153–61.
[48] Wittkampf FH, Vonken EJ, Derksen R, et al. Pulmonary vein ostium geometry: analysis by magnetic resonance angiography. Circulation 2003;107:21–3.
[49] Wellens HJ. Pulmonary vein ablation in atrial fibrillation: hype or hope? Circulation 2000;102(21):2562–4.
[50] Cabrera JA, Sanchez-Quintana D, Farre J, et al. Ultrasonic characterization of the pulmonary venous wall: echographic and histological correlation. Circulation 2002;106:968–73.
[51] Guerra PG, Thibault B, Dubuc M, et al. Identification of atrial tissue in pulmonary veins using intravascular ultrasound. J Am Soc Echocardiogr 2003;16(9):982–7.
[52] Pappone C, Santinelli V. Remote navigation and ablation of atrial fibrillation. J Cardiovasc Electrophysiol 2007;18(1):S18–20.
[53] Pappone C, Vicedomini G, Manguso F, et al. Robotic magnetic navigation for atrial fibrillation ablation. J Am Coll Cardiol 2006;47(7):1390–400.
[54] Withering W. An account of the foxglove and some of its medical uses, with practical remarks on dropsy, and other diseases. In: Willius FA, Keys TE, editors. Classics of cardiology, 1New York: Dover Publications Inc.; 1941. p. 231–52.
[55] Fischermann K, Schleisner P. [Quinidine sulphate therapy of chronic auricular fibrillation in patients over fifty]. Nord Med 1950;43(17):705–6.
[56] Zagatti G, Benzoni A, Caturelli G. [Cordarone in the maintenance of sinus rhythm: prevention of paroxysmal atrial fibrillation and of supraventricular paroxysmal tachycardia]. Arch Maragliano Patol Clin 1974;30(2):245–9 [in Italian].
[57] Santos AL, Aleixo AM, Landeiro J, et al. Conversion of atrial fibrillation to sinus rhythm with amiodarone. Acta Med Port 1979;1:15–23.
[58] Kimura E, Mashima S, Tanaka T. Clinical evaluation of antiarrhythmic effects of disopyramide by multiclinical controlled double-blind methods. Int J Clin Pharmacol Ther Toxicol 1980;18(8):338–43.
[59] Vaughan Williams EM. A classification of antiarrhythmic actions reassessed after a decade of new drugs. J Clin Pharmacol 1984;24:129–47.
[60] Rinkenberger RL, Naccarelli GV, Berns E, et al. Efficacy and safety of class IC antiarrhythmic agents for the treatment of coexisting supraventricular and ventricular tachycardia. Am J Cardiol 1988;62(6):44D–55D.
[61] Preliminary report: effect of encainide and flecainide on mortality in a randomized trial of arrhythmia suppression after myocardial infarction. The Cardiac Arrhythmia Suppression Trial (CAST) Investigators. N Engl J Med 1989;321(6):406–12.

[62] Alboni P, Botto GL, Baldi N, et al. Outpatient treatment of recent-onset atrial fibrillation with the "pill-in-the-pocket" approach. N Engl J Med 2004;351(23):2384–91.

[63] Simon A, Berman E. Long-term sotalol therapy in patients with arrhythmias. J Clin Pharmacol 1979;19(8–9 Pt 2):547–56.

[64] Teo KK, Harte M, Horgan JH. Sotalol infusion in the treatment of supraventricular tachyarrhythmias. Chest 1985;87(1):113–8.

[65] Rasmussen HS, Allen MJ, Blackburn KJ, et al. Dofetilide, a novel class III antiarrhythmic agent. J Cardiovasc Pharmacol 1992;20(2):S96–105.

[66] Nabih MA, Prcevski P, Fromm BS, et al. Effect of ibutilide, a new class III agent, on sustained atrial fibrillation in a canine model of acute ischemia and myocardial dysfunction induced by microembolization. Pacing Clin Electrophysiol 1993;16(10):1975–83.

[67] Wyse DG, Waldo AL, DiMarco JP, et al. A comparison of rate control and rhythm control in patients with atrial fibrillation. N Engl J Med 2002;347(23):1825–33.

[68] Hagens VE, Ranchor AV, Van Sonderen E, et al. Effect of rate or rhythm control on quality of life in persistent atrial fibrillation. Results from the Rate Control Versus Electrical Cardioversion (RACE) Study. J Am Coll Cardiol 2004;43(2):241–7.

[69] Weintraub G, Sprecace G. Paroxysmal atrial fibrillation and cerebral embolism with apparently normal heart. N Engl J Med 1958;259(18):875–6.

[70] Fisher CM. The use of anticoagulants in cerebral thrombosis. Neurology 1958;8(5): 311–32.

[71] Gage BF, Waterman AD, Shannon W, et al. Validation of clinical classification schemes for predicting stroke: results from the National Registry of Atrial Fibrillation. JAMA 2001; 285(22):2864–70.

[72] Lown B, Amarasingham R, Neuman J. New method for terminating cardiac arrhythmias: use of synchronized capacitor discharge. JAMA 1962;182:548–55.

[73] Lown B, Perlroth MG, Kaidbey S, et al. Cardioversion" of atrial fibrillation. A report on the treatment of 65 episodes in 50 patients. N Engl J Med 1963;269:325–31.

[74] Winters WL Jr, McDonough MT, Hafer J, et al. Diazepam. A useful hypnotic drug for direct-current cardioversion. JAMA 1968;204:926–8.

[75] DeSilva RA, Lown B. Cardioversion for atrial fibrillation—indications and complications. In: Kulbertus HE, Olsson SB, Schlepper M, editors. Atrial fibrillation. Hassle: Mondal; p. 231–239.

[76] Wikland B, Edhag O, Eliasch H. Atrial fibrillation and flutter treated with synchronized DC shock. A study on immediate and long term results. Acta Med Scand 1967;182: 665–71.

[77] Fisher RD, Mason DT, Morrow AG. Restoration of normal sinus rhythm after mitral valve replacement. Correlations with left atrial pressure and size. Circulation 1968;37(2): 173–7.

[78] Hoglund C, Rosenhamer G. Echocardiographic left atrial dimension as a predictor of maintaining sinus rhythm after conversion of atrial fibrillation. Acta Med Scand 1985; 217:411–5.

[79] Futral AA, McGuire LB. Reversion of chronic atrial fibrillation. JAMA 1967;199:885–8.

[80] Kleiger R, Lown B. Cardioversion and digitalis.II. Clinical studies. Circulation 1966;33: 878–87.

[81] Manning WJ, Leeman DE, Gotch PJ, et al. Pulse Doppler evaluation of atrial mechanical function after electrical cardioversion of atrial fibrillation. J Am Coll Cardiol 1989;13: 617–23.

[82] Kerber RE, Jensen SR, Grayzel J, et al. Elective cardioversion: influence of paddle-electrode location and size on success rates and energy requirements. N Engl J Med 1981; 305:658–62.

[83] Siaplaouras S, Buob A, Rotter C, et al. Randomized comparison of anterolateral versus anteroposterior electrode position for biphasic external cardioversion of atrial fibrillation. Am Heart J 2005;150(1):150–2.

[84] Wellens HJ, Lau CP, Luderitz B, et al. Atrioverter: an implantable device for the treatment of atrial fibrillation. Circulation 1998;98(16):1651–6.

[85] Scheinman MM, Morady F, Hess DS, et al. Catheter-induced ablation of the atrioventricular junction to control refractory supraventricular arrhythmias. JAMA 1982;248: 851–5.

[86] Haissaguerre M, Marcus FI, Fischer B, et al. Radiofrequency catheter ablation in unusual mechanisms of atrial fibrillation: report of three cases. J Cardiovasc Electrophysiol 1994; 5(9):743–51.

[87] Yiu KH, Lau CP, Lee KL, et al. Emerging energy sources for catheter ablation of atrial fibrillation. J Cardiovasc Electrophysiol 2006;17(3):S56–61.

[88] Wazni OM, Marrouche NF, Martin DO, et al. Radiofrequency ablation vs antiarrhythmic drugs as first-line treatment of symptomatic atrial fibrillation: a randomized trial. JAMA 2005;293(21):2634–40.

[89] Swartz J, Pellersels G, Silvers J. A catheter-based approach to atrial fibrillation in humans. Circulation 1994;18(4, Part II):I-335.

[90] Olgin JE, Kalman JM, Chin M, et al. Electrophysiological effects of long, linear atrial lesions placed under intracardiac ultrasound guidance. Circulation 1997;96(8): 2715–21.

[91] Lesh MD, Guerra P, Roithinger FX, et al. Novel catheter technology for ablative cure of atrial fibrillation. J Interv Card Electrophysiol 2000;4(1):127–39.

[92] Cox JL, Schuessler RB, D'Agostino HJ Jr, et al. The surgical treatment of atrial fibrillation. III. Development of a definitive surgical procedure. J Thorac Cardiovasc Surg 1991;101(4): 569–83.

[93] Cox JL, Boineau JP, Schuessler RB, et al. Five-year experience with the maze procedure for atrial fibrillation. Ann Thorac Surg 1993;56(4):814–23.

[94] Cox JL, Boineau JP, Schuessler RB, et al. Electrophysiologic basis, surgical development, and clinical results of the maze procedure for atrial flutter and atrial fibrillation. Adv Card Surg 1995;6:1–67.

[95] Cox JL, Boineau JP, Schuessler RB, et al. Modification of the maze procedure for atrial flutter and atrial fibrillation. I. Rationale and surgical results. J Thorac Cardiovasc Surg 1995; 110(2):473–84.

[96] Kamata J, Kawazoe K, Izumoto H, et al. Predictors of sinus rhythm restoration after Cox maze procedure concomitant with other cardiac operations. Ann Thorac Surg 1997;64(2): 394–8.

[97] Cox JL. Atrial transport function after the Maze procedure for atrial fibrillation: a 10-year clinical experience. Am Heart J 1998;136(6):934–6.

[98] Kim KB, Huh JH, Kang CH, et al. Modifications of the Cox-Maze III procedure. Ann Thorac Surg 2001;71(3):816–22.

[99] Damiano RJ, Voeller RK. Surgical and minimally invasive ablation for atrial fibrillation. Curr Treat Options Cardiovasc Med 2006;8(5):371–6.

[100] Patwardhan AM, Dave HH, Tamhane AA, et al. Intraoperative radiofrequency microbipolar coagulation to replace incisions of Maze III procedure for correcting atrial fibrillation in patients with rheumatic valvular disease. Eur J Cardiothorac Surg 1997; 12:627–33.

[101] Calkins H, Hall J, Ellenbogen K, et al. A new system for catheter ablation of atrial fibrillation. Am J Cardiol 1999;83:227D–36D.

[102] Yii M, Yap CH, Nixon I, et al. Modification of the Cox-Maze III procedure using bipolar radiofrequency ablation. Heart Lung Circ 2007;16(1):37–49.

[103] Sternik L, Ghosh P, Luria D, et al. Mid-term results of the 'hybrid maze': a combination of bipolar radiofrequency and cryoablation for surgical treatment of atrial fibrillation. J Heart Valve Dis 2006;15(5):664–70.

[104] Defauw JJ, Guiraudon GM, van Hemel NM, et al. Surgical therapy of paroxysmal atrial fibrillation with the "corridor" operation. Ann Thorac Surg 1992;53(4):564–70.

[105] Velimirovic DB, Petrovic P, Djukic P, et al. Corridor procedure—surgical option for treat-ment of chronic atrial fibrillation in patients undergoing mitral valve replacement. Cardio-vasc Surg 1997;5(3):320–7.

[106] Skanes AC, Klein GJ, Guiraudon G, et al. Hybrid approach for minimally-invasive operative therapy of arrhythmias. J Interv Card Electrophysiol 2003;9(2):289–94.

[107] Guiraudon G, Jones DL, Skanes AC, et al. En bloc exclusion of the pulmonary vein region in the pig using off pump, beating, intra-cardiac surgery: a pilot study of minimally invasive surgery for atrial fibrillation. Ann Thorac Surg 2005;80(4):1417–23.

ELSEVIER
SAUNDERS

THE MEDICAL
CLINICS
OF NORTH AMERICA

Med Clin N Am 92 (2008) 17–40

Status of the Epidemiology of Atrial Fibrillation

William B. Kannel, MD, MPH, FACC[a,b,c,*],
Emelia J. Benjamin, MD, ScM[a,b,c,d]

[a]Boston University, The Framingham Heart Study, 73 Mount Wayte Avenue, Framingham,
MA 01702, USA
[b]National Heart Lung and Blood Institute, The Framingham Heart Study,
73 Mount Wayte Avenue, Framingham, MA 01702, USA
[c]Boston University School of Medicine, Boston University Medical Center,
88 East Newton Street, Boston, MA 02118, USA
[d]Boston University School of Public Health, Boston University Medical Center,
88 East Newton Street, Boston, MA 02118, USA

Atrial fibrillation (AF), a common and serious cardiac rhythm disturbance, is responsible for substantial morbidity and mortality in the population. Currently approximately 2.3 million people in the United States are diagnosed with AF and, based on the United States census, this number is expected to rise to 5.6 million by 2050. It doubles in prevalence with each decade of age, reaching almost 9% at ages 80 to 89 years. It has increased in prevalence over the decades, reaching epidemic proportions. This alarming increase in prevalence is explained incompletely by an increase in the population prevalence of elderly individuals, valve disease, heart failure, or myocardial infarction. New-onset AF also doubles with each decade of age, independent of the prevalence of known predisposing conditions.

Based on Framingham Study data, men have a 1.5-fold greater risk for developing AF than women after adjustment for age and predisposing conditions. Of the standard cardiovascular risk factors, hypertension, diabetes, and obesity are significant independent predictors of AF. Because of its high prevalence, hypertension is responsible for more AF in the population (14%) than any other risk factor.

Funding: N01-HC 25195; RO1 HL076784; 1R01 AG028321; 6R01-NS 17950.

* Corresponding author. Boston University/Framingham Study, 73 Mount Wayte Avenue, Framingham, MA 01702-5827.

E-mail address: billkannel@yahoo.com (W.B. Kannel).

0025-7125/08/$ - see front matter © 2008 Elsevier Inc. All rights reserved.
doi:10.1016/j.mcna.2007.09.002

Adjusting for cardiovascular risk factors, heart failure, valvular heart disease, and myocardial infarction substantially increase the likelihood of AF. Echocardiographic predictors of AF include left atrial enlargement, left ventricular (LV) fractional shortening, LV wall thickness, and mitral annular calcification, offering prognostic information for AF beyond traditional clinical risk factors. Novel risk factors for AF include reduced vascular compliance, atherosclerosis, insulin resistance, environmental factors, inflammation, and natriuretic peptides. There is emerging evidence that genetic variation also contributes to risk for AF.

The chief hazard of AF is a four- to fivefold increase in embolic stroke, assuming great importance in advanced age, when it becomes a dominant factor. The attributable risk for stroke associated with AF increases steeply with age to 23.5% at ages 80 to 89. AF is associated with a doubling of mortality in both genders.

Before the Framingham Study report in 1982, there were many misconceptions about AF [1]. Its prognosis was believed to be dependent on the underlying cardiac condition, not AF per se. AF unassociated with overt cardiovascular disease was considered a benign condition. Risk for embolism was not considered excessive unless AF was intermittent or associated with mitral stenosis. The Framingham Study report established that AF further increased stroke risk associated with coronary heart disease and heart failure [1].

AF is responsible for substantial morbidity and mortality in the general population, chiefly from stroke, and leads to more hospital admissions than any other dysrhythmia [2–4]. In addition to often disabling symptoms and impaired quality of life, AF can precipitate heart failure and trigger potentially fatal ventricular dysrhythmias. Reflecting this widespread epidemic of AF, data from United States, Scottish, and Danish studies reported a two- to 2.5-fold increase in hospitalization rates for AF between the 1980s and 1990s [5–7].

AF doubles in prevalence with each decade of age and is becoming increasingly prevalent in the population. The reason for the alarming increase is largely unexplained. There is a need for new strategies to prevent AF and improve its treatment. Although newer pharmacologic and nonpharmacologic therapies are being developed, more effective measures are needed to treat AF safely and prevent its occurrence and its cardiovascular consequences.

Incidence, prevalence, and lifetime risk

AF is a highly prevalent sustained dysrhythmia. It is the most common cardiac rhythm disturbance treated in clinical practice, accounting for approximately one third of hospitalizations for cardiac dysrhythmias. Currently, it is estimated to affect more than 6 million patients in Europe and approximately 2.3 million in the United States, and this number continues to grow rapidly because of the increasing proportion of the aging population with and without underlying heart disease. Reports from the Cardiovascular Health Study and the Framingham Study indicate that the incidence of AF per 1000 person-years in subjects under age 64 is 3.1 in men and 1.9 in women, rising sharply to approximately 19.2 per 1000 person-years in those ages 65 to 74 and is as high as 31.4 to 38 in octogenarians [8,9].

The estimated prevalence of AF in the general population is 0.4% to 1%, increasing with advancing age [10,11]. AF is uncommon before 60 years of age, but the prevalence increases markedly thereafter, afflicting approximately 10% of the population by 80 years of age [11]. The median age of patients who have AF is approximately 75 with approximately 70% between 65 and 85 years of age. Approximately one third of all patients who have AF are age 80 or older and it is estimated that by 2050 half will be in this age group [11].

Many studies of the incidence and prevalence of AF in the United Sates, Europe, and Australia have produced reasonably consistent findings [10]. For reasons that largely are unexplained, the age-adjusted prevalence of AF in the United States is greater in men than in women, in a large cross-sectional study of adults enrolled in the Kaiser Permanente health maintenance organization and in the Framingham Study. Likewise, in the large population-based Rotterdam Study, the prevalence of AF increased with age and was higher in men than in women in each age group, but the high lifetime risk for AF differed little between genders [12].

Because of the more than half-century surveillance of the Framingham Study cohort, it was possible to determine the lifetime risk for developing AF, which is 1 in 4 for men and women ages 40 and older [13]. These lifetime risks for AF remain high (1 in 6), even in the absence of antecedent predisposing conditions, such as heart failure or myocardial infarction (Table 1). Prospective data from the Rotterdam Study also found a high lifetime AF risk (22%–24% at age 40) similar to North American epidemiologic data [12]. The substantial lifetime risks underscore the major public health burden posed by AF and the need for further investigation into predisposing conditions, preventive strategies, and more effective therapies.

Most of the literature on the epidemiology of AF is based on white individuals residing in North America or Europe [14]. Based on limited data, the age-adjusted risk for developing AF in African Americans is reported to be less than half of that in whites. AF also is less common in African American than in white patients who have heart failure [8,15–17].

Secular trends

The prevalence of AF has increased over the past few decades, although studies have varied as to whether or not the increasing prevalence is restricted to men or both genders. In the Copenhagen City Heart Study, the

Table 1
Lifetime risk for atrial fibrillation in the absence of antecedent or concurrent diagnosis of congestive heart failure or myocardial infarction

Index age, years	Men	Women
Lifetime risk for atrial fibrillation without antecedent or concurrent congestive heart failure		
40	20.5	17.0
50	20.5	17.3
60	20.3	17.4
70	19.1	17.0
80	17.6	15.9
Lifetime risk for atrial fibrillation without antecedent or concurrent congestive heart failure or myocardial infarction		
40	16.3	15.6
50	16.6	15.9
60	16.8	16.1
70	16.5	15.9
80	16.0	14.8

All values are percentages.
Data from Lloyd-Jones DM, Wang TJ, Leip E, et al. Lifetime risk for development of atrial fibrillation: The Framingham Heart Study. Circulation 2004;110:1042–6.

prevalence in men more than doubled from the 1970s to the 1990s, whereas the prevalence in women remained unchanged [18]. Other studies, however, show that it is increasing in both genders [19,20]. The alarming increase in numbers of patients who have AF in the general population is not the result of increasing use of ECGs in the community, because in the Framingham Study cohort, ECGs are obtained routinely on each examination; there was an age-adjusted secular increase in prevalence of AF on clinic ECGs [5]. Also, in the Rochester population, use of the ECG increased by only 9% to 12%, over a 30-year period, whereas there was a two- to threefold increase in the prevalence of AF [21]. In Denmark, standardizing by age and 10-year age group, the AF incidence rates approximately doubled for men and women (197 per 100,000 in 1980 and 448 per 100,000 in 1999) [20].

A more credible explanation of the increasing prevalence of AF over time is that the elderly population of today has a higher prevalence of predisposing conditions for AF, such as diabetes, obesity, heart failure, coronary and valvular heart disease, and prior cardiac surgery. This trend, brought about by advances in the treatment of cardiovascular disease, has produced a population of elderly survivors containing more candidates for AF than formerly. The Rochester study, however, observed only modest increases in the prevalence of these predisposing conditions over a 3-decade period that did not seem to explain more than partially the observed magnitude of the increase in prevalence of AF [21].

United States census projections for the next 50 years estimate that approximately 3 million Americans will have AF by the year 2020, increasing to 5.6 million by the year 2050, with more than half of those affected aged 80 or older [11,22–24]. The magnitude of these projections may be underestimated because many episodes of AF are undetected.

Public health burden and cost

AF, first described in 1909, has acquired increasing clinical and public health importance as a result of an expanding elderly population containing more vulnerable candidates [6]. Data from a National Hospital Discharge Survey indicate that hospital admissions resulting from AF increased two- to threefold from 1985 to 1999. During this period, hospitalizations listing AF increased from under 800,000 to more than 2 million, predominantly in the elderly and men. Coyne and colleagues [25], assessing direct costs of treating AF in the United States, list AF as one of the principal discharge diagnoses for 350,000 hospitalizations, and 5 million office visits in 2001. The total costs in 2005 dollars were estimated at $6.65 billion, including $2.93 billion for hospitalizations.

Data from the United States and the United Kingdom indicate that AF is a costly public health problem [26]. Many factors contribute to the high cost of AF, with hospitalizations constituting the major contributor (52%), followed by drugs (23%), consultations (9%), further investigations (8%), loss of work (6%), and paramedical procedures (2%). Globally, the annual cost per patient is close to $3600. Considering the prevalence of AF, the total economic burden is huge [17].

Clinical manifestations

AF may cause palpitations, fatigue, lightheadedness, and dyspnea on exertion by precipitating cardiac failure. If there is underlying coronary artery disease, it can initiate or aggravate angina from the associated rapid heart rate. AF often goes undetected, however, because of lack of symptoms. It frequently is detected first by routine ECG examination, in the course of a myocardial infarction or stroke, on implanted pacemakers, or ambulatory ECG monitoring. AF was diagnosed incidentally in 12% of patients having an ECG for unrelated reasons in the Cardiovascular Health Study [8] and in 45% of patients in the Stroke Prevention in Atrial Fibrillation Trials [27]. In a study of patients who had paroxysmal AF, there were 12 times as many asymptomatic as symptomatic episodes of AF and 38% of the patients who had implanted pacemakers who experienced AF for more than 48 hours were unaware of it [28]. The low prevalence of AF in the absence of clinical and subclinical cardiovascular disease in the Cardiovascular Health Study of the elderly (1.6%) suggests that "lone atrial fibrillation" is fairly uncommon in the elderly [15].

Prognosis

AF is associated with an increased long-term risk for stroke, heart failure, and all-cause mortality, particularly in women [29]. The mortality rate of patients who have AF is approximately double that of patients in normal sinus rhythm and linked to the severity of underlying heart disease [30–32]. Approximately two thirds of the 3.7% mortality over 8.6 months in the Activité Liberale la Fibrillation Auriculaire (ALFA) Study was attributed to cardiovascular causes [33]. AF independently predicts, however, excess mortality and is associated with an increased incidence of embolic stroke, accounting for between 75,000 and 100,000 strokes per year in the United States [3]. AF is in itself a powerful risk factor for stroke among patients of advanced age. The epidemic of AF in the twenty-first century is occurring in conjunction with a rising prevalence of heart failure, obesity, type 2 diabetes mellitus, and the prediabetic metabolic syndrome [34].

The Framingham Study shows that AF and heart failure often coexist and that each may have an adverse impact on the other [35]. The decreased survival associated with AF occurs across a wide age range, partially attributable to the vulnerability of patients who have AF to development of heart failure. The differences in mortality reported among studies may be influenced by the proportion of deaths from heart failure and thromboembolism. In large trials of heart failure, AF is a strong independent risk factor for mortality and major morbidity. In the Carvedilol or Metoprolol European Trial (COMET), there was no difference in all-cause mortality in subjects who had AF at entry, but mortality increased in those who developed AF during follow-up [36]. In the Valsartan Heart Failure Trial (Val-HeFT) cohort of patients who had chronic heart failure, development of AF was associated with significantly worse outcomes [37]. Heart failure promotes AF, AF aggravates failure, and persons who have either share a poor prognosis. Thus, managing AF in conjunction with heart failure is a major challenge requiring more trial data to guide and optimize its management.

The most feared consequence of AF is stroke, the risk for which is increased four- to fivefold. AF assumes greater importance as a stroke hazard with advancing age and by the ninth decade becomes a dominant factor. The attributable risk for stroke associated with AF increases steeply from 1.5% at ages 50 to 59 to 23.5% at ages 80 to 89. AF is associated with a doubling of mortality in both genders, which is decreased to 1.5- from 1.9-fold after adjusting for associated cardiovascular conditions. The decreased survival associated with AF occurs across a wide age range.

In the distant past, paroxysmal AF was considered more dangerous than persistent chronic AF, the former postulated as more likely to embolize. The Framingham Study found chronic sustained AF to be at least as dangerous [1]. Analyses of pooled data from five randomized controlled trials suggest that paroxysmal and chronic AF have similar risks for stroke [38]. Several studies suggest, however, higher mortality in persistent versus chronic AF [39–41].

Risk factors

Age and gender

As discussed previously, AF increases with age, doubling in prevalence and incidence with each decade of age, even accounting for known predisposing conditions. Based on 38-year follow-up data from the Framingham Study, men had a 1.5-fold greater risk for developing AF than women after adjustment for age and predisposing conditions. The reason for the male preponderance of risk currently is unexplained [42].

Aging is accompanied by multiple cardiac abnormalities, including gradual loss of nodal fibers and increased fibrous and adipose tissue in the sinoatrial node, decreased ventricular compliance from myocardial fibrosis resulting in atrial dilatation that predisposes to AF, and extensive senile amyloid infiltration of the sinoatrial node that may occur [43–45]. In patients who have AF, aging is associated with left atrial enlargement and reduced left atrial appendage flow velocity, both of which predispose to left atrial thrombus formation [17]. Prothrombin activation fragment and thrombin generation also increase with age in the general population and in persons who have AF, suggesting an age-related prothrombotic diathesis. Age seems to be a more potent risk factor for AF if it is combined with other risk factors [17]. Also, aging reflects longer exposure to predisposing conditions for AF, and even in advanced age, some are clearly more vulnerable to the development of AF than others.

Cardiovascular risk factors

Of the major cardiovascular risk factors investigated by the Framingham study [9], hypertension and diabetes were significant independent predictors of AF, adjusting for age and other predisposing conditions (Table 2). Cigarette smoking was a significant risk factor in women adjusting only for age (odds ratio [OR] 1.4) but was just short of significance on adjustment for other risk factors. Neither obesity nor alcohol intake appeared to be independently associated with short-term risk (pooled logistic regression) of AF incidence in either gender. In other studies, however, with sufficient power and of individuals who consume alcohol at sufficiently high amounts, it seems that alcohol abuse is related to occurrence of AF [46,47]. As discussed later, obesity is associated with long-term risk for AF (Cox model), which seems to be mediated partially by left atrial enlargement.

For men and women, respectively, diabetes conferred a 1.4- and 1.6-fold risk and hypertension a 1.5- and 1.4-fold risk, after adjusting for other

Table 2
Cardiovascular risk factors for atrial fibrillation; 38-year follow-up: Framingham Study

Risk factors	Odds ratios			
	Age adjusted		Risk factor adjusted	
	Men	Women	Men	Women
Diabetes	1.7*	2.1**	1.4***	1.6*
ECG LV Hypertrophy	3.0**	3.8**	1.4	1.3
Hypertension	1.8**	1.7**	1.5*	1.4***
Cigarettes	1.0	1.4***	1.1	1.4
BMI	1.03	1.02	—	—
Alcohol	1.01	0.95	—	—

*P<.01; **P<.001; ***P<.05.
Data from Benjamin EJ, Levy D, Vaziri SM, et al. Independent risk factors for atrial fibrillation in a population-based cohort: the Framingham heart study. JAMA 1994;271:840–4.

associated conditions. Because of its high prevalence, hypertension was responsible for more AF in the population [14%] than any other risk factor [9,42].

Increased pulse pressure, a reflection of aortic stiffness, increases the cardiac load and, in the Framingham Study, increases AF risk [48]. Cumulative 20-year AF incidence rates were 5.6% for subjects who had a pulse pressure 40 mm Hg or less (25th percentile) and 23.3% for those who had a pulse pressure greater than 61 mm Hg (75th percentile). In models adjusted for age, gender, baseline and time-dependent change in mean arterial pressure, and clinical risk factors for AF (body mass index [BMI], smoking, valvular disease, diabetes, ECG LV hypertrophy, hypertension treatment, and prevalent myocardial infarction or heart failure), pulse pressure was associated with increased risk for AF (adjusted hazard ratio [HR], 1.26 per 20–mm Hg increment; 95% confidence interval [CI], 1.12–1.43; P = .001).

In contrast, mean arterial pressure was unrelated to incident AF. Systolic pressure was related to AF (HR 1.14 per 20–mm Hg increment; 95% CI, 1.04−1.25; P = .006). When diastolic pressure was added, however, the model fit improved and the diastolic relation was inverse (adjusted HR 0.87 per 10–mm Hg increment), consistent with a pulse pressure effect. Furthermore, the association between pulse pressure and AF persisted in models that adjusted for baseline left atrial dimension, LV mass, and LV fractional shortening (adjusted HR 1.23; 95% CI, 1.09–1.39; P = .001). It seems that pulse pressure is an important risk factor for incident AF. Further research is needed to determine whether or not interventions that reduce pulse pressure can help retard the growing incidence of AF.

Diabetes also was a significant independent predictor of AF in four other studies, associated with an average relative risk (RR) of 1.8, but in two other studies, it was not [17]. Because the strength of diabetes as a predictor seems to be greater in lower-risk patients who have AF, it is speculated that it also may be associated with noncardioembolic strokes. Diabetes is a less powerful independent predictor than prior stroke or transient ischemic attack (TIA), hypertension, or age, but further analysis is needed to refine its predictive value for thromboembolism in patients who have AF. The reduction in stroke in warfarin-treated patients who had diabetes was below average in two studies [17].

Thyroid disease

Hyperthyroidism long has been implicated as a condition predisposing to AF. The prevalence of AF reported in patients at time of diagnosis of overt hyperthyroidism varies widely from 2% to 30% [49–52]. Approximately 10% to 15% of persons who have overt hyperthyroid disease and AF are reported to have an arterial embolic event [52–54]. Studies also suggest that subclinical abnormalities in thyroid stimulating hormone levels have detrimental effects on the cardiovascular system. In one small study based on samples from a central reference laboratory, AF developed in 3 of 32 subjects who had subclinical hyperthyroidism over 2 years of follow-up compared with none in 35 who had normal thyrotropins [55].

Although AF is an acknowledged manifestation of hyperthyroidism, older people in whom AF is common do not often have clinically overt hyperthyroidism. It was not established firmly that subclinical hyperthyroidism imposed a risk for AF until the Framingham Study investigated this hypothesis. The Framingham Study examined prospectively the incidence of AF in relation to serum thyrotropin concentrations over 10 years in study participants over age 60. A low-serum thyrotropin (<0.1 mU per liter) was associated with a threefold higher risk for developing AF over a decade after adjusting for other known risk factors [56].

The increased AF risk for hyperthyroidism was confirmed in the Cardiovascular Health Study of community dwellers ages 65 years or older for whom baseline serum thyroid-stimulating hormone levels were measured, and the relationship between baseline thyroid status and incident AF, incident cardiovascular disease, and mortality in older men and women not taking thyroid medication was determined [57]. Eighty-two percent of participants (n = 2639) had normal thyroid function, 15% (n = 496) had subclinical hypothyroidism, 1.6% (n = 51) had overt hypothyroidism, and 1.5% (n = 47) had subclinical hyperthyroidism. After exclusion of those who had prevalent AF, individuals who had subclinical hyperthyroidism had a greater incidence of AF compared with those who had normal thyroid function (67 events versus 31 events per 1000 person-years [adjusted HR 1.98; CI, 1.29–3.03]). No differences were seen in the subclinical hyperthyroidism and euthyroidism groups for incident coronary heart disease, stroke, cardiovascular death, or all-cause mortality. Likewise, there were no differences in the subclinical hypothyroidism or overt hypothyroidism groups and the euthyroidism group for cardiovascular outcomes or mortality. These data show an association between subclinical hyperthy-roidism and development of AF but do not support the hypothesis that un-recognized subclinical hyperthyroidism or subclinical hypothyroidism is associated with other cardiovascular disorders that might predispose to AF.

Cardiovascular conditions

Persons who develop AF usually are elderly and more likely than persons of the same age to have coronary disease, valvular heart disease, heart failure, echocardiographic abnormalities, or LV hypertrophy [9,42]. Approximately 20% of men and 30% of women have valvular heart disease, approximately a quarter of both genders have heart failure, and 26% of men and 13% of women have prevalence myocardial infarctions. These overt cardiac conditions impose a substantial risk of AF. Adjusting for other rel-evant conditions, heart failure was associated with a 4.5- and 5.9-fold risk and valvular heart disease a 1.8- and 3.4-fold risk for AF in men and women, respectively. Myocardial infarction significantly increased the risk factor–adjusted likelihood of AF by 40% in men only (Table 3).

Echocardiographic abnormalities

Valvular heart disease, echocardiographic enlargement of the left atrial dimension, and abnormal mitral or aortic valve function were associated independently with increased prevalence and incidence of AF in the Cardio-vascular Health Study [8,15]. Based on Framingham Study data, echocar-diographic predictors of AF include left atrial enlargement (39% increase in risk per 5-mm increment), LV fractional shortening (34% per 5% decre-ment), and LV wall thickness (28% per 4-mm increment) (Table 4). These echocardiographic features offer prognostic information for AF beyond the traditional clinical risk factors [42,58].

Table 3
Odds of developing atrial fibrillation for specified cardiac conditions in Framingham Study; subjects ages 55 to 94 years; based on 38 years' follow-up

Cardiac conditions	Odds ratios			
	Age adjusted		Risk factor adjusted	
	Men	Women	Men	Women
Myocardial infarction	2.2*	2.4*	1.4**	1.2
Heart failure	6.1***	8.1***	4.5***	5.9***
Valve disease	2.2***	3.6***	1.8*	3.4***

$*P < .01$; $**P < .05$; $***P < .001$.

Data from Benjamin EJ, Levy D, Vaziri SM, et al. Independent risk factors for atrial fibril-lation in a population-based cohort: the Framingham heart study. JAMA 1994;271:840–4.

Table 4
Echocardiographic predictors of atrial fibrillation: Framingham study; subjects ages 50 to 59 years

Echocardiographic features	Atrial fibrillation risk
Left atrial diameter, mm	39% increase per 5 mm
Fractional shortening, %	34% increase per −5%
Left ventricular wall thickness	28% increase per 4 mm
Two or more of above versus none	17% versus 3.7%

Data from Vaziri SM, Larson MG, Benjamin EJ, et al. Echocardiographic predictors of nonrheumatic atrial fibrillation. The Framingham Heart Study. Circulation 1994;89:724–30.

Mitral annular calcification is associated with adverse cardiovascular disease outcomes and stroke in longitudinal and community-based cohorts. Prospective data are limited on its association with AF. The Framingham Study investigated the association between mitral annular calcification and long-term risk for AF (more than 16 years of follow-up) in participants in the original cohort attending routine examinations between 1979 and 1981 [59]. The age- and gender-adjusted incidence rate of AF was 362 per 10,000 person-years in subjects who had mitral annular calcification compared with 185 per 10,000 person-years in those who did not have it. In multivariable-adjusted analyses, mitral annular calcification was associated with 1.6-fold increased risk for AF. This association was attenuated somewhat on further adjustment for left atrial size (HR 1.4; 95% CI, 0.9–2.0), suggesting that the association between mitral annular calcification and incident AF is mediated only partially through left atrial enlargement [59].

In a double-blind, randomized, parallel-group study of 8831 men and women who had hypertension and ECG LV hypertrophy enrolled in the Losartan Intervention for Endpoint Reduction in Hypertension Study, the occurrence of new-onset AF was investigated in relation to in-treatment regression or continued absence of ECG LV hypertrophy [60]. Quantified regression of ECG LV hypertrophy was associated with a reduced likelihood of new-onset AF, independent of blood pressure lowering and treatment.

Novel risk factors

Many novel risk factors for AF have been identified, some modifiable and some not. These include inflammatory markers, the obesity-induced metabolic syndrome, insulin resistance, thrombogenic tendencies, sleep apnea, decreased arterial compliance, left atrial volume, and diastolic dysfunction.

Inflammation

The suspicion that inflammation contributes to some types of AF is supported by the frequent occurrence of AF after cardiac surgery (25%

to 40%), genetic studies, and the association of AF with pericarditis and myocarditis. The time course of AF after cardiac surgery parallels activation of the complement system and release of proinflammatory cytokines [61,62].

C-reactive protein, a sensitive marker of inflammation, is a predictor of adverse cardiac events recently linked to AF [63–65]. In the Cardiovascular Health Study, a large, population-based study of cardiovascular disease in the elderly, C-reactive protein was associated independently with the presence of AF at baseline and predicted patients at increased risk for developing future AF [66]. It is not clear whether or not indices of inflammation should be regarded as direct risk factors for AF by causing an atrial inflammatory state or whether or not these are markers for the underlying atherosclerotic vascular disease.

Insulin resistance and the metabolic syndrome

Concurrently, the prevalence of obesity, diabetes, and the metabolic syndrome has reached major proportions around the world. In a retrospective analysis of the incidence of AF in relation to BMI in consecutive cardiac surgery patients, obesity was reported to be an important determinant of new-onset AF after cardiac surgery [67]. It is unclear to what extent cardiovascular risk factors mediate the association between obesity and AF. In a population-based Veterans Administration case-control study of subjects who had new-onset AF and controls identified through medical record review of inpatient and outpatient visits, the association of AF with BMI seemed mediated partially by diabetes but minimally through other cardiovascular risk factors [68].

Obesity is associated with atrial enlargement and ventricular diastolic dysfunction, which are established predictors of AF. The Framingham Study investigated the association between BMI and the long-term risk for developing new onset of AF in a prospective, community-based observational cohort [69]. During a mean follow-up of 13.7 years, age-adjusted incidence rates for AF increased across the three BMI categories (normal, overweight, and obese) in men (9.7, 10.7, and 14.3 per 1000 person-years) and women (5.1, 8.6, and 9.9 per 1000 person-years). In multivariable models adjusted for cardiovascular risk factors and interim myocardial infarction or heart failure, a 4% increase in AF risk per 1-unit increase in BMI was observed in men and women. The adjusted HRs for AF associated with obesity were 1.5 for men and women, compared with individuals who had normal BMI. After adjustment for echocardiographic left atrial diameter in addition to clinical risk factors, BMI no longer was associated with AF risk. It was concluded that obesity is an important, potentially modifiable risk factor for AF, the excess risk of which seems to be mediated chiefly by left atrial dilatation. These prospective data suggest that interventions to promote normal weight may reduce the population burden of AF.

The inter-relations between obesity, diabetes, and the metabolic syndrome strongly suggests an insulin-resistant state. In a prospective analysis of consecutive hospitalized patients who were in sinus rhythm and who did not have obvious structural heart disease, paroxysmal AF or atrial flutter occurred in 9% of the patients who had metabolic syndrome but only 4% of patients who did not have the syndrome ($P = .02$). Multivariate logistic regression analysis indicated that the metabolic syndrome was a significant risk factor that was independent of left atrial diameter or age (OR 2.8; $P < .01$). Among the five components of the metabolic syndrome, BMI was associated the most strongly with AF/atrial flutter (OR 3.0, $P = .02$). It was concluded that the metabolic syndrome was associated strongly with AF/atrial flutter in patients who did not have structural heart diseases and that obesity may be an important underlying mechanism [70].

A community-based, cross-sectional observational study conducted in a primary health care facility in Sweden explored the prevalence of AF in patients who had hypertension and type 2 diabetes mellitus seeking possible mechanisms for its development. An association of AF with combined hypertension and type 2 diabetes mellitus was found that remained significant when adjusted for other cardiovascular disease risk factors. BMI AF risk was attenuated by adjustment for ischemic ECG findings and lost significance with adjustment for insulin resistance (OR 1.3 [0.5–3.1]). It was suggested that AF may be associated with the combined occurrence of type 2 diabetes mellitus and hypertension because of insulin resistance [71].

Given the evidence that the metabolic syndrome is proinflammatory and that AF is linked to inflammation, the relations of these risk factors to incident AF merits further investigation. The finding that new-onset AF is related significantly to BMI in multivariate analysis, adjusting for age and gender, also has some credibility because obesity is an independent predictor of diastolic dysfunction, also a major determinant of AF [72].

Stature

Data from a multicenter registry of patients who had impaired LV function (National Registry to Advance Heart Health) were used to investigate the influence of stature on AF in high-risk patients who had reduced LV systolic function [73]. Because left atrial size is associated strongly with stature, it was hypothesized that height and body surface area are risk factors for AF, independent of other known associations. The study was based on 25,268 patients (mean age 66 years) consisting mostly of white men (72%) who had ischemic cardiomyopathy (72%) and who had a mean LV ejection fraction of 31%.

A history of AF was present in 7027 patients (27.8%). AF prevalence increased significantly between the lowest and highest height quartiles (32% relative increase, $P < .0001$). In multivariable analysis, the effect of height on AF risk persisted after adjusting for age, gender, race, LV ejection fraction, heart failure class and etiology, hypertension, diabetes, and medication use. In patients who have LV dysfunction, increasing stature seems to portend a higher risk for AF after accounting for other traditional risk factors for the arrhythmia. This association may account for some of the higher prevalence of AF in men [73]. Height also is observed to be associated with an increased risk for incident AF in the community (HR 1.03 per cm [1.02–1.05]) [8].

Plasma natriuretic peptides

Obesity-promoted natriuretic peptides are secreted from cardiomyocytes. They play a fundamental role in cardiovascular remodeling, volume homeostasis, and response to ischemia. Investigation of the relation of B-type natriuretic peptide and N-terminal proatrial natriuretic peptide by the Framingham Study shows these natriuretic peptides to be associated with an increased risk for AF and its predisposing cardiovascular conditions, such as heart failure and stroke (Table 5) [74].

Sleep apnea

There is a well-documented relationship between obesity and sleep apnea, but the prevalence of sleep-disordered breathing also is substantial in those who are nonobese. A high recurrence of AF in patients undergoing cardioversion is reported and AF recurrences are more common in untreated than treated obstructive sleep apnea. Patients undergoing cardioversion are reported to have a 49% prevalence of sleep apnea compared with a 39% frequency among other cardiac patients who do not have AF that is not attributable other predisposing conditions [75,76]. Mechanisms postulated include hypoxia, hypercarbia, autonomic imbalance, stretching of the atrium, and LV wall stress. Increased right-sided cardiac pressure stimulates atrial natriuretic peptide release that is noted in AF. Prospective studies of the relationship of sleep-disordered breathing with AF are needed, taking

Table 5
Plasma B-type natriuretic peptides and risk for cerebrovascular disease: Framingham Study

Cardiovascular disease event	Percent increase in cardiovascular disease per SD increment	Multivariable hazard ratio for BNP >80th percentile[a]
Heart failure	77%	3.1*
Atrial fibrillation	66%	1.9**
Stroke/TIA	53%	2.0**
First CV event	28%	1.8**
Death	27%	1.6**

[a] Adjusted for age, diabetes, blood pressure, smoking, creatinine, LV mass, and systolic function; 80th percentile B-type natriuretic peptide (BNP): women 23.3 pg/mL, men 20 pg/mL.
    Peptide levels not significantly related to coronary heart disease.
    *$P<.01$; **$P<.05$.
    Data from Wang TJ, Larson MG, Levy D, et al. Plasma natriuretic peptide levels and the risk of cardiovascular events and death. N Engl J Med 2004;350:655–63.

into account the sleep apnea relationship to obesity, metabolic syndrome, coronary artery disease, heart failure, and stroke [77,78].

Diastolic dysfunction

Diastolic dysfunction is a common accompaniment of aging, hypertension, obesity, diabetes, heart failure, and coronary artery disease in the elderly. Elderly patients in sinus rhythm at the time of an echocardiographic examination developed AF at a 1% rate with mild diastolic dysfunction compared with 12% with moderate diastolic dysfunction and 20% severe diastolic dysfunction. Diastolic dysfunction provides additional predictive information for development of AF over that obtained from the clinical risk factors. As left atrial volumes increase, diastolic function deteriorates, providing predictive information for the development of AF and stroke [79,80]. Furthermore, left atrial volume is a predictor of other cardiovascular events, including myocardial infarction, stroke, and coronary revascularization, all of which predispose to AF [81,82].

Atrial fibrillation as a stroke risk factor

AF is an established major independent risk factor for embolic stroke or TIA; AF is associated with a four- to fivefold greater risk than in the unaffected population [3]. There also is evidence, however, that a stroke may precipitate the occurrence of AF because of its hemodynamic and autonomic consequences. Approximately half of all elderly patients who have AF have hypertension as a major risk factor for stroke. Hypertension is a powerful independent predictor of stroke in AF and an important risk factor for developing AF. The strong association between AF, hypertension, and stroke could depend on reduced aortic compliance, LV hypertrophy, diastolic dysfunction, and left atrial dilatation, giving rise to stasis and thrombus formation [27,83,84].

AF accounts for approximately 45% of all embolic strokes. The risk for stroke in placebo-treated patients in randomized warfarin trials is reported as 4.5% per year [83,85]. A collaborative analysis of five randomized trials by the Atrial Fibrillation Investigators identified five major risk factors for stroke in patients who have AF, namely, prior stroke or TIA, a history of hypertension, advanced age, a history of heart failure, and diabetes (Table 6) [84]. The risk for stroke increases at least fivefold in patients who have clinical risk factors, and this is in marked contrast to the low risk for stroke in younger patients who do not have clinical risk factors. Other factors, such as female gender, systolic blood pressure over 160 mm Hg, and LV dysfunction, are linked variably to stroke.

In patients 80 to 89 years old, 36% of strokes occur in those who have AF. The annual risk for stroke for octogenarians who have AF is in the range of 3% to 8% per year, depending on associated stroke risk factors

Table 6
Risk factors for ischemic stroke and systemic embolism in patients who have nonvalvular atrial fibrillation

Risk factors	Relative risk
Previous stroke or TIA	2.5
Diabetes	1.7
History of hypertension	1.6
Heart failure	1.4
Advanced age (continuous, per decade)	1.4

As a group, patients who have AF carry an approximately fivefold increased risk for thromboembolism compared with patients in sinus rhythm. Relative risk refers to comparison of patients who have AF to patients who do not have these risk factors.

Data from Mukamal KJ, Tolstrup JS, Friberg J, et al. Alcohol consumption and risk of atrial fibrillation in men and women: the Copenhagen City Heart Study. Circulation 2005;112:1736–42. From Atrial Fibrillation Investigators. Risk factors for stroke and efficacy of antithrombotic treatment in atrial fibrillation: analysis of pooled data from five randomized controlled studies. Arch Intern Med 1994;154:1449–57.

[3]. The powerful impact of age and clinical risk factors on the risk for stroke in patients who have AF suggests that vigorous control of accompanying risk factors should be undertaken to lower the risk.

Ischemic stroke and systemic arterial occlusion in AF generally are attributed to embolism of thrombus from the left atrium; however, up to 25% of strokes in patients who have AF may be the result of intrinsic cerebrovascular diseases, other cardiac sources of embolism, or atherosclerotic pathology in the proximal aorta [17,83]. Although 12% harbor carotid artery stenosis, carotid atherosclerosis is not substantially more prevalent in patients who have AF and who have stroke and seems to be a minor contributing factor [86,87].

Genetic influences

Familial occurrence of AF has been recognized for many years but was considered uncommon. The Framingham Study found that parental AF increases the future risk for offspring AF approximately two- to threefold after excluding persons who have predisposing conditions, an observation supporting a genetic susceptibility to developing this dysrhythmia (Fig. 1) [88]. In such families who have AF, familial linkage studies are beginning to explore the genetics of AF, particularly in younger persons [89–91].

Purported genetically determined constitutional factors, such as blood pressure, obesity, and greater stature, predispose to AF. It is uncertain how these constitutional factors promote AF, but metabolic disorders and genetic factors seem to be implicated.

Identification of a gene defect linked to chromosome 10q in a Spanish family, nearly half the members of which had AF, supports the hypothesis of familial AF [90,92]. The majority of patients who have AF in these

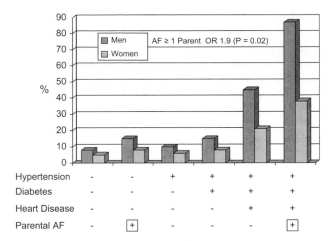

Hypertension	-	-	+	+	+	+
Diabetes	-	-	-	+	+	+
Heart Disease	-	-	-	-	+	+
Parental AF	-	+	-	-	-	+

Fig. 1. Risk of AF by parental AF status: Framingham Offspring Cohort. (*Data from* Fox CS, Parise H, D'Agostino Sr RB, et al. Parental atrial fibrillation as a risk factor for atrial fibrillation in offspring. JAMA 2004;291:2851–5.)

families are younger, however, than age 65, suggesting that the postulated genes causing AF may not be involved directly in the elderly.

The National Heart Lung and Blood Institute (NHLBI) is sponsoring several projects to examine the genetic contribution to AF and other cardiovascular phenotypes in the community. Two studies in particular will genotype 1000s of candidate genes (Candidate gene Association Resource [CARE] project) and a 550K genome–wide scan of genetic polymorphisms (SNP Health Association Resource [SHARe]) with thousands of participants across many of the NHLBI's cohort studies. The data from these studies will be available for analysis to investigators who have approved projects and ethical oversight. The aggregate results of these studies will be posted on the Web (http://www.ncbi.nlm.nih.gov/projects/gap/cgi-bin/study.cgi?id=phs000007). Over the next decade, the advent of large-scale genotyping efforts undoubtedly will lead to major advances in understanding the contribution of common complex genetic variation to AF in the community.

Multivariable risk assessment

Multivariable risk assessment of the stroke risk for patients who have AF is desirable for selecting those who most and least need aggressive anticoagulant therapy. The number needed to treat to prevent one event is related inversely to the level of risk. Estimating the risk for stroke for individual patients who have AF is crucial for the decision to prescribe anticoagulation therapy, but the threshold risk warranting anticoagulation is controversial. Patients who have a stroke risk of 2% per year or less do not benefit substantially from oral anticoagulation, and it would require treating 100 or more patients for 1 year to prevent a single stroke [17]. For high-risk patients with AF who have stroke rates of 6% per year or greater, the comparable needed-to-treat number is 25 or fewer, strongly favoring anticoagulation. For patients at intermediate stroke risk (annual rate 3% to 5%), opinion about routine anticoagulation remains divided.

AF is a major component of the Framingham stroke risk prediction algorithm [3]. Framingham Study investigators sought to stratify risk further and elucidate which individuals who had AF were at particularly increased risk for stroke or stroke and death [93]. Their multivariable analysis examined risk factors for stroke among 705 patients who had recently detected AF, excluding those who had sustained ischemic stroke, TIA, or death within 30 days of diagnosis (Fig. 2). The significant predictors of ischemic stroke in subjects who had AF were age (RR 1.3 per decade), female gender (RR 1.9), prior stroke or TIA (RR 1.9), and diabetes (RR 1.8). Systolic blood pressure became a significant predictor of stroke if warfarin was included in a time-dependent Cox proportional hazards model. With a scoring system based on age, gender, systolic hypertension, diabetes, and prior stroke or TIA, the proportion of patients classified as low risk varied from 14.3% to 30.6% depending on whether or not selected stroke rate thresholds were less than 1.5% per year or less than 2% per year.

Preventive measures

AF remains a substantial global health burden requiring detection of candidates likely to develop it for preventive management. The disappointing

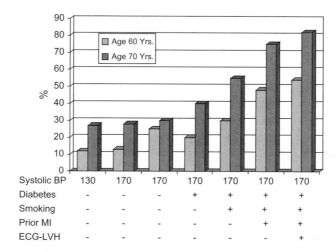

Fig. 2. Five-year stroke/death risk in AF Framingham Study. (*Data from* Wang TJ, Massaro JM, Levy D, et al. A risk score for predicting stroke or death in individuals with new onset atrial fibrillation in the community. The Framingham Heart Study. JAMA 2003;290:1049.)

results of antidysrhythmic therapy for AF require a therapeutic approach that focuses treatment on the underlying myocardial pathology leading to the occurrence of the AF. Many risk factors for AF are shared by other cardiac conditions that in turn predispose to the occurrence of AF. The premordial prevention of the risk factors jointly would prevent their emergence and in turn the AF they promote. Identification of modifiable risk factors specific for AF enables intervention early in the course of the disease when preventative or corrective strategies are most efficient. Improvement of the multivariable risk profile to prevent a stroke, coronary disease, or cardiovascular disease in general should carry a bonus of prevention of AF.

For example, angiotensin-converting enzyme inhibitors and angiotensin receptor blockers, which are recommended for hypertensive cardiovascular disease, seem to reduce the rate of recurrence of AF after cardioversion and protect against development of AF in patients who have LV dysfunction [94–96]. They also may inhibit the proinflammatory and sympathetic effects of angiotensin and interfere with the triggers and substrate of AF [17].

Warfarin anticoagulant therapy is highly effective for prevention of stroke in patients who have AF, reducing the risk by 62% [27,83]. Meta-analysis, according to the principle of intention to treat, shows that adjusted-dose oral anticoagulation is highly efficacious for prevention of all stroke (ischemic and hemorrhagic), with a risk reduction of 62% (95% CI, 48%–72%) versus placebo [83]. This reduction was similar for primary and secondary prevention and for disabling and nondisabling strokes. Using "on-treatment analysis" (excluding patients not on oral anticoagulation at the time of stroke), the preventive efficacy of oral anticoagulation exceeded 80%. Despite this, a survey of treatment for patients who had cerbrovascular disease indicates that only 50% are being treated to recommended standards of care. The deficits found in adherence to recommended processes for basic care for cardiovascular disease in general and AF in particular pose serious threats to the health of the American public. Strategies to reduce these deficits in care urgently are urgently needed.

Summary

We are confronted with a rapidly growing epidemic of AF, the scope of which urgently demands improved prevention and treatment of this condition and its predisposing cardiovascular substrate. The cardiovascular conditions associated with AF justifiably are considered risk factors rather than risk markers. It also is likely that AF and the left atrial enlargement associated with it are direct causes of embolic stroke, requiring early detection and treatment. AF now is a global health burden requiring targeted screening to detect persons likely to develop this condition.

The disappointing results of therapy to suppress or eliminate the rhythm disturbance have focused greater attention on treatment to prevent or delay myocardial changes leading to the occurrence of the AF. Many risk factors associated with AF also predispose to cardiovascular diseases that beget the development of AF, so their eradication theoretically should confer a substantial public health and health care benefit. Identification and treatment of modifiable risk factors specific for AF in high-risk candidates for the condition would enable early intervention, when preventative or corrective measures are most effective. In addition, advances in identifying genetic and biologic markers of risk for AF and its complications will provide pathophysiologic insights and enable better risk stratification for more personalized and targeted therapy.

References

[1] Kannel WB, Abbott RD, Savage DD, et al. Epidemiologic features of chronic atrial fibrillation: the Framingham Study. N Engl J Med 1982;306:1018–22.
[2] Benjamin EJ, Wolf PA, D'Agostino RB, et al. Impact of atrial fibrillation on risk of death: the Framingham study. Circulation 1999;98:946–52.
[3] Wolf PA, Abbot RD, Kannel WB. Atrial fibrillation as independent risk factor for stroke: the Framingham study. Stroke 1991;22:983–8.
[4] Bialy D, Lehnmann MH, Schumacher DN, et al. Hospitalization for arrhythmias in the United States. Importance of atrial fribrillation [abstract]. J Am Coll Cardiol 1992;19:41A.
[5] Wolf PA, Benjamin EJ, Belanger AJ, et al. Secular trends in the prevalence of atrial fibrillation: the Framingham study. Am Heart J 1996;131:790–5.
[6] Stewart S, MacIntyre K, MacLeod MM, et al. Trends in hospital activity, morbidity and case fatality related to atrial fibrillation in Scotland, 1986–1996. Eur Heart J 2001;22:693–701.
[7] Frost L, Engholm G, Møller H, et al. Decrease in mortality in patients with a hospital diagnosis of atrial fibrillation in Denmark during the period 1980–1993. Eur Heart J 1999;20: 1592–9.
[8] Psaty BM, Manolio TA, Kuller LH, et al. Incidence of and risk factors for atrial fibrillation in older adults. Circulation 1997;96:2455–61.
[9] Benjamin EJ, Levy D, Vaziri SM, et al. Independent risk factors for atrial fibrillation in a population-based cohort: the Framingham heart study. JAMA 1994;271:840–4.
[10] Feinberg WM, Blackshear JL, Laupacis A, et al. Prevalence, age distribution and gender of patients with atrial fibrillation: analysis and implications. Arch Intern Med 1995;155:469–73.
[11] Go AS, Hylek EM, Phillips KA, et al. Prevalence of diagnosed atrial fibrillation in adults: national implications for rhythm management and stroke prevention: the anticoagulation and risk factors in atrial fibrillation (ATRIA) Study. JAMA 2001;285:2370–5.
[12] Heeringa J, van der Kuip DA, Hofman A, et al. Prevalence, incidence and lifetime risk of atrial fibrillation: the Rotterdam study. Eur Heart J 2006;27:949–53.
[13] Lloyd-Jones DM, Wang TJ, Leip E, et al. Lifetime risk for development of atrial fibrillation: The Framingham Heart Study. Circulation 2004;110:1042–6.
[14] Ryder KM, Benjamin EJ. Epidemiology and significance of atrial fibrillation. Am J Cardiol 1999;84:131R–8R.
[15] Furberg CD, Psaty BM, Manolio TA, et al. Prevalence of atrial fibrillation in elderly subjects (the Cardiovascular Health Study). Am J Cardiol 1994;74:236–41.
[16] Ruo B, Capra AM, Jensvold NG, et al. Racial variation in the prevalence of atrial fibrillation among patients with heart failure: the epidemiology, practice, outcomes, and costs of heart failure (EPOCH) study. J Am Coll Cardiol 2004;43:429–35.
[17] Fuster V, Ryden LE, Cannom DS, et al. ACC/AHA/ESC 2006 Guidelines for the Management of Patients with Atrial Fibrillation: a report of the American College of Cardiology/

American Heart Association Task Force on Practice Guidelines and the European Society of Cardiology Committee for Practice Guidelines (Writing Committee to Revise the 2001 Guidelines for the Management of Patients With Atrial Fibrillation): developed in collaboration with the European Heart Rhythm Association and the Heart Rhythm Society. Circulation 2006;114:e257–354.

[18] Friberg J, Scharling H, Gadsboll N, et al. Sex-specific increase in the prevalence of atrial fibrillation (The Copenhagen City Heart Study). Am J Cardiol 2003;92:1419–23.

[19] DeWilde S, Carey IM, Emmas C, et al. Trends in the prevalence of diagnosed atrial fibrillation, its treatment with anticoagulation and predictors of such treatment in UK primary care. Heart 2006;92:1064–70.

[20] Frost L, Vestergaard P, Mosekilde L, et al. Trends in incidence and mortality in the hospital diagnosis of atrial fibrillation or flutter in Denmark, 1980–1999. Int J Cardiol 2005;103:78–84.

[21] Tsang TS, Petty GW, Barnes ME, et al. The prevalence of atrial fibrillation in incident stroke cases and matched population controls in Rochester, Minnesota: changes over three decades. J Am Coll Cardiol 2003;42:93–100.

[22] Gillum R. Trends in acute myocardial infarction and coronary heart disease death in the United States. J Am Coll Cardiol 1994;23:1273–7.

[23] McGovern PG, Jacobs DR Jr, Shahar E, et al. Trends in acute coronary heart disease mortality, morbidity, and medical care from 1985 through 1997: the Minnesota Heart Survey. Circulation 2001;104:19–24.

[24] Wattigney WA, Mensah GA, Croft JB. Increasing trends in hospitalization for atrial fibrillation in the United States, 1985 through 1999: implications for primary prevention. Circulation 2003;108:711–6.

[25] Coyne KS, Paramore C, Grandy S, et al. Assessing the direct costs of treating nonvalvular atrial fibrillation in the United States. Value Health 2006;9:348–56.

[26] Stewart S, Murphy N, Walker A, et al. Cost of an emerging epidemic: an economic analysis of atrial fibrillation in the UK. Heart 2004;90:286–92.

[27] The SPAF III Writing Committee for the Stroke Prevention in Atrial Fibrillation Investigators. The SPAF III Writing Committee for the Stroke Prevention in Atrial Fibrillation Investigators. Patients with nonvalvular atrial fibrillation at low risk of stroke during treatment with aspirin: stroke prevention in atrial fibrillation III study. JAMA 1998;279:1273–7.

[28] Israel CW, Gronefeld G, Ehrlich JR, et al. Long-term risk of recurrent atrial fibrillation as documented by an implantable monitoring device: implications for optimal patient care. J Am Coll Cardiol 2004;43:47–52.

[29] Stewart S, Hart CL, Hole DJ, et al. A population-based study of the long-term risks associated with atrial fibrillation: 20-year follow-up of the Renfrew/Paisley study. Am J Med 2002;113:359–64.

[30] Kannel WB, Abbott RD, Savage DD, et al. Coronary heart disease and atrial fibrillation: the Framingham Study. Am Heart J 1983;106:389–96.

[31] Krahn AD, Manfreda J, Tate RB, et al. The natural history of atrial fibrillation: incidence, risk factors, and prognosis in the Manitoba Follow-Up Study. Am J Med 1995;98:476–84.

[32] Flegel KM, Shipley MJ, Rose G. Risk of stroke in non-rheumatic atrial fibrillation [published erratum appears in Lancet 1987;1:878]. Lancet 1987;1:526–9.

[33] Levy S, Maarek M, Coumel P, et al. Characterization of different subsets of atrial fibrillation in general practice in France: the ALFA study. The College of French Cardiologists. Circulation 1999;99:3028–35.

[34] Braunwald E. Shattuck lecture—cardiovascular medicine at the turn of the millennium: triumphs, concerns, and opportunities. N Engl J Med 1997;337:1360–9.

[35] Wang TJ, Larson MG, Levy D, et al. Temporal relations of atrial fibrillation and congestive heart failure and their joint influence on mortality: the Framingham Heart Study. Circulation 2003;107:2920–5.

[36] Swedberg K, Olsson LG, Charlesworth A, et al. Prognostic relevance of atrial fibrillation in patients with chronic heart failure on long-term treatment with beta-blockers. Eur Heart J 2005;26:1303–8.

[37] Maggioni AP, Latini R, Carson PE, et al. Valsartan reduces the incidence of atrial fibrillation in patients with heart failure: results from the Valsartan Heart Failure Trial (Val-HeFT). Am Heart J 2005;149:1–10.

[38] Atrial Fibrillation Investigators. Risk factors for stroke and efficacy of antithrombotic treatment in atrial fibrillation: analysis of pooled data from five randomized controlled studies. Arch Intern Med 1994;154:1449–57.

[39] Le Heuzey JY, Paziaud O, Piot O, et al. Cost of care distribution in atrial fibrillation patients: the COCAF study. Am Heart J 2004;147:121–6.

[40] Keating RJ, Gersh BJ, Hodge DO, et al. Effect of atrial fibrillation pattern on survival in a community-based cohort. Am J Cardiol 2005;96:1420–4.

[41] Ruigomez A, Johansson S, Wallander MA, et al. Predictors and prognosis of paroxysmal atrial fibrillation in general practice in the UK. BMC Cardiovasc Disord 2005;5:20.

[42] Kannel WB, Wolf PA, Benjamin EJ, et al. Prevalence, incidence, prognosis, and predisposing conditions for atrial fibrillation: population-based estimates. Am J Cardiol 1998;82: 2N–9N.

[43] Falk RH. Etiology and complications of atrial fibrillation: insights from pathology studies. Am J Cardiol 1998;82:10N–7N.

[44] Manyari DE, Patterson C, Johnson D, et al. Atrial and ventricular arrhythmias in asymptomatic elderly subjects. Correlation with left atrial size and left ventricular mass. Am Heart J 1990;119:1069–76.

[45] Lie JT, Hammond PI. Pathology of the senescent heart: anatomic observations on 237 autopsy studies of patients 90 ~ 105 years old. Mayo Clin Proc 1998;63:552–64.

[46] Mukamal KJ, Tolstrup JS, Friberg J, et al. Alcohol consumption and risk of atrial fibrillation in men and women: the Copenhagen City Heart Study. Circulation 2005;112: 1736–42.

[47] Djousse L, Levy D, Benjamin EJ, et al. Long-term alcohol consumption and the risk of atrial fibrillation in the Framingham Study. Am J Cardiol 2004;93:710–3.

[48] Mitchell GF, Vasan RS, Keyes MJ, et al. Pulse pressure and risk of new onset atrial fibrillation. JAMA 2007;297:709–15.

[49] White PD, Aub JC. The electrocardiogram in thyroid disease. Arch Intern Med 1918;22: 766–9.

[50] Sandler G, Wilson GM. The nature and prognosis of heart disease in thyrotoxicosis: a review of 150 patients with [131]I. Q J Med 1959;52:347–69.

[51] Peterson P, Hansen JM. Stroke in thyrotoxicosis with atrial fibrillation. Stroke 1988;19:15–8.

[52] Nordyke RA, Gilbert FI, Harada AS. "Graves" disease: influence of age on clinical findings. Arch Intern Med 1988;148:626–31.

[53] Presti CF, Hart RG. Thyrotoxicosis, atrial dfibrillation and embolism revisted. Am Heart J 1989;117:976–7.

[54] Singer DE. Randomized trials of warfarin for atrial fibrillation. N Engl J Med 1992;327: 1451–3.

[55] Tenerz A, Forberg R, Jansson R. Is a more acive attitude warranted in patients with subclinical thyrotoxicosis? J Intern Med 1990;228:229–33.

[56] Sawin CT, Geller A, Wolf PA, et al. Low serum thyrotropin concentrations as a risk factor for atrail fibrillation in older persons. N Engl J Med 1994;331:1249–52.

[57] Cappola AR Fried LP, Arnold AM, et al. Thyroid status, cardiovascular risk and mortality in older adults. JAMA 2006;295:1033–41.

[58] Vaziri SM, Larson MG, Benjamin EJ, et al. Echocardiographic predictors of nonrheumatic atrial fibrillation. The Framingham Heart Study. Circulation 1994;89:724–30.

[59] Fox CS, Parise H, Vasan R, et al. Mitral annular calcification is a predictor for incident atrial fibrillation. Atherosclerosis 2004;173:291–4.

[60] Okin PM, Wachtell K, Devereux RB, et al. Regression of electrocardiographic left ventricular hypertrophy and decreased incidence of new-onset atrial fibrillation in patients with hypertension. JAMA 2006;296:1242–8.

[61] Falk RH. Atrial fibrillation. N Engl J Med 2001;344:1067–78.

[62] Bruins P, Velthuis H, Yazdanbakhsh AP, et al. Activation of the complement system during and after cardiopulmonary bypass surgery: postsurgery activation involves C-reactive protein and is associated with postoperative arrhythmia. Circulation 1997;96:3542–8.

[63] Boss CJ, Lip GY. The role of inflammation in atrial fibrillation. Int J Clin Pract 2005;59(8): 870–2.

[64] Dernellis J, Panaretou M. C-reactive protein and paroxysmal atrial fibrillation: evidence of the implication of an inflammatory process in paroxysmal atrial fibrillation. Acta Cardiol 2001;56:375–80.

[65] Chung MK, Martin DO, Sprecher D, et al. C-reactive protein elevation in patients with atrial arrhythmias: inflammatory mechanisms and persistence of atrial fibrillation. Circulation 2001;104:2886–91.

[66] Aviles RJ, Martin DO, Apperson-Hansen C, et al. Inflammation as a risk factor for atrial fibrillation. Circulation 2003;108:3006–10.

[67] Zacharias A, Schwann TA, Riordan CJ, et al. Obesity and risk of new-onset atrial fibrillation after cardiac surgery. Circulation 2005;112:3247–55.

[68] Dublin S, French B, Glazer NL, et al. Risk of new-onset atrial fibrillation in relation to body mass index. Arch Intern Med 2006;166:2322–8.

[69] Wang TJ, Parise H, Levy D, et al. Obesity and the risk of new onset atrial fibrillation. Am J Med 1995;98(5):476–84.

[70] Umetani K, Kodama Y, Nakamura T, et al. High prevalence of paroxysmal atrial fibrillation and/or atrial flutter in metabolic syndrome. Circ J 2007;71:252–5.

[71] Östgren CJ, Merlo J, Råstam L, et al. For Skaraborg Hypertension and Diabetes Project. Atrial fibrillation and its association with type 2 diabetes and hypertension in a Swedish community. Diabetes Obes Metab 2004;6:367–74.

[72] Powell BD, Redfield MM, Bybee KA, et al. Association of obesity with left ventricular remodeling and diastolic dysfunction in patients without coronary artery disease. Am J Cardiol 2006;98:116–20.

[73] Hanna IR, Heeke B, Bush H. The relationship between stature and the prevalence of atrial fibrillation in patients with left ventricular dysfunction. J Am Coll Cardiol 2006;47:1683–8.

[74] Wang TJ, Larson MG, Levy D, et al. Plasma natriuretic peptide levels and the risk of cardiovascular events and death. N Engl J Med 2004;350:655–63.

[75] Kanagala R, Murali NS, Friedman PA, et al. Obstructive sleep apnea and the recurrence of atrial fibrillation. Circulation 2003;107:2589–94.

[76] Gami AS, Pressman G, Caples SM, et al. Association of atrial fibrillation and obstructive sleep apnea. Circulation 2004;110:364–7.

[77] Shamsuzzaman AS, Gersh BJ, Somers VK. Obstructive sleep apnea: implications for cardiac and vascular disease. JAMA 2003;290:1906–14.

[78] Krieger J, Laks L, Wilcox I, et al. Atrial natriuretic peptide release during sleep in patients with obstructivesleep apnea before and after treatment with nasal continuous positive airway pressure. Clin Sci 1989;77:407–11.

[79] Redfield MM, Jacobsen SJ, Burnett JC Jr, et al. Burden of systolic and diastolic ventricular dysfunction in the community: appreciating the scope of the heart failure epidemic. JAMA 2003;289:194–202.

[80] Tsang TS, Gersh BJ, Appleton CP. Left ventricular diastolic dysfunction as a predictor of the first diagnosed nonvalvular atrial fibrillation in 840 elderly men and women. J Am Coll Cardiol 2002;40:1636–44.

[81] Benjamin EJ, D'Agostino RB, Belanger AJ, et al. Left atrial size and the risk of stroke and death. The Framingham Heart Study. Circulation 1995;92:835–41.

[82] Douglas P. The left atrium: a biomarker of chronic diastolic dysfunction and cardiovascular disease risk. J Am Coll Cardiol 2003;42:1206–7.

[83] Gersh BJ, Tsang TSM, Barnes ME, et al. The changing epidemiology of non-valvular atrial fibrillation: the role of novel risk factors. Eur Heart J Suppl 2005;7:C5–11.

[84] Risk factors for stroke and efficacy of antithrombotic therapy in atrial fibrillation. Analysis of pooled data from five randomized, controlled trials. Arch Intern Med 1994;154:1449–57.

[85] Krahn AD, Manfreda J, Tate RB, et al. The natural history of atrial fibrillation: incidence, risk factors, and prognosis in the Manitoba follow-up study. JAMA 1994;98:476–84.

[86] Kanter MC, Tegeler CH, Pearce LA, et al. Carotid stenosis in patients with atrial fibrillation. Prevalence, risk factors, and relationship to stroke in the Stroke Prevention in Atrial Fibrillation Study. Arch Intern Med 1994;154:1372–7.

[87] Hart RG, Halperin JL. Atrial fibrillation and stroke: concepts and controversies. Stroke 2001;32:803–8.

[88] Fox CS, Parise H, D'Agostino RB Sr, et al. Parental atrial fibrillation as a risk factor for atrial fibrillation in offspring. JAMA 2004;291:2851–5.

[89] Darbar D, Herron KJ, Ballew JD, et al. Familial atrial fibrillation is a genetically heterogeneous disorder. J Am Coll Cardiol 2003;41:2185–92.

[90] Mestroni L. Genomic medicine in atrial fibrillation. J Am Coll Cardiol 2003;41:2193–6.

[91] Crenshaw BS, Ward SR, Granger CB, et al. Atrial fibrillation in the setting of acute myocardial infarction: the GUSTO-I experience. J Am Coll Cardiol 1997;30:406–13.

[92] Chen YH, Xu SJ, Bendahhou S. KCNQ1 gain-of-function mutation in familial atrial fibrillation. Science 2003;299:251–4.

[93] Wang TJ, Massaro JM, Levy D, et al. A risk score for predicting stroke or death in individuals with new onset atrial fibrillation in the community: the Framingham Heart Study. JAMA 2003;290:1049–56.

[94] Vermes E, Tardif JC, Bourassa MG. Enalapril decreases the incidence of atrial fibrillation in patients with left ventricular dysfunction: insight from the studies of left ventricular dysfunction (SOLVD) trials. Circulation 2003;107:2926–31.

[95] Klein HU, Goette A. Blockade of atrial angiotensin II type 1 receptors: a novel antiarrhythmic strategy to prevent atrial fibrillation? J Am Coll Cardiol 2003;41:2205–6.

[96] Rowan SB, Bailey DN, Bublitz CE, et al. Trends in anticoagulation for atrial fibrillation in the U.S.: an analysis of the national ambulatory medical care survey database. J Am Coll Cardiol 2007;49:1561–5.

THE MEDICAL
CLINICS
OF NORTH AMERICA

Med Clin N Am 92 (2008) 41–51

Genetics of Atrial Fibrillation

Patrick T. Ellinor, MD, PhD[a],[*],
B. Alexander Yi, MD, PhD[b],
Calum A. MacRae, MB, ChB, PhD[c]

[a]Cardiac Arrhythmia Service and Cardiovascular Research Center, Massachusetts General
Hospital, 55 Fruit Street, and Harvard Medical School, Boston, MA 02114, USA
[b]Cardiology Division, Massachusetts General Hospital, 55 Fruit Street, Bigelow 852,
and Harvard Medical School, Boston, MA 02114, USA
[c]Cardiology Division and Cardiovascular Research Center, Massachusetts General Hospital,
55 Fruit Street, and Harvard Medical School, Boston, MA 02114, USA

Atrial fibrillation (AF) is the most common cardiac arrhythmia. It affects over 2 million Americans, a number that will more than double by 2020 [1]. The clinic visits, hospitalizations, medications, and procedures necessary to treat AF cost in excess of $6.4 billion per year [2]. It accounts for one third of all strokes in patients older than 65 [2] and is associated with an increased mortality [3,4]. While often associated with hypertension and structural heart disease, it is also seen in the setting of acute illness and in those who have undergone thoracic surgery. Traditionally, AF has not been considered a genetic condition; however, a number of recent studies have demonstrated that some forms of the arrhythmia, and in particular lone AF, have a substantial genetic basis [5–8]. Mutations in several ion channels have been identified in individuals and families with AF [9–13], but appear to be rare causes of the arrhythmia [14,15]. In the course of this review we will discuss the heritability of AF, the methods used to identify the causal genes underlying an inherited disorder, and our current understanding of the specific genes implicated to date in AF.

Atrial fibrillation is a heritable condition

A genetic predisposition for AF has until recently not been well appreciated. It has long been reported that AF develops in some individuals at a relatively young age despite the absence of any evidence of structural heart

* Corresponding author.
E-mail address: pellinor@partners.org (P.T. Ellinor).

0025-7125/08/$ - see front matter © 2008 Elsevier Inc. All rights reserved.
doi:10.1016/j.mcna.2007.09.005   *medical.theclinics.com*

disease and without any apparent etiology, although these families were typically considered rare [16].

In 2003, Fox and coworkers [7] prospectively studied more than 5000 individuals whose parents were enrolled in the Framingham Heart Study. Over a 19-year follow-up period, they found that AF in the offspring was independently associated with parental AF, particularly if the subset was limited to those younger than 75 and if those with antecedent heart disease were excluded. Having a parent with AF approximately doubled the 4-year risk of developing AF even after adjustment for risk factors such as hypertension, diabetes mellitus, or myocardial infarction.

A genetic predisposition for AF in the general population was also demonstrated in a study of Icelandic individuals by Arnar and colleagues in 2006 [5]. After identifying more than 5000 Icelanders with AF and then assessing relatedness from a nationwide genealogical database, 80% of those with AF were related within four meioses to another individual with AF. First-degree relatives of those with AF had a 1.77 higher relative risk for AF compared with the general population. The relative risk was 4.67 when only patients younger than 60 were considered.

The heritability of AF has also been examined in more selected patient populations. In a chart review of more than 2000 patients referred to the arrhythmia clinic for AF, investigators at the Mayo Clinic found that 5% had a family history of AF. This number was as high as 15% among patients with lone AF [8]. In 2005, in a study with prespecified ascertainment, we found that nearly 40% of individuals with lone AF referred to the Arrhythmia Service at Massachusetts General Hospital had at least one relative with the arrhythmia, and a substantial number reported having multiple relatives with AF [6]. In over 90% of cases, AF in the relatives could be verified. To obtain a crude index of heritability, we determined that prevalence of AF among each class of relative compared with the prevalence of age- and sex-matched subjects. We found a significantly increased relative risk of AF among family members ranging from 2 fold in fathers to nearly 70 fold in male siblings.

Genetic studies in atrial fibrillation

Once a condition is found to be heritable, there are several techniques that are commonly used to identify the genetic basis of a disease, namely, linkage analysis, candidate gene resequencing, and association studies. We will discuss each of these methods in turn as they have been applied to AF.

Linkage analysis

The genes that underlie simple monogenic disorders with a Mendelian pattern of inheritance can be identified using linkage analysis. When passed from generation to generation, genetic markers that lie close together on the same chromosome are likely to be transmitted en bloc in proportion to their proximity to each other. A genome-wide search for groups of markers that cosegregate with the disease as it travels through the family is performed to identify the approximate location of a genetic disease locus. Linkage studies report a logarithm of the odds or LOD score that reflects the likelihood of two markers or a marker and disease cosegregating when compared with chance alone. An LOD score of 3 or more (or odds of greater than a 1000:1) is considered to be statistically significant. Traditionally, restriction enzyme sites and microsatellite repeats have been used as genetic markers, but more recently, it has become possible to use single nucleotide polymorphisms or SNPs [17]. The ease of use in genotyping have made SNPs the most widely used genetic markers today.

Linkage analysis can be used to narrow the search for a causative gene to a chromosomal locus or relatively small region of the human genome associated with disease; however, this minimal genetic interval may still contain hundreds of genes spread over millions of base pairs. Once a genetic locus is identified, online data from human genome databases that have been developed as a direct result of the Human Genome Project are used to identify candidate genes within the genetic locus. These individual genes are then sequenced in affected individuals in an attempt to identify sequence variants that correlate with the disease. Once a base pair change is identified, it is then important to differentiate between a mutation and a genetic polymorphism or more common variant in the genome. For a sequence alteration to be considered a mutation, it must segregate with the disease, have a plausible mechanism, and not be found in healthy controls. Ultimately, the mutation should be sufficient to cause the phenotype, either in a human kindred or in a genetic model organism.

There are several genetic loci that have been reported in large kindreds with Mendelian AF: on chromosomes 5, 6, and 10 (Table 1) [9,18,19]. In one such family of Chinese descent, Chen and coworkers [9] identified a mutation in KCNQ1, a potassium channel that underlies the slow repolarizing current in cardiomyocytes known as I_{Ks} (Fig. 1). From a four-generation family with AF, they were able to map the disease locus to a 12-megabase region on the short arm of chromosome 11. The KCNQ1 gene was located within this region and sequencing of the gene revealed a serine to glycine missense mutation at position 140 (S140G) in affected family members. The S140G mutation is located in the first transmembrane-spanning segment [20] at the outer edges of the voltage-sensing domain and far from the pore-forming region of the potassium channel structure. Unlike the mutations in KCNQ1 associated with the long QT syndrome, which typically result in a loss of channel function, the S140G mutation resulted in a gain of channel function. In cultured cells, expression of the S140G mutant channel resulted in dramatically enhanced potassium channel currents and markedly altered potassium channel gating kinetics, changes that would be

Table 1
Genes and loci implicated in atrial fibrillation

Genes

Chromosome	Gene name	Effect	Inheritance	Reference
11p15.5	KCNQ1/KvLQT1	Increases I_{Ks}; expected to shorten APD	AD	[9]
21q22.1	KCNE2/MiRP1	Increases I_{Ks}	AD	[10]
17q23.1-24.2	KCNJ2	Increases I_{K1}; expected to shorten APD	AD	[11]
12p13	KCNA5	Loss of I_{Kur}; expected to prolong APD	AD	[12]
1q21.1	GJA5/Connexin 40	Reduced gap junction conductance	Acquired	[13]

Genetic Loci

Chromosome	Gene	Comments	Inheritance	Reference
5p13	Unknown	Associated with sudden death	AR	[37]
6q14-q16	Unknown	Overlaps with locus for DCM	AD	[19]
10q22-q24	Unknown	Overlaps with locus for DCM	AD	[18]
10p11-q21	Unknown		AD	[38]

Abbreviations: AD, autosomal dominant; AR, autosomal recessive; DCM, dilated cardiomyopathy.

predicted to increase I_{Ks}. Such an increase would be expected to lead to a shortening of the action potential duration and thus make atrial myocytes vulnerable to reentry and subsequent AF (see Fig. 1).

While the identification of this mutation provided an initial inroad into the pathogenesis of AF, this family also illustrates our limited understanding of the role of the KCNQ1 channel in atrial versus ventricular repolarization. Specifically, it remains unclear why a mutation that results in an in vitro gain of function in KCNQ1 is associated with delayed ventricular repolarization (as manifest by a prolonged QT interval on their electrocardiograms) in more than half of the individuals with the S140G mutation.

Other gain of function mutations in KCNQ1 have been associated with the short QT syndrome [21]. Hong and colleagues [22] reported an unusual case of AF detected in utero and confirmed by an electrocardiogram at birth. The child's electrocardiogram also displayed a short QT interval. Based on this association, the investigators sequenced the KCNQ1 gene and found a valine to methionine mutation in position 141 (adjacent to the mutation described by Chen and colleagues). Like the S140G mutation, V141M mutant channels when expressed in vitro displayed a markedly enhanced current density and altered gating kinetics.

Candidate gene studies

A candidate gene can be any gene that is hypothesized to cause a disease. In the case of linkage analysis, a gene may be considered a candidate gene

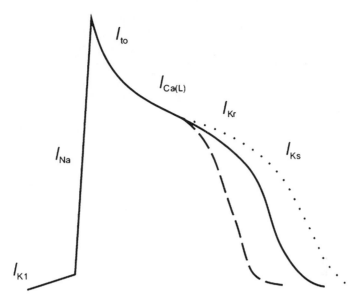

Fig. 1. Both gain of function and loss of function mutations in I_{Ks} have been associated with AF. Mutations in KCNQ1 and KCNE2 increase the current I_{Ks}, which is predicted to shorten the action potential (*dashed line*) in cardiac myocytes and render atrial myocytes susceptible to reentrant arrhythmias. Mutations in KCNA5 (Kv1.5) that are predicted to prolong the action potential duration (*dotted line*) have also been associated with AF.

based on its location within the region of interest, as well on the basis of any other information suggesting that the gene may play a role in the disease process in question. Based on the work relating KCNQ1 to AF, investigators have considered other potassium channels as potential candidate genes for AF and begun screening these genes in cohorts with AF.

Otway and colleagues [23] examined 50 kindreds with AF and amplified the genes for KCNQ1 and KCNE1-3, accessory subunits of KCNQ1. They found a single mutation in KCNQ1 in only one family—an arginine to cysteine change at amino acid position 14 (R14C) in KCNQ1. Unlike the S140 G mutation discovered by Chen and colleagues, R14C had no significant effect on KCNQ1/KCNE1 current amplitudes in cultured cells at baseline; however, upon exposure to hypotonic solution, mutant channels exhibited a marked increase in current density compared to the wild-type channels. Interestingly, of those who carried the R14C mutation, only those with left atrial dilatation had AF leading the authors to propose a "two-hit" hypothesis of AF. These investigators also identified a mutation in KCNE2 in two of the kindreds. Like the S140 G mutation in KCNQ1, the mutation in KCNE2 (R27C) also dramatically increased the amplitude of I_{Ks} [10].

Finally, the relationship between potassium channels and AF extends beyond I_{Ks}. Xia and colleagues [11] identified a mutation in KCNJ2, an inward rectifier potassium channel that underlies the I_{K1} current, in one kindred with AF. This V93I variant also led to a gain of function in the KCNJ2 channel. A loss of function mutation in another small family with AF has also been identified in KCNA5 or IKur, the ultrarapid repolarizing potassium channel found predominately in the atria [14].

To date, the significance of these potassium channel mutations in other populations AF is unknown. We have screened our cohort with lone atrial fibrillation for mutations in KCNQ1, KCNJ2, and KCNE1-5 and were unable to find any mutations in those genes [14]. These findings suggest that potassium channels are an uncommon cause of AF and there is much more to be learned about the diversity of molecular pathways that lead to this arrhythmia.

The genes encoding the connexins, gap-junction proteins that mediate the spread of action potentials between cardiac myocytes, have also been examined as potential candidates for AF. Prior work has shown that mice with null alleles of *GJA5*, the gene for connexin40, exhibit atrial reentrant arrhythmias [24]. Based on these results, Gollob and coworkers [13] considered this gene as a potential candidate in individuals with idiopathic AF who underwent pulmonary vein isolation surgery. An analysis of DNA isolated from their cardiac tissue showed that 4 of the 15 subjects had mutations in *GJA5* that markedly interfered with the electrical coupling between cells. In three of the patients, DNA isolated from their lymphocytes lacked the same mutation in *GJA5,* suggesting that the connexin40 mutations arose after fertilization, possibly during cardiac embryogenesis. One of the four individuals carried in the mutation in both cardiac tissue and in their lymphocytes arguing that, in this instance, the mutation was transmitted in the germline; however, more information about the transmission of AF in relatives of this individual was not available.

Association studies

Although traditional methods such as linkage analysis can be applied to families where the phenotype and pattern of inheritance are consistent with a monogenic disorder, the mode of transmission for AF is less clear. Association studies have been used in an attempt to identify the genetic basis of AF and other apparently complex traits. In an association study, the frequency of a single nucleotide polymorphism or SNP in individuals with a disease is compared with that in control populations. Over the past 10 years, many case control association studies have been performed in subjects with AF. These studies have typically tested a small number of variants and have been directed at candidate genes previously believed to be involved in AF. Examples include genes in the renin-angiotensin system [25,26], interleukins [27], signaling molecules [28], gap junction proteins [29] and ion channels [30–32] (summarized in Table 2). Unfortunately, these studies have been limited by a low prior probability of any polymorphism truly being associated with AF. Further complicating these analyses are the small

Table 2
Polymorphisms associated with atrial fibrillation

Gene	Variant	Cases	Controls	OR	P value	Replicated?	Comments	Reference
Connexin 40	−44A, +71 G	173	232	1.514	<.006	No		[29]
Angiotensinogen	M235T	250	250	2.5	<.001	No		[25]
Angiotensinogen	G-6A	250	250	3.3	.005	No		[25]
Angiotensinogen	G-217A	250	250	2.0	.002	No		[25]
Mink	38 G	108	108	1.8	.024	No		[30]
GNB3	C825T	291	292	0.46	.02	No		[28]
KCNE5	97T	158	96	0.52	.007	No		[31]
Interleukin 6	−174 G/C	26	84	3.25	.006	No	In postoperative CABG patients	[27]
CETP	Taq1B	97	97	0.35	.05	No		[39]
KCNE4	E145D	142	238	1.66	.044	No		[32]
ACE	D/D	51	289	1.5	.16	No	In patients with CHF	[26]
ENOS	894T/T	51	289	3.2	.001	No	In patients with CHF	[26]
SCN5A	H558R	157	314	1.6	.002	No	Lone AF	[38]
–	rs2200733	3,913	22,092	1.72	3.3×10^{-41}	Yes	Identified in GWAS	[35]
–	rs10033464	3,913	22,092	1.39	6.9×10^{-11}	Yes	Identified in GWAS	[35]

Abbreviations: AF, atrial fibrillation; CABG, coronary artery bypass graft; CHF, congestive heart failure; GWAS, genome-wide association studies.

sample sizes and a lack of replication in distinct populations, as well as phenotypic and genetic heterogeneity.

In recent years, genome-wide association studies (GWAS) have been
made possible by advancements in genotyping technology that allow investigators to assay hundreds of thousands of SNPs spread over the entire human
genome. The studies are typically done using a case-control study design
similar to that used in epidemiology [33]. Genome-wide association studies
attempt to identify novel genetic polymorphisms that are significantly more
or less common in a group with a disease as compared with a control group.
Since the markers are spread over the entire genome, these experiments are
unbiased with no weight given to previously known candidate genes. Such
studies have been used successfully in the past year to identify potential novel
pathways for diabetes, macular degeneration, and repolarization.

While GWAS have the potential to identify new pathways for disease,
they also have a number of limitations. In particular, with hundreds of thousands of individual associations being tested, these studies have a high likelihood of producing a false-positive result. There is still discussion within the
field of what the threshold P value should be for genome-wide significance
[34]. False-positive results can also emerge from population stratification or
the failure to properly control for ethnicity, thus resulting in over- or under-
representation of spurious ethnic specific markers. Although there have been
proposed variations in study design in an effort to eliminate false associations, ultimately replication of the results in other populations may be the
best test of whether a result is a true positive [33].

The biological significance of the identified variants is another concern.
Most variants found in genetic association studies have been associated
with relatively weak effects, eg, relative risks on the order of approximately
1.3 to 1.5. While these variants associated with a disease may generate new
ideas about disease pathogenesis, understanding the biological mechanism
for most of these variants remains difficult.

Recently, a team led by the researchers at deCODE genetics reported the
results of a genome-wide association study for AF. Gudbjartsson and colleagues examined over 300,000 SNPs and identified two polymorphisms at
a locus on the long arm of chromosome 4 (4q25) that demonstrated a highly
significant association ($P = 3.3 \times 10^{-41}$) with AF [35]. A strength of this
work is that the investigators were able to replicate their original findings
in other populations in Sweden, the United States, and Hong Kong. Neither
variant was correlated with obesity, hypertension, or myocardial infarction,
suggesting that the genetic variants are not associated with AF by affecting
those risk factors.

How do the variants on chromosome 4 lead to AF? At present, the mechanism of action of these variants is unclear. Interestingly, these SNPs lie
upstream from a gene that could plausibly play a role in the pathogenesis
of AF: the paired-like homeodomain transcription factor 2, *PITX2*. This
gene is known to play a role in the development of the left atrium [36–39]

and has been shown to be involved in suppression of pacemaker cells outside the sinus node in early development [40]. Further work should help clarify the mechanism underlying the association of these markers with AF.

Refining genetic studies of atrial fibrillation

To continue to improve on the utility of genetic studies for AF we will need to overcome a number of obstacles. A critical step in any genetic study is the ability to correctly assign the diagnosis. While on first pass this may seem straightforward, it can be challenging in AF, a condition that can be asymptomatic, paroxysmal, and have an onset later in life. Further complicating studies of AF are the genotypic and phenotypic heterogeneity. Rather than a single entity, AF may represent the final common pathway for a number of distinct pathogenic insults such as heart failure, hypertension, or thyroid abnormalities.

To address these challenges, we will have to continue to improve upon the characterization and classification of AF. The identification of endophenotypes or subtle, heritable traits that cosegregate with AF may help to refine ongoing genetic studies. For AF, endophenotypes such as specific P-wave morphologies, pulmonary venous anatomy as assessed by computed tomography or magnetic resonance imaging, or biomarkers that are heritable and easily detectable may be helpful.

Summary

In summary, recent studies of AF have identified mutations in a series of ion channels; however, these channels appear to be relatively rare causes of AF. Recent genome-wide association studies for AF have identified novel variants associated with the disease, although the mechanism of action for these variants remains unknown. Ultimately, a greater understanding of the genetics of AF should yield insights into novel pathways, therapeutic targets, and diagnostic testing for this common arrhythmia.

Acknowledgment

This work was supported by National Institutes of Health awards to P.T.E. (HL71632) and C.A.M. (HL75431).

References

[1] Go AS, Hylek EM, Phillips KA, et al. Prevalence of diagnosed AF in adults: national implications for rhythm management and stroke prevention: the AnTicoagulation and Risk Factors in AF (ATRIA) Study. JAMA 2001;285(18):2370–5.
[2] Coyne KS, Paramore C, Grandy S, et al. Assessing the direct costs of treating nonvalvular AF in the United States. Value Health 2006;9(5):348–56.

[3] Benjamin EJ, Wolf PA, D'Agostino RB, et al. Impact of AF on the risk of death: the Framingham Heart Study. Circulation 1998;98(10):946–52.

[4] Gajewski J, Singer RB. Mortality in an insured population with AF. JAMA 1981;245(15): 1540–4.

[5] Arnar DO, Thorvaldsson S, Manolio TA, et al. Familial aggregation of AF in Iceland. Eur Heart J 2006;27(6):708–12.

[6] Ellinor PT, Yoerger DM, Ruskin JN, et al. Familial aggregation in lone AF. Hum Genet 2005;118(2):179–84.

[7] Fox CS, Parise H, D'Agostino RB Sr., et al. Parental AF as a risk factor for AF in offspring. JAMA 2004;291(23):2851–5.

[8] Darbar D, Herron KJ, Ballew JD, et al. Familial AF is a genetically heterogeneous disorder. J Am Coll Cardiol 2003;41(12):2185–92.

[9] Chen YH, Xu SJ, Bendahhou S, et al. KCNQ1 gain-of-function mutation in familial AF. Science 2003;299(5604):251–4.

[10] Yang Y, Xia M, Jin Q, et al. Identification of a KCNE2 gain-of-function mutation in patients with familial AF. Am J Hum Genet 2004;75(5):899–905.

[11] Xia M, Jin Q, Bendahhou S, et al. A Kir2.1 gain-of-function mutation underlies familial AF. Biochem Biophys Res Commun 2005;332(4):1012–9.

[12] Olson TM, Alekseev AE, Liu XK, et al. Kv1.5 channelopathy due to KCNA5 loss-of-function mutation causes human AF. Hum Mol Genet 2006;15(14):2185–91.

[13] Gollob MH, Jones DL, Krahn AD, et al. Somatic mutations in the connexin 40 gene (GJA5) in AF. N Engl J Med 2006;354(25):2677–88.

[14] Ellinor PT, Moore RK, Patton KK, et al. Mutations in the long QT gene, KCNQ1, are an uncommon cause of AF. Heart 2004;90(12):1487–8.

[15] Ellinor PT, Petrov-Kondratov VI, Zakharova E, et al. Potassium channel gene mutations rarely cause AF. BMC Med Genet 2006;7:70.

[16] Wolff L. Familial auricular fibrillation. N Engl J Med 1943;229:396–8.

[17] The International HapMap Consortium. A haplotype map of the human genome. Nature 2005;437(7063):1299–320.

[18] Brugada R, Tapscott T, Czernuszewicz GZ, et al. Identification of a genetic locus for familial AF. N Engl J Med 1997;336(13):905–11.

[19] Ellinor PT, Shin JT, Moore RK, et al. Locus for AF maps to chromosome 6q14-16. Circulation 2003;107(23):2880–3.

[20] Schenzer A, Friedrich T, Pusch M, et al. Molecular determinants of KCNQ (Kv7) K+ channel sensitivity to the anticonvulsant retigabine. J Neurosci 2005;25(20):5051–60.

[21] Bellocq C, van Ginneken ACG, Bezzina CR, et al. Mutation in the KCNQ1 gene leading to the short QT-interval syndrome. Circulation 2004;109:2394–7.

[22] Hong K, Piper DR, Diaz-Valdecantos A, et al. De novo KCNQ1 mutation responsible for AF and short QT syndrome in utero. Cardiovasc Res 2005;68(3):433–40.

[23] Otway R, Vandenberg JI, Guo G, et al. Stretch-sensitive KCNQ1 mutation: a link between genetic and environmental factors in the pathogenesis of AF? J Am Coll Cardiol 2007;49(5): 578–86.

[24] Hagendorff A, Schumacher B, Kirchhoff S, et al. Conduction disturbances and increased atrial vulnerability in connexin 40-deficient mice analyzed by transesophageal stimulation. Circulation 1999;99:1508–15.

[25] Tsai CT, Lai LP, Lin JL, et al. Renin-angiotensin system gene polymorphisms and AF. Circulation 2004;109(13):1640–6.

[26] Bedi M, McNamara D, London B, et al. Genetic susceptibility to AF in patients with congestive heart failure. Heart Rhythm 2006;3(7):808–12.

[27] Gaudino M, Andreotti F, Zamparelli R, et al. The -174G/C interleukin-6 polymorphism influences postoperative interleukin-6 levels and postoperative AF. Is AF an inflammatory complication? Circulation 2003;108(Suppl 1):II195–9.

[28] Schreieck J, Dostal S, von Beckerath N, et al. C825T polymorphism of the G-protein beta3 subunit gene and AF: association of the TT genotype with a reduced risk for AF. Am Heart J 2004;148(3):545–50.

[29] Juang JM, Chern YR, Tsai CT, et al. The association of human connexin 40 genetic polymorphisms with AF. Int J Cardiol 2007;116(1):107–12.

[30] Lai LP, Su MJ, Yeh HM, et al. Association of the human minK gene 38G allele with AF: evidence of possible genetic control on the pathogenesis of AF. Am Heart J 2002;144(3): 485–90.

[31] Ravn LS, Hofman-Bang J, Dixen U, et al. Relation of 97T polymorphism in KCNE5 to risk of AF. Am J Cardiol 2005;96(3):405–7.

[32] Zeng Z, Tan C, Teng S, et al. The single nucleotide polymorphisms of I(Ks) potassium channel genes and their association with af in a chinese population. Cardiology 2006;108(2): 97–103.

[33] Risch NJ. Searching for genetic determinants in the new millennium. Nature 2000;405(6788): 847–56.

[34] Hunter DJ, Kraft P. Drinking from the fire hose–statistical issues in genomewide association studies. N Engl J Med 2007;357(5):436–9.

[35] Gudbjartsson DF, Arnar DO, Helgadottir A, et al. Variants conferring risk of AF on chromosome 4q25. Nature 2007;448(7151):353–7.

[36] Franco D, Campione M. The role of Pitx2 during cardiac development. Linking left-right signaling and congenital heart diseases. Trends Cardiovasc Med 2003;13:157–63.

[37] Oberti C, Wang L, Li L, et al. Genome-wide linkage scan identifies a novel genetic locus on chromosome 5p13 for neonatal AF associated with sudden death and variable cardiomyopathy. Circulation 2004;110(25):3753–9.

[38] Volders PG, Zhu Q, Timmermans C, et al. Mapping a novel locus for familial AF on chromosome 10p11-q21. Heart Rhythm 2007;4(4):469–75.

[39] Asselbergs FW, Moore JH, van den Berg MP, et al. A role for CETP TaqIB polymorphism in determining susceptibility to AF: a nested case control study. BMC Med Genet 2006;7:39.

[40] Mommersteeg MT, Hoogaars WM, Prall OW, et al. Molecular pathway for the localized formation of the sinoatrial node. Circ Res 2007;100(3):354–62.

THE MEDICAL
CLINICS
OF NORTH AMERICA

Med Clin N Am 92 (2008) 53–63

New Concepts in Atrial Fibrillation: Mechanism and Remodeling

Chung-Chuan Chou, MD[a],*, Peng-Sheng Chen, MD[b]

[a]The Second Section of Cardiology, Chang Gung Memorial Hospital and Chang Gung
University College of Medicine, 199 North Tung-Hwa Road, Taipei 10591, Taiwan
[b]Krannert Institute of Cardiology and the Division of Cardiology,
Department of Medicine, Indiana University School of Medicine, 1801 North Capitol Avenue,
E475, Indianapolis, IN 46202, USA

Atrial fibrillation (AF) is a complex disease with many possible mechanisms [1]. Many studies indicate that the arrhythmogenic foci within the thoracic veins are AF initiators. Once initiated, AF alters atrial electrical and structural properties (atrial remodeling) in a way that promotes its own maintenance and recurrences and may alter the response to antiarrhythmic drugs. The exact mechanisms by which the initiators trigger AF remained elusive, however. One possible immediate trigger is the paroxysmal autonomic nervous system (ANS) discharge. In normal dogs, sympathetic nerve stimulation rarely triggers AF. In dogs that undergo chronic rapid atrial pacing, however, sympathetic stimulation can lead to rapid repetitive activations in the isolated canine pulmonary vein (PV) and vein of Marshall preparations [2,3]. Sharifov and colleagues [4] reported that a combined isoproterenol and acetylcholine infusion is more effective than acetylcholine alone in the induction of AF. Clinically, alterations of autonomic tone, involving the sympathetic and parasympathetic nervous systems, are implicated in initiating paroxysmal AF [5]. These results suggest that simultaneous sympathetic and parasympathetic (sympathovagal) discharge is particularly profibrillatory. Also, there is evidence for heightened atrial sympathetic innervation in patients who have persistent AF [6], suggesting that potential autonomic substrate modification may serve as part of remodeled atrial substrate for AF maintenance.

* Corresponding author.
  E-mail address: 2867@adm.cgmh.org.tw (C-C. Chou).

0025-7125/08/$ - see front matter © 2008 Elsevier Inc. All rights reserved.
doi:10.1016/j.mcna.2007.08.008

Patterns of activation at the pulmonary vein and pulmonary vein–left atrial junction during sustained atrial fibrillation

AF is characterized by the coexistence of multiple activation wavelets within the atria. The mechanisms by which multiple wavefronts occur have been debated actively for many years. The focal source hypothesis states that a single rapidly focal driver underlies the mechanisms of AF. Alternatively, the multiple wavelet hypothesis posits that heterogeneous dispersion of repolarization is responsible for wavebreaks and the generation of multiple wavelets that sustain AF [7]. Zipes and Knope [8], Spach and colleagues [9], and Scherlag and colleagues [10] provided the first pieces of evidence to support the importance of thoracic veins in the generation of electrical activity. The importance of these original works was proved by Haissaguerre and colleagues [11], who demonstrated the critical role of PV in the generation and maintenance of AF in humans. Hamabe and colleagues [12] reported that the PV–left atrial (LA) junction has segmental muscle disconnection and differential muscle narrowing in dogs. These changes combined with the complex fiber orientations within the PV provide robust anatomic bases for generating conduction disturbances at the PV-LA junction and complex intra-PV conduction patterns, to facilitate reentry formation. High-density (1-mm resolution) computerized mapping techniques have demonstrated that rapid PV focal discharge [13–15] and PV-LA junction microreentry [15] are present during sustained AF induced by rapid LA pacing. Fig. 1 shows an example. Fig. 1A shows the activation snapshots of right superior PV during sustained AF, showing three consecutive focal discharges (6081 ms, 6203 ms, and 6316 ms). The focal discharge wavefronts met lines of functional conduction block (dotted lines), followed by the formation of complete reentry loops (6409 ms to 6595 ms). The wavefronts from LA also encountered a functional line of block, followed by the formation of reentry. After infusion of ibutilide (see Fig. 1B), a typical class III antiarrhythmic drug that is effective in prolonging the effective refractory period of atria, focal discharges (6344 ms and 6582 ms) and reentrant wavefronts activated (6035 ms to 6296 ms) at slower rates during AF. The conducted wavefronts between the PV and LA were reduced significantly by ibutilide. The overall incidence of focal discharge in the PVs was not suppressed, however. A high dose of ibutilide may terminate all reentrant activity completely, thereby converting AF to PV tachycardia before conversion to sinus rhythm. These findings suggest that sustained AF is the result of a combination of PV focal discharge and PV-LA reentrant activity.

A recent computational simulation study [16] showed that upregulation of the L-type Ca^{2+} current steepened restitution curves of the action potential duration (APD) and the conduction velocity. Spontaneous firing of ectopic foci, coupled with sinus activity, produced dynamic spatial dispersion of repolarization, including discordant alternans, which facilitated unidirectional conduction block and initiated reentrant atrial flutter or AF. The size

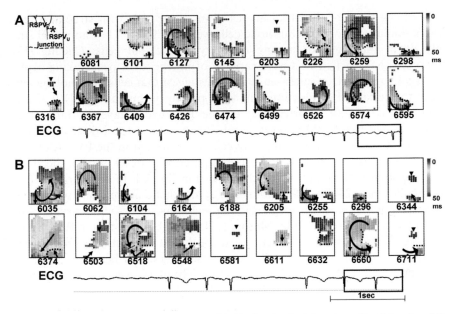

Fig. 1. Patterns of activation during sustained AF in dog that had chronic rapid atrial pacing. (*A*) Snapshots of focal discharge and reentrant activation patterns within right super PV at baseline AF. Asterisk in the left upper corner indicates the anatomic location of focal discharge at the proximal right superior PV. Black horizontal dotted line indicates the PV-LA junction. The number below each snapshot represents the time in milliseconds, with the beginning of data acquisition as time zero. In snapshots, red color represents the wavefront; black arrows, the direction of wave propagation; black dotted line, line of block; arrowhead, site of focal discharge. The color bar on the right shows the time scale (0 to 50 ms). (*B*) Snapshots of focal discharge and reentrant activation patterns within right superior PV after ibutilide infusion (0.02 mg/kg). A rectangle toward the end of the ECG tracings shows the time period corresponding to the snapshots in (*A*) and (*B*). (*From* Chou CC, Shou S, Tan AY, et al. High-density mapping of pulmonary veins and left atrium during ibutilide administration in a canine model of sustained atrial fibrillation. Am J Physiol Heart Circ Physiol 2005;289:H2706; with permission.)

of vulnerable window was larger for PV ectopic foci than the right atrial foci. These findings imply that the ectopic beats originated from PV are more likely to trigger AF than ectopic beats from elsewhere in the atria.

Anatomic and neural substrates in the pulmonary veins

Zipes and Knope [8] conclude that not only did atrial muscle extend for some distance into the thoracic veins but also that these muscle sleeves received vagal innervation. It was possible that the autonomic nerves and atrial muscles in the PVs were important in triggering AF. Subsequent works demonstrated significant heterogeneity of the cell types within the PV muscle sleeves. Masani [17] showed that node-like cells were present in the myocardial layer of the PV of rats. Among the ordinary myocardial cells resembling those of the atrial myocardium, clear cells with structural features similar to those of sinus node cells were identified. They appeared singly or in small groups among ordinary myocardial cells. Cheung [18] reported that isolated PVs were capable of independent pacemaking activity. Light and electron microscope studies suggest that cells morphologically akin to specialized conduction cells were present in human PVs [19]. Chou and colleagues [20] reported that canine PVs had a layer of large pale periodic acid–Schiff (PAS)-positive cells at the site of focal discharge, supporting the notion that Purkinje-like cells were present in the PVs. A distinguishing feature of the sinus node, as compared with other parts of the atria, is the presence of rich autonomic innervation [21–23]. In comparison, Tan and colleagues [24] identified abundant sympathetic nerve fibers within the PV using immunohistochemical staining techniques. These findings are consistent with those reported by Masani [17], who observed that in PVs, nerve fibers containing small and large vesicles with and without dense cores were juxtaposed to the node-like cells. The close interaction between the nerve structures and the specialized muscle cells might play a role in the generation of ectopic activities.

Cardiac autonomic innervation

Kawashima [25] performed detailed anatomic studies of human cardiac autonomic innervation. The cardiac sympathetic ganglia include a superior cervical ganglion, which communicates with C_{1-3}, and the cervicothoracic (stellate) ganglion, which communicates with C_{7-8}–T_{1-2}. In addition, the thoracic ganglia (as low as the seventh thoracic ganglion) also contribute to the sympathetic innervation to the heart. The superior, middle, and inferior cardiac nerves from these ganglia innervate the heart by following a simple course along the brachiocephalic trunk, common carotid, and subclavian arteries. Alternatively, the thoracic cardiac nerves in the posterior mediastinum have to follow a complex course to reach the heart in the middle mediastinum. The parasympathetic innervation comes from the vagus nerve and is divided into superior, middle, and inferior branches. Although both sides of the autonomic branches run through the ventral and dorsal aspects of the aortic arch, the right autonomic cardiac nerves tend to follow a ventral course.

Many investigators have studied the macroscopic and microscopic anatomy of cardiac autonomic nerves within the atria. Among those who focused on PV autonomic nerves, Armour and colleagues [26] provided a detailed map of autonomic nerve distributions in human hearts. They found that autonomic nerves were concentrated in "ganglionic plexi" around great vessels, such as the PVs. Chiou and colleagues [27] determined that these nerves converged functionally onto fat pads located around the superior vena cava–aortic junction and that catheter ablation of this fat pad effectively denervated many regions of the atria but preserved innervation of the ventricle. On a more microscopic scale, Chevalier and colleagues

[28] discovered several gradients of PV autonomic innervation, with nerves more abundant in the proximal PV than distal PV and more abundant in the epicardium than endocardium. The PV-LA junction is rich in autonomic innervation [24]. Stimulation of the ganglionic plexi at the PV-LA junction can convert PV focal discharge into AF [29], and radiofrequency ablation at these sites potentially can result in successful denervation and prevent AF inducibility [30].

Vagal influences on cardiac electrophysiology

It is well known that vagal nerve stimulation and acetylcholine infusion can result in significant changes of cardiac electrophysiology, including heterogeneous effects on atrial refractory period [31], on pacemaker activity and atrioventricular conduction [32], and on induction of AF [33]. Cervical vagal stimulation shortens the atrial effective refractory period primarily in the high right atrium and facilitates induction of AF by single premature extrastimulus [34]. Coumel and colleagues [35] reported that vagal activity might predispose patients to develop paroxysmal atrial arrhythmias. The investigators studied 18 human cases and discovered sinus slowing often preceded the onset of atrial arrhythmias in these mostly middle-aged male. The investigators proposed that vagal activation might induce shortening of the APD, which in turn facilitates reentrant atrial arrhythmias.

Sympathetic activation and the "Ca_i-transient triggering" hypothesis

Two recent works have enhanced the understanding of the mechanisms by which sympathovagal activation facilitates the onset of paroxysmal AF. Burashnikov and Antzelevitch [36] infused acetylcholine to abbreviate atrial APD and permit rapid pacing in isolated coronary-perfused canine right atrium, which led to Ca_i accumulation. If this is coupled with a long pause (such as that occurred after AF), then a large Ca^{2+} release from the sarcoplasmic reticulum could induce late phase 3 early after-depolarizations (EADs) and extrasystoles that initiated AF. This novel late phase 3 EAD mechanism is observed only in association with marked APD abbreviation. Patterson and colleagues [37] showed that simultaneous infusion of norepinephrine and acetylcholine during rapid pacing facilitated the development of EADs and triggered atrial tachycardias. They also measured tension development and discovered that the persistent diastolic elevation of tension was associated with EADs. Assuming that tension is a good measure of Ca_i, then diastolic Ca_i elevation underlies the mechanisms of EADs. The investigators named this phenomenon, "Ca_i transient triggering," and suggested that increased forward Na-Ca exchanger current might contribute to the generation of EADs.

The muscle sleeves of thoracic veins are capable of developing automaticity and triggered activity during sympathetic stimulation [38]. Ryanodine at low concentrations (0.5–2 μmol/L) causes a Ca^{2+}-independent Ca_i release and facilitates the development of pacemaker activity in rabbit PVs [39]. The importance of Ca_i transient in atrial arrhythmogenesis is supported by a study that used isolated, Langendorff-perfused canine PV-LA preparations and two cameras to map membrane potential and Ca_i simultaneously [20]. Rapid PV firing was induced by rapid atrial pacing, low-dose ryanodine and isoproterenol infusion, and the rise of Ca_i preceded the action potential upstroke during focal discharge. There was clustering of PAS-positive large cells around the PV focal discharge sites. To determine further the interaction between sympathetic nerves and the PAS-positive cells, Tan and colleagues [40] performed a study in normal dogs. After sinus node crushing, left stellate ganglion stimulation caused PV tachycardias. The focus of tachycardia was determined by multichannel computerized mapping. PAS staining at the site of PV ectopy showed abundant pale-looking, glycogen-rich, specialized conducting (Purkinje's) cells. In addition, immunostaining showed abundant sympathetic (tyrosine hydroxylase positive) nerves at those sites. These preliminary results support the notion that sympathetic simulation induced PV focal discharge from sites with juxtapositioning of specialized conducting cells and autonomic nerves.

Structural anatomy of the atrial and pulmonary vein autonomic nerves

Pappone and colleagues [41] hypothesized that the induction of bradycardia was the result of vagal nerve stimulation, whereas the abolition of bradycardia with continued RF application suggests vagal denervation. The distribution of adrenergic and cholinergic nerves in this region were not delineated, however, so it is unclear whether or not sympathetic nerves also were eliminated during RF application. Tan and colleagues [24] performed immunostaining of 192 PV-LA segments harvested from 32 veins of eight human autopsied hearts using antityrosine hydroxylase antibodies to label adrenergic nerves and anticholine acetyltransferase antibodies to label cholinergic nerves. Nerve densities were analyzed along the longitudinal and circumferential axes of the PV-LA junction. Longitudinally, adrenergic and cholinergic nerve densities were highest in the LA within 5 mm from the PV-LA junction versus further distally in the PV or more proximally in the LA proper. Circumferentially, both nerve densities were higher in the superior aspect of LSPV, anterosuperior aspect of RSPV, and inferior aspects of both inferior PVs than diametrically opposite and higher in the epicardial than endocardial half of the tissue. Significantly, no area of discrete adrenergic or cholinergic predominance was noted. Rather, both nerve types have similar macroscopic distributions in and around PVs. Additionally, confocal microscopy of dual-stained sections showed that at cellular levels, up to 25% of all nerve fiber bundles contained both adrenergic and cholinergic nerves, more than 90% of ganglia contain both adrenergic and cholinergic elements within the same ganglion, and up to 30% of ganglion cell bodies may express adrenergic and cholinergic enzymes simultaneously within its neuroplasm. These data indicate that adrenergic and cholinergic nerves are highly colocated not only at tissue but also at cellular levels.

Implications of neural anatomy of the pulmonary vein

If both sympathetic and parasympathetic nerves are costimulated/ablated, why is bradycardia the dominant response elicited during ganglionic stimulation/ablation rather than tachycardia? Several explanations are proposed. First, complex extracardiac neural pathways [27,42] involved in the generation of bradycardic reflexes during stimulation/ablation around the PVs project to vagal nuclei centrally but do not involve sympathetic tracts generally [42]. Second, a paracrine mechanism might be in operation, as ganglion cells predominantly are cholinergic [24] and release mostly acetylcholine when stimulated/ablated. Third, adrenergic nerves are distributed more widely than cholinergic nerves [24,43]. Hence, radiofrequency ablation may eliminate a greater proportion of cholinergic nerves than that of adrenergic nerves, disrupting sympathovagal balance. Clinical reports [30,41] show that autonomic reflexes are elicited most commonly within approximately 1 cm of PV-LA junction. The anatomic colocalization of adrenergic and cholinergic innervations implies that it virtually would be impossible to eliminate only sympathetic or parasympathetic nerves selectively during catheter ablation of AF. The coexistence of adrenergic and cholinergic phenotypes within ganglionic cell neuroplasm also suggests that when ganglion cells are stimulated, adrenergic and cholinergic mediators may be released simultaneously, affecting cellular electrophysiology in ways that may predispose to triggered activity [37].

Sympathetic nerve recordings in animal models of paroxysmal atrial fibrillation

Barrett and colleagues [44] first reported successful recording of renal sympathetic nerve activity in conscious rabbits continuously for more than 7 days. The renal sympathetic nerve activity may not predict the cardiac sympathetic nerve activity, however. To record cardiac sympathetic nerve activity, Jung and colleagues [45] used Data Sciences International transmitters to record stellate ganglion nerve activity, 24 hours a day, 7 days a week, for an average of 41.5 (±16.6) days in normal ambulatory dogs. The results showed a circadian variation of sympathetic outflow. Normal dogs rarely develop paroxysmal AF, however. To test the hypothesis that spontaneous ANS discharges can serve as triggers of paroxysmal AF, it is necessary to develop an animal model of paroxysmal AF. Wijffels and colleagues [46] previously demonstrated that intermittent rapid pacing could induce progressively increased electrophysiologic remodeling, leading to persistent AF. Rapid atrial pacing also causes significant neural remodeling characterized by heterogeneous increase of sympathetic innervation [47] and extensive nerve sprouting [48]. In a preliminary study, Tan and colleagues [49] implanted Data Sciences International transmitters to directly record left stellate ganglion nerve activity, left vagal nerve activity, and LA local bipolar electrograms or surface ECG simultaneously in ambulatory dogs over several weeks. Intermittent rapid atrial pacing was performed and ANS activity monitored when the pacemaker was turned off. Paroxysmal atrial tachycardia and paroxysmal AF were documented and simultaneous sympathovagal discharges were the most common triggers of paroxysmal atrial tachycardia and paroxysmal AF in this study. These preliminary results support the hypothesis that ANS activity is important in the generation of paroxysmal AF.

Autonomic nervous system and atrial fibrillation in human patients

Several observations suggest the ANS plays an important role in the initiation and maintenance of AF in humans. Most patients who have idiopathic paroxysmal AF seem vagally dependent, with a heightened susceptibility to vasovagal cardiovascular response. In contrast, in most patients who have organic heart diseases, the paroxysmal AF episodes seem more sympathetically dependent [50]. A shift toward an increase in sympathetic tone or toward a loss of vagal tone has been observed before postoperative paroxysmal AF [51], before the onset of atrial flutter [52] and before paroxysmal AF occurring during sleep [53]; whereas a shift toward vagal predominance was observed in young patients who had lone AF and nocturnal episodes of paroxysmal AF [54]. More recently, a primary increase in adrenergic drive followed by marked modulation toward vagal predominance immediately before the onset of paroxysmal AF was observed [5,55,56]. The ANS activity in all these studies was evaluated indirectly, however, by the analysis of heart rate variability parameters on continuous ECG recordings. Heart rate variability measures changes in the relative degree of ANS, not the absolute level of sympathetic or parasympathetic discharges. It is necessary, therefore, to perform direct recording of sympathetic and vagal nerve activity to prove or disprove these observations in ambulatory animals.

Neural modulation as a potential therapeutic strategy

The effectiveness of autonomic modulation as an adjunctive therapeutic strategy to catheter ablation of AF is inconsistent. Although favorable results have been obtained by Nakagawa and colleagues and Pappone and colleagues [30,41], others found no beneficial [57] or deleterious [58] outcomes in patients who had denervation compared with those who did not, a finding underlined by animal studies by Hirose and colleagues [34], where partial vagal denervation of the high right atrium was found to increase inducibility of AF. These conflicting studies suggest that the interactions between the ANS and AF are more complex than currently understood. Perhaps a degree of individual variability accounts for these discrepancies, with some patients having more pronounced autonomic triggers than others. As an illustration, Scanavacca and colleagues [59] recently found that in a small number of patients who had "autonomic" paroxysmal AF, denervation alone without substrate modification in the atria was effective in preventing AF recurrence in 2 of 11 patients, these two patients having the most pronounced and persistent changes in heart rate variability. In summary, the evidence to date suggests that autonomic modulation does have an adjunctive role to play in catheter AF ablation, especially when applied selectively. Further mechanistic and clinical studies are warranted before a wider application can be recommended.

References

[1] Allessie MA, Boyden PA, Camm AJ, et al. Pathophysiology and prevention of atrial fibrillation. Circulation 2001;103:769–77.

[2] Chen YJ, Chen SA, Chang MS, et al. Arrhythmogenic activity of cardiac muscle in pulmonary veins of the dog: implication for the genesis of atrial fibrillation. Cardiovasc Res 2000; 48:265–73.

[3] Doshi RN, Wu T-J, Yashima M, et al. Relation between ligament of Marshall and adrenergic atrial tachyarrhythmia. Circulation 1999;100:876–83.

[4] Sharifov OF, Fedorov VV, Beloshapko GG, et al. Roles of adrenergic and cholinergic stimulation in spontaneous atrial fibrillation in dogs. J Am Coll Cardiol 2004;43:483–90.

[5] Bettoni M, Zimmermann M. Autonomic tone variations before the onset of paroxysmal atrial fibrillation. Circulation 2002;105:2753–9.

[6] Gould PA, Yii M, McLean C, et al. Evidence for increased atrial sympathetic innervation in persistent human atrial fibrillation. Pacing Clin Electrophysiol 2006;29:821–9.

[7] Moe GK, Abildskov JA. Atrial fibrillation as a self-sustaining arrhythmia independent of focal discharge. Am Heart J 1959;58:59–70.

[8] Zipes DP, Knope RF. Electrical properties of the thoracic veins. Am J Cardiol 1972;29: 372–6.

[9] Spach MS, Barr RC, Jewett PH. Spread of excitation from the atrium into thoracic veins in human beings and dogs. Am J Cardiol 1972;30:844–54.

[10] Scherlag BJ, Yeh BK, Robinson MJ. Inferior interatrial pathway in the dog. Circ Res 1972; 31:18–35.

[11] Haissaguerre M, Jais P, Shah DC, et al. Spontaneous initiation of atrial fibrillation by ectopic beats originating in the pulmonary veins. N Engl J Med 1998;339:659–66.

[12] Hamabe A, Okuyama Y, Miyauchi Y, et al. Correlation between anatomy and electrical activation in canine pulmonary veins. Circulation 2003;107:1550–5.

[13] Zhou S, Chang C-M, Wu T-J, et al. Nonreentrant focal activations in pulmonary veins in canine model of sustained atrial fibrillation. Am J Physiol Heart Circ Physiol 2002;283: H1244–52.

[14] Chou CC, Zhou S, Miyauchi Y, et al. Effects of procainamide on electrical activity in thoracic veins and atria in canine model of sustained atrial fibrillation. Am J Physiol Heart Circ Physiol 2004;286:H1936–45.

[15] Chou CC, Zhou S, Tan AY, et al. High density mapping of pulmonary veins and left atrium during ibutilide administration in a canine model of sustained atrial fibrillation. Am J Physiol Heart Circ Physiol 2005;289:H2704–13.

[16] Gong Y, Xie F, Stein KM, et al. Mechanism underlying initiation of paroxysmal atrial flutter/atrial fibrillation by ectopic foci. A Simulation Study. Circulation 2007;115:2094–102.

[17] Masani F. Node-like cells in the myocardial layer of the pulmonary vein of rats: an ultra-structural study. J Anat 1986;145:133–42.
[18] Cheung DW. Electrical activity of the pulmonary vein and its interaction with the right atrium in the guinea-pig. J Physiol 1981;314:445–56.
[19] Perez-Lugones A, McMahon JT, Ratliff NB, et al. Evidence of specialized conduction cells in human pulmonary veins of patients with atrial fibrillation. J Cardiovasc Electrophysiol 2003; 14:803–9.
[20] Chou C-C, Nihei M, Zhou S, et al. Intracellular calcium dynamics and anisotropic reentry in isolated canine pulmonary veins and left atrium. Circulation 2005;111:2889–97.
[21] Crick SJ, Sheppard MN, Anderson RH, et al. A quantitative study of nerve distribution in the conduction system of the guinea pig heart. J Anat 1996;188:403–16.
[22] Crick SJ, Wharton J, Sheppard MN, et al. Innervation of the human cardiac conduction system. A quantitative immunohistochemical and histochemical study. Circulation 1994;89: 1697–708.
[23] Miyauchi Y, Zhou S, Okuyama Y, et al. Altered atrial electrical restitution and heteroge-neous sympathetic hyperinnervation in hearts with chronic left ventricular myocardial infarction: implications for atrial fibrillation. Circulation 2003;108:360–6.
[24] Tan AY, Li H, Wachsmann-Hogiu S, et al. Autonomic innervation and segmental muscular disconnections at the human pulmonary vein-atrial junction: implications for catheter abla-tion of atrial-pulmonary vein junction. J Am Coll Cardiol 2006;48:132–43.
[25] Kawashima T. The autonomic nervous system of the human heart with special reference to its origin, course, and peripheral distribution. Anat Embryol (Berl) 2005;209:425–38.
[26] Armour JA, Murphy DA, Yuan BX, et al. Gross and microscopic anatomy of the human intrinsic cardiac nervous system. Anat Rec 1997;247:289–98.
[27] Chiou C-W, Eble JN, Zipes DP. Efferent vagal innervation of the canine atria and sinus and atrioventricular nodes–the third fat pad. Circulation 1997;95:2573–84.
[28] Chevalier P, Tabib A, Meyronnet D, et al. Quantitative study of nerves of the human left atrium. Heart Rhythm 2005;2:518–22.
[29] Scherlag BJ, Yamanashi W, Patel U, et al. Autonomically induced conversion of pulmonary vein focal firing into atrial fibrillation. J Am Coll Cardiol 2005;45:1878–86.
[30] Nakagawa H, Scherlag BJ, Wu R, et al. Addition of selective ablation of autonomic ganglia to pulmonary vein antrum isolation for treatment of paroxysmal and persistent atrial fibril-lation [abstract]. Circulation 2006;110:III-459.
[31] Zipes DP, Mihalick MJ, Robbins GT. Effects of selective vagal and stellate ganglion stimu-lation of atrial refractoriness. Cardiovasc Res 1974;8:647–55.
[32] Spear JF, Moore EN. Influence of brief vagal and stellate nerve stimulation on pacemaker activity and conduction within the atrioventricular conduction system of the dog. Circ Res 1973;32:27–41.
[33] Goldberger AL, Pavelec RS. Vagally-mediated atrial fibrillation in dogs: conversion with bretylium tosylate. Int J Cardiol 1986;13:47–55.
[34] Hirose M, Leatmanoratn Z, Laurita KR, et al. Partial vagal denervation increases vulnera-bility to vagally induced atrial fibrillation. J Cardiovasc Electrophysiol 2002;13:1272–9.
[35] Coumel P, Attuel P, Lavallee J, et al. The atrial arrhythmia syndrome of vagal origin. Arch Mal Coeur Vaiss 1978;71:645–56.
[36] Burashnikov A, Antzelevitch C. Reinduction of atrial fibrillation immediately after termina-tion of the arrhythmia is mediated by late phase 3 early afterdepolarization-induced trig-gered activity. Circulation 2003;107:2355–60.
[37] Patterson E, Lazzara R, Szabo B, et al. Sodium-calcium exchange initiated by the Ca2+ tran-sient: an arrhythmia trigger within pulmonary veins. J Am Coll Cardiol 2006;47:1196–206.
[38] Wit AL, Cranefield PF. Triggered and automatic activity in the canine coronary sinus. Circ Res 1977;41:434–45.
[39] Honjo H, Boyett MR, Niwa R, et al. Pacing-induced spontaneous activity in myocardial sleeves of pulmonary veins after treatment with ryanodine. Circulation 2003;107:1937–43.

[40] Tan AY, Zhou S, Jung B-C, et al. In-vivo sympathetic nerve stimulation induces ectopic beats and focal atrial tachycardia from thoracic veins in dogs: insights from sympathetic nerve recording and high density mapping [abstract]. J Am Coll Cardiol 2006;47(1S):3A.

[41] Pappone C, Santinelli V, Manguso F, et al. Pulmonary vein denervation enhances long-term benefit after circumferential ablation for paroxysmal atrial fibrillation. Circulation 2004;109: 327–34.

[42] Aviado DM, Guevara AD. The Bezold-Jarisch reflex. A historical perspective of cardiopulmonary reflexes. Ann N Y Acad Sci 2001;940:48–58.

[43] Marron K, Wharton J, Sheppard MN, et al. Distribution, morphology, and neurochemistry of endocardial and epicardial nerve terminal arborizations in the human heart. Circulation 1995;92:2343–51.

[44] Barrett CJ, Ramchandra R, Guild SJ, et al. What sets the long-term level of renal sympathetic nerve activity: a role for angiotensin II and baroreflexes? Circ Res 2003;92:1330–6.

[45] Jung B-C, Dave AS, Tan AY, et al. Circadian variations of stellate ganglion nerve activity in ambulatory dogs. Heart Rhythm 2005;3:78–85.

[46] Wijffels MC, Kirchhof CJ, Dorland R, et al. Atrial fibrillation begets atrial fibrillation. A study in awake chronically instrumented goats. Circulation 1995;92:1954–68.

[47] Jayachandran JV, Sih HJ, Winkle W, et al. Atrial fibrillation produced by prolonged rapid atrial pacing is associated with heterogeneous changes in atrial sympathetic innervation. Circulation 2000;101:1185–91.

[48] Chang C-M, Wu T-J, Zhou S-M, et al. Nerve sprouting and sympathetic hyperinnervation in a canine model of atrial fibrillation produced by prolonged right atrial pacing. Circulation 2001;103:22–5.

[49] Tan AY, Zhou S, Gholmieh G, et al. Spontaneous autonomic nerve activity and paroxysmal atrial tachyarrhythmias [abstract]. Heart Rhythm 2006;3(1S):184.

[50] Huang JL, Wen ZC, Lee WL, et al. Changes of autonomic tone before the onset of paroxysmal atrial fibrillation. Int J Cardiol 1998;66:275–83.

[51] Dimmer C, Tavernier R, Gjorgov N, et al. Variations of autonomic tone preceding onset of atrial fibrillation after coronary artery bypass grafting. Am J Cardiol 1998;82:22–5.

[52] Wen ZC, Chen SA, Tai CT, et al. Role of autonomic tone in facilitating spontaneous onset of typical atrial flutter. J Am Coll Cardiol 1998;31:602–7.

[53] Coccagna G, Capucci A, Bauleo S, et al. Paroxysmal atrial fibrillation in sleep. Sleep 1997;20: 396–8.

[54] Herweg B, Dalal P, Nagy B, et al. Power spectral analysis of heart period variability of preceding sinus rhythm before initiation of paroxysmal atrial fibrillation. Am J Cardiol 1998;82: 869–74.

[55] Zimmermann M, Kalusche D. Fluctuation in autonomic tone is a major determinant of sustained atrial arrhythmias in patients with focal ectopy originating from the pulmonary veins. J Cardiovasc Electrophysiol 2001;12:285–91.

[56] Amar D, Zhang H, Miodownik S, et al. Competing autonomic mechanisms precede the onset of postoperative atrial fibrillation. J Am Coll Cardiol 2003;42:1262–8.

[57] Lemery R, Birnie D, Tang AS, et al. Feasibility study of endocardial mapping of ganglionated plexuses during catheter ablation of atrial fibrillation. Heart Rhythm 2006;3:387–96.

[58] Cummings JE, Gill I, Akhrass R, et al. Preservation of the anterior fat pad paradoxically decreases the incidence of postoperative atrial fibrillation in humans. J Am Coll Cardiol 2004; 43:994–1000.

[59] Scanavacca M, Pisani CF, Hachul D, et al. Selective atrial vagal denervation guided by evoked vagal reflex to treat patients with paroxysmal atrial fibrillation. Circulation 2006; 114:876–85.

THE MEDICAL
CLINICS
OF NORTH AMERICA

Med Clin N Am 92 (2008) 65–85

Diagnosis and Management of Typical Atrial Flutter

Navinder S. Sawhney, MD, Gregory K. Feld, MD*

*Clinical Cardiac Electrophysiology Program, Division of Cardiology,
University of California Medical Center, 4169 Front Street,
San Diego, CA 92103, USA*

Type 1 atrial flutter (AFL) is a common atrial arrhythmia that may cause significant symptoms and serious adverse effects, including embolic stroke, myocardial ischemia and infarction, and, rarely, a tachycardia-induced cardiomyopathy resulting from rapid atrioventricular conduction. The electrophysiologic substrate underlying type 1 AFL is shown to be a combination of slow conduction velocity in the cavotricuspid isthmus (CTI) plus anatomic or functional conduction block along the crista terminalis and eustachian ridge. This electrophysiologic milleu allows for a long enough reentrant path length relative to the average tissue wavelength around the tricuspid valve annulus to allow for sustained reentry.

As a result of its well-defined anatomic substrate and its relative pharmacologic resistance, radiofrequency catheter ablation has emerged since its first description in 1992 as a safe and effective first-line treatment of type 1 AFL. Although several techniques are described for ablating type 1 AFL, the most widely accepted and successful is an anatomically guided approach targeting the CTI. Recent technologic developments, including 3-D electroanatomic contact and noncontact mapping and the use of large-tip ablation electrode catheters with high-power generators, have produced nearly uniform efficacy without increased risk. This article reviews the electrophysiology of human type 1 AFL and techniques currently used for its diagnosis and management.

---

* Corresponding author. Division of Cardiology, University of California, San Diego, 200 West Arbor Drive, San Diego, CA 92103-9000.
E-mail address: gfeld@ucsd.edu (G.K. Feld).

0025-7125/08/$ - see front matter © 2008 Elsevier Inc. All rights reserved.
doi:10.1016/j.mcna.2007.08.005
medical.theclinics.com

Atrial flutter terminology

Because of the variety of terms used to describe AFL in humans, including type 1 AFL and type 2 AFL, typical and atypical AFL, counterclockwise and clockwise AFL, isthmus and nonisthmus dependent flutter, the Working Group of Arrhythmias of the European Society of Cardiology and the North American Society of Pacing and Electrophysiology convened and published a consensus document in 2001 in an attempt to develop a generally accepted standardized terminology for AFL [1]. The consensus terminology derived from this working group to describe CTI-dependent, right atrial macroreentry tachycardia in the counterclockwise or clockwise direction around the tricuspid valve annulus was "typical" and "reverse typical" AFL [1]. For the purposes of this article, these two arrhythmias are referred to specifically as typical and reverse typical AFL when described individually, but as type 1 AFL when referred to jointly.

Pathophysiologic mechanisms of type 1 atrial flutter

The development of successful radiofrequency catheter ablation techniques for human type 1 AFL largely was dependent on the delineation of its electrophysiologic mechanism. Through the use of advanced electrophysiologic techniques, including intraoperative and transcatheter activation mapping [2–7], type 1 AFL was determined to be the result of a macroreentrant circuit rotating in a counterclockwise (typical) or clockwise (reverse typical) direction in the right atrium around the tricuspid valve annulus, with an area of relatively slow conduction velocity in the low posterior right atrium (Fig. 1A, B). The predominate area of slow conduction in the AFL reentry circuit has been shown to be in the CTI, through which conduction times may reach 80 to 100 milliseconds, accounting for one third to one half of the AFL cycle length [8–10]. The CTI is bounded anatomically by the inferior vena cava and eustachian ridge posteriorly and the tricuspid valve annulus anteriorly (see Fig. 1A, B), both of which form lines of conduction block or barriers delineating a protected zone of slow conduction in the reentry circuit [7,11–13]. The presence of conduction block along the eustachian ridge has been confirmed by demonstrating double potentials along its length during AFL. Double potentials also have been recorded along the crista terminalis, suggesting that it too forms a line of block separating the smooth septal right atrium from the trabeculated right atrial free wall. Such lines of block, which may be functional or anatomic, are necessary to create an adequate path length for reentry to be sustained and to prevent short-circuiting of the reentrant wavefront [12–14]. The medial CTI is contiguous with the interatrial septum near the coronary sinus ostium and the lateral CTI is contiguous with the low lateral right atrium near the inferior vena cava (Fig. 1). These areas correspond electrophysiologically to the exit and entrance to the zone of slow conduction, depending on whether or not

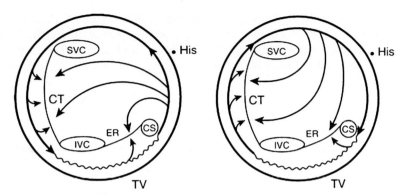

Fig. 1. Schematic diagrams demonstrating the activation patterns in the typical (*A*) and reverse typical (*B*) forms of human type 1 AFL, as viewed from below the tricuspid valve annulus (TV) looking up into the right atrium. In the typical form of AFL, the reentrant wavefront rotates counterclockwise in the right atrium, whereas in the reverse typical form reentry is clockwise. The eustachian ridge (ER) and crista terminalis (CT) form lines of block and that an area of slow conduction (*wavy line*) is present in the isthmus between the inferior vena cava (IVC) and eustachian ridge and the tricuspid valve annulus. CS, coronary sinus ostium; His, His' bundle; SVC, superior vena cava. (*Adapted from* Feld GK, Srivatsa U, Hoppe B. Ablation of isthmus dependent atrial flutters. In: Huang SS, Wood MA, editors. Catheter ablation of cardiac arrhythmias. Philadelphia: Elsevier; 2006. p. 197; with permission.)

the direction of reentry is counterclockwise or clockwise in the right atrium. The path of the reentrant circuit outside the confines of the CTI consists of a broad activation wavefront in the interatrial septum and right atrial free wall around the crista terminalis and the tricuspid valve annulus [11–14].

The slower conduction velocity in the CTI, relative to the interatrial septum and right atrial free wall, may be caused by anisotropic fiber orientation in the CTI [2,8–10,15,16]. This also may predispose to development of unidirectional block during rapid atrial pacing and account for the observation that typical (counterclockwise) AFL more likely is induced when pacing is performed from the coronary sinus ostium and, conversely, reverse typical (clockwise) AFL more likely is induced when pacing from the low lateral right atrium [17,18]. This hypothesis is supported further by direct mapping in animal studies, demonstrating that the direction of rotation of the reentrant wavefront during AFL is dependent on the direction of the paced wavefront producing unidirectional block at the time of its induction [7]. In humans, the predominate clinical presentation of type 1 AFL is the typical variety, likely because the triggers for AFL commonly arise from the left atrium in the form of premature atrial contractions or nonsustained atrial fibrillation [19]. Triggers arising from the left atrium or pulmonary veins usually conduct to the right atrium via the coronary sinus or interatrial septum, thus entering the CTI from medial to lateral, which results in clockwise unidirectional block in the CTI with resultant initiation of counterclockwise typical AFL.

The development of abnormal dispersion or shortening of atrial refractoriness as a result of atrial electrical remodeling may increase the likelihood of developing regional conduction block and abnormal shortening of tissue wavelength responsible for initiating and sustaining reentry in AFL [20,21].

ECG diagnosis of type 1 atrial flutter

The surface 12-lead ECG is helpful in establishing a diagnosis of type 1 AFL, in particular the typical form. In typical AFL, an inverted saw-tooth F wave pattern is observed in the inferior ECG leads II, III, and aVF, with a low-amplitude biphasic F waves in leads I and aVL, an upright F wave in precordial lead V1, and an inverted F wave in lead V6. In contrast, in reverse typical AFL, the F-wave pattern on the 12-lead ECG is less specific, often with a sine wave pattern in the inferior ECG leads (Fig. 2A, B). The determinants of F-wave pattern on ECG largely are dependent on the activation pattern of the left atrium, resulting from reentry in the right atrium, with inverted F waves inscribed in the inferior ECG leads in typical AFL as a result of activation of the left atrium initially posterior near the coronary sinus and upright F waves inscribed in the inferior ECG leads in reverse typical AFL as a result of activation of the left atrium initially anterior near Bachmann's bundle [22,23]. Because the typical and reverse typical forms of type 1 AFL use the same reentry circuit, but in opposite directions, their rates usually are similar.

Medical therapy versus catheter ablation

Class III antiarrhythmic drugs (eg, N-acetylprocainamide, sotalol, and dofetilide), by selectively lengthening the cardiac action potential, have demonstrated efficacy in converting AFL and maintaining normal sinus rhythm [24,25]. Experimental studies demonstrate that the mechanism by which the class III antiarrhythmic drugs convert and suppress AFL is their predominate effect of prolongation of action potential duration, resulting in prolongation of atrial effective refractory period and wavelength in excess of the path length of the AFL circuit [24,26]. In contrast, the class 1c antiarrhythmic drugs commonly used for treatment of atrial fibrillation have a significant incidence of atrial proarrhythmic effect, promoting the development of AFL because they depress conduction velocity and shorten atrial wavelength [26,27]. Despite an 80% clinical efficacy with the class III drug, ibutilide (Corvert), in converting AFL to sinus rhythm [28], long-term recurrence rates of AFL are high (70%–90%) despite maintenance on antiarrhythmic drugs [29,30], and, therefore, catheter ablation is considered a first-line approach for many patients who have AFL given the high acute and chronic efficacy of the procedure (>90%) and low complication rates [31]. Prospective trials that have randomized patients to

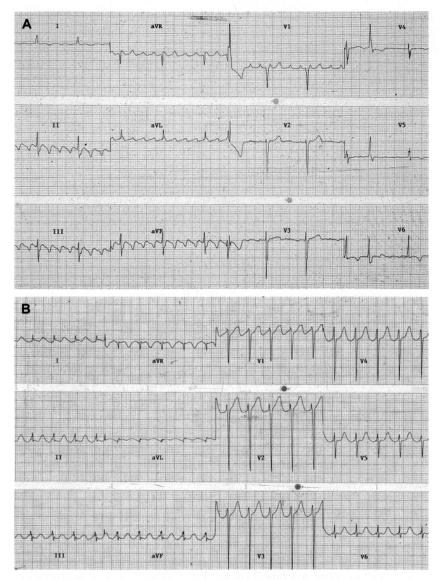

Fig. 2. (*A*) 12-Lead electrocardiogram recorded from a patient with typical AFL. Note the typical saw-toothed pattern of inverted F waves in the inferior leads II, III, and aVF. Typical AFL also is characterized by flat to biphasic F waves in I and aVL, respectively, an upright F wave in V1 and an inverted F wave in V6. (*B*) 12-Lead electrocardiogram recorded from a patient who had the reverse typical AFL. The F wave in the reverse typical form of AFL has a less distinct sine wave pattern in the inferior leads. In this case, the F waves are upright in the inferior leads II, III, and aVF; biphasic in leads I, aVL, and V1; and upright in V6. (*From* Feld GK, Srivatsa U, Hoppe B. Ablation of isthmus dependent atrial flutters. In: Huang SS, Wood MA, editors. Catheter ablation of cardiac arrhythmias. Philadelphia: Elsevier; 2006. p. 201; with permission.)

medical therapy versus first-line catheter ablation show that patients who received ablation as a first-line strategy had significantly better maintenance of sinus rhythm, fewer hospitalizations, better quality of life (QOL), and fewer overall complications compared with antiarrhythmic drug therapy [30,32].

Despite the excellent acute results and long-term outcome after radiofrequency catheter ablation for freedom from type 1 AFL, development of AFL is high in this population of patients; up to 30% of these patients may develop AFL over a 5-year period, especially if there is a pre-existing history of AFL or underlying heart disease [30,32–34]. Ablation of the CTI may reduce or in rare cases eliminate recurrences of atrial fibrillation, however, and CTI ablation also is effective in patients undergoing pharmacologic treatment for atrial fibrillation with antiarrhythmic drug-induced type 1 AFL (the so-called "hybrid approach"). Ablation of the CTI also may be required in patients undergoing ablation for AFL who have a history of type 1 AFL [35].

Electrophysiologic mapping of type 1 atrial flutter

Despite the usefulness of the 12-lead ECG in making a presumptive diagnosis of typical AFL, an electrophysiologic study with mapping and entrainment must be performed to confirm the underlying mechanism if radiofrequency catheter ablation is to be performed successfully. This is true particularly in the case of reverse typical AFL, which is much more difficult to diagnose on 12-lead ECG. For the electrophysiologic study of AFL, activation mapping may be performed using standard multielectrode catheters or one of the currently available 3-D computerized activation mapping systems. For standard multielectrode catheter mapping, catheters are positioned in the right atrium, His' bundle region, and coronary sinus. To elucidate the endocardial activation sequence most precisely, a Halo 20-electrode mapping catheter (Biosense-Webster, Diamond Bar, California) is used most commonly in the right atrium positioned around the tricuspid valve annulus (Fig. 3). Recordings obtained during AFL from all electrodes are analyzed to determine the right atrial activation sequence. In patients presenting to the laboratory in sinus rhythm, it is necessary to induce AFL to confirm its mechanism. Induction of AFL is accomplished by atrial programmed stimulation or burst pacing. Preferred pacing sites are the coronary sinus ostium or low lateral right atrium. Burst pacing at cycle lengths between 180 and 240 milliseconds typically is the most effective method to induce AFL. Induction of AFL typically occurs after the onset of unidirectional block in the CTI isthmus, either during pacing or after a short period of atrial fibrillation [17,18].

During electrophysiologic study, a diagnosis of either typical or reverse typical AFL is suggested by observing a counterclockwise or clockwise activation pattern in the right atrium around the tricuspid valve annulus.

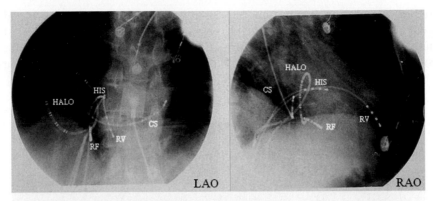

Fig. 3. LAO and RAO fluoroscopic projections showing the intra-cardiac positions of the right ventricular (RV), His' bundle (HIS), coronary sinus (CS), Halo (HALO), and mapping/ablation catheter (RF). The Halo catheter is positioned around the tricuspid valve annulus, with the proximal electrode pair at the 1 o'clock position and the distal electrode pair at the 7 o'clock position in the LAO view. The mapping/ablation catheter is positioned in the subeustachian isthmus, midway between the interatrial septum and low lateral right atrium, with the distal 8-mm ablation electrode near the tricuspid valve annulus. (*From* Feld GK, Srivatsa U, Hoppe B. Ablation of isthmus dependent atrial flutters. In: Huang SS, Wood MA, editors. Catheter ablation of cardiac arrhythmias. Philadelphia: Elsevier; 2006. p. 202; with permission.)

For example, as seen in Fig. 4A in a patient who had typical AFL, the atrial electrogram recorded at the coronary sinus ostium is timed with the initial down stroke of the F wave in the inferior surface ECG leads, followed by caudal-to-cranial activation in the interatrial septum to the His bundle atrial electrogram, then cranial-to-caudal activation in the right atrial free wall from proximal to distal on the Halo catheter, and finally to the ablation catheter in the CTI, indicating that the underlying mechanism is a counter-clockwise macroreentry circuit with electrical activity encompassing the entire tachycardia cycle length. In a patient who had reverse typical AFL, the mirror image of this activation pattern is seen (shown in Fig. 4B.)

Radiofrequency catheter ablation of type 1 atrial flutter

Radiofrequency catheter ablation of type 1 AFL is performed with a steerable mapping/ablation catheter with a large distal ablation electrode positioned in the right atrium via a femoral vein [3,5–7,36–38]. The typical radiofrequency generator used by most laboratories is capable of automatically adjusting applied power to achieve an operator programmable tissue-electrode interface temperature. Tissue temperature is monitored via a thermistor or thermocouple embedded in the distal ablation electrode. Programmable temperature with automatic power control is important because successful ablation requires a stable temperature of at least 50°C to 60°C and occasionally 70°C. Temperatures in excess of 70°C may cause tissue vaporization (steam pops), tissue charring, and formation of blood coagulum on the ablation electrode resulting in a rise in impedance that limits energy delivery and lesion formation, and may lead to complications, such as cardiac perforation or embolization. Several of mapping/ablation

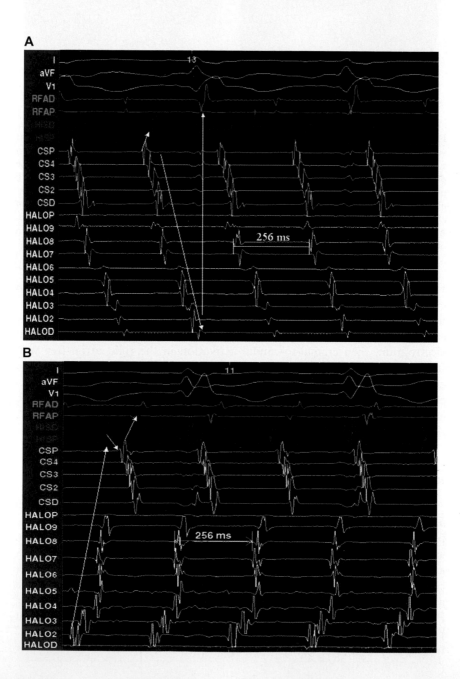

catheters with different shapes and curve lengths currently are available from several commercial manufacturers. The authors prefer to use a larger curve catheter (K2 or mid-distal large curve, EP Technologies, San Jose, California), with or without a preshaped guiding sheath, such as an SR-0, SL-1, or ramp sheath (Daig, Minnetonka, Minnesota), to ensure that the ablation electrode reaches the tricuspid valve annulus.

Recently, radiofrequency ablation catheters with saline-cooled ablation electrodes or large distal ablation electrodes (ie, 8–10 mm) have been approved by the Food and Drug Administration for ablation of type 1 AFL (EP Technologies, San Jose, California, and Biosense-Webster, Diamond Bar, California). During ablation with saline-cooled catheters, the use of lower power and temperature settings is recommended to avoid steam pops, because higher intramyocardial tissue temperatures are produced than measured at the tissue-electrode interface because of the electrode cooling effect of saline perfusion [39–41]. Typically, a maximum power of 35 to 40 W and temperature of 43° to 45°C should be used initially, although studies have reported use of up to 50 W and 60°C for ablation of AFL without higher than expected complication rates [39–42]. In contrast, the large-tip (8–10 mm) ablation catheters require a higher power, up to 100 W, to achieve target temperatures of 50°C to 70°C because of the greater energy dispersive effects of the larger ablation electrode. This also requires the use of two grounding pads applied to patients' skin to avoid skin burns [31,41,43,44].

The preferred target for type 1 AFL ablation is the CTI, which, when using standard multipolar electrode catheters for mapping and ablation, is localized with a combined fluoroscopically and electrophysiologically guided approach [3,5–7,31,36 42,44]. Typically, a steerable mapping/ablation catheter is positioned, initially fluoroscopically (Fig. 3) in the CTI with the distal ablation electrode on or near the tricuspid valve annulus in the right anterior oblique (RAO) view, and midway between the septum and low right atrial free wall (6 o'clock or 7 o'clock position) in the left

---

Fig. 4. Endocardial electrograms from the mapping/ablation, Halo, CS, and His' bundle catheters, and surface ECG leads I and aVF, demonstrating a counterclockwise rotation of activation in the right atrium in a patient who had typical AFL (*A*) and a clockwise rotation of activation in the right atrium in a patient with reverse typical AFL (*B*). The AFL cycle length was 256 milliseconds for counterclockwise and clockwise forms. Arrows demonstrate activation sequence. HALO D–HALO P tracings arc 10 bipolar electrograms recorded from the distal (low lateral right atrium) to proximal (high right atrium) poles of the 20-pole Halo catheter positioned around the tricuspid valve annulus with the proximal electrode pair at the 1 o'clock position and the distal electrode pair at the 7 o'clock position. CSP, electrograms recorded from the coronary sinus catheter proximal electrode pair positioned at the ostium of the coronary sinus; HISP, electrograms recorded from the proximal electrode pair of the His' bundle catheter; RF, electrograms recorded from the mapping/ablation catheter positioned with the distal electrode pair in the CTI. (*From* Feld GK, Srivatsa U, Hoppe B. Ablation of isthmus dependent atrial flutters. In: Huang SS, Wood MA, editors. Catheter ablation of cardiac arrhythmias. Philadelphia: Elsevier; 2006. p. 203; with permission.)

anterior oblique (LAO) view. The distal ablation electrode position then is adjusted toward or away from the TV annulus based on the ratio of atrial and ventricular electrogram amplitude recorded by the bipolar ablation electrode. An optimal AV ratio typically is 1:2 or 1:4 at the tricuspid valve annulus (seen in Fig. 4A) on the distal radiofrequency ablation electrode (RFAD). After positioning the ablation catheter on or near the tricuspid valve annulus, it is withdrawn slowly a few millimeters at a time (usually the length of the distal ablation electrode) pausing for 30 to 60 seconds at each location during a continuous or interrupted energy application. Electrogram recordings may be used in addition to fluoroscopy to ensure that the ablation electrode is in contact with viable tissue in the CTI throughout each energy application. Ablation of the entire CTI may require several sequential 30- to 60-second energy applications during a stepwise catheter pullback or a prolonged energy application of up to 120 seconds or more during a continuous catheter pullback. The catheter should be withdrawn gradually until the distal ablation electrode records no atrial electrogram, indicating it has reached the inferior vena cava or until the ablation electrode is noted to abruptly slip off the eustachian ridge fluoroscopically. Radiofrequency energy application should be interrupted immediately when the catheter has reached the inferior vena cava, because ablation in the venous structures is known to cause significant pain to patients.

Procedure endpoints for radiofrequency catheter ablation of type 1 atrial flutter

Ablation may be performed during sustained AFL or during sinus rhythm. If performed during AFL, the first endpoint is its termination during energy application. Despite termination of AFL however, it is common to find that CTI conduction persists. After the entire CTI ablation is completed, electrophysiologic testing should be performed. Pacing then should be done at a cycle length of 600 milliseconds (or greater depending on sinus cycle length) to determine if there is bidirectional conduction block in the CTI (Fig. 5A, B, Fig. 6A, B). Bidirectional conduction block in the CTI is confirmed by demonstrating a change from a bidirectional wavefront with collision in the right atrial free wall or interatrial septum before ablation to a strictly cranial to caudal activation sequence after ablation during pacing from the coronary sinus ostium or low lateral right atrium, respectively [45–47]. The presence of bidirectional conduction block in the CTI also is supported strongly by recording widely spaced double potentials [48,49] at the site of linear ablation during pacing from the low lateral right atrium or coronary sinus ostium. If ablation is done during sinus rhythm, pacing also can be done during energy application to monitor for the development of conduction block in the CTI. The use of this endpoint for ablation may be associated with a significantly lower recurrence rate of type 1 AFL during long-term follow-up [45–47,50]. Programmed stimulation and burst pacing should be repeated over the course of at least 30 minutes to ensure that bidirectional CTI block has been achieved and that neither typical nor reverse typical AFL can be reinduced [3,5–7, 31,36–40,42–44,51].

If AFL is not terminated during the first attempt at CTI ablation, the activation sequence and isthmus dependence of the AFL should be reconfirmed and ablation repeated. During repeat ablation, it may be necessary to use a slightly higher power or ablation temperature or to rotate the ablation catheter away from the initial line of energy application, either medially or laterally in the CTI, to create new or additional lines of block. In addition, if ablation initially is attempted using a standard 4- to 5-mm tip electrode and fails, repeat ablation with a larger-tip 8- to 10-mm electrode catheter or cooled-tip ablation catheter may be successful [31,39–44].

Outcomes and complications of catheter ablation of type 1 atrial flutter

Early reports [3–5,7] of radiofrequency catheter ablation of AFL revealed high initial success rates but with recurrence rates up to 20% to 45% (Table 1). As experience with radiofrequency catheter ablation of AFL has increased, however, both acute success rates, defined as termination of AFL and bidirectional isthmus block, and chronic success rates, defined as no recurrence of type 1 AFL, have risen to 85% to 95%. Contributing in large degree to these improved results has been the introduction of bidirectional conduction block in the CTI as an endpoint for successful radiofrequency catheter ablation of AFL [31,36–44]. In the most recent studies using either large-tip (8–10 mm) electrode ablation catheters with high-power radiofrequency generators or cooled-tip electrode ablation catheters with standard radiofrequency generators, acute success rates as high as 100% and chronic success rates as high as 98% are reported [31,41,44]. Randomized comparisons of internally cooled, externally cooled, and large-tip ablation catheters suggest a slightly better acute and chronic success rate with the externally cooled ablation catheters compared with internally cooled ablation catheters or large-tip ablation catheters [39,40,42,44,51].

In nearly all the large-scale studies where CTI ablation successfully has eliminated recurrence of type 1 AFL and where QOL has been assessed, there have been statistically significant improvements in QOL due to reduced symptoms and antiarrhythmic medication use [30,31,51].

Radiofrequency catheter ablation of the CTI for type 1 AFL is relatively safe, but serious complications can occur, including heart block, cardiac perforation and tamponade, and thromboembolic events, including pulmonary embolism and stroke. In recent large-scale studies, major complications have been observed in approximately 2.5% to 3.0% of patients [31,44,51]. In the studies of large-tip ablation electrode catheters, there did not seem to be any relationship between complication rates and the use of higher power (ie, >50 W) for ablation of the CTI. Anticoagulation with warfarin before ablation must be considered in patients who have chronic type 1 AFL to help decrease the risk for thromboembolic complications, such as stroke [52]. This may be important particularly in those patients who have depressed left ventricular function, mitral valve disease, and left atrial enlargement with spontaneous contrast (ie, smoke) on echocardiography. As an alternative, the use of transesophageal echocardiography to rule out left atrial clot before ablation may be acceptable, but subsequent anticoagulation with warfarin still is recommended as atrial stunning may occur after conversion of AFL, as it does with atrial fibrillation [52].

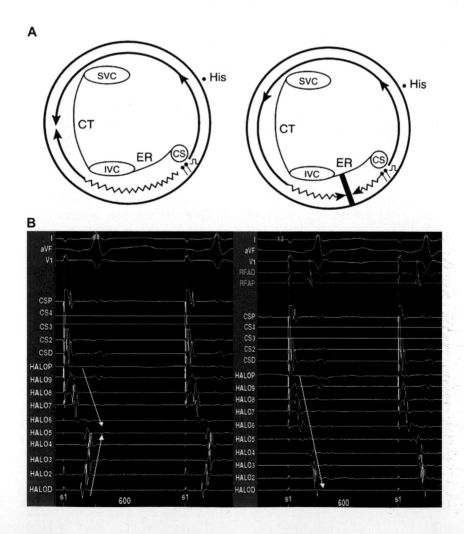

Role of computerized 3-D mapping in diagnosis and ablation of type 1 atrial flutter

The 3-D electroanatomic CARTO (BioSense-Webster) or noncontact EnSite (Endocardial Solutions, St. Paul, Minnesota) activation mapping systems, although certainly not required for successful ablation of type 1 AFL, have specific advantages that have made them a widely used and accepted technology. Although it is not within the scope of this article to describe the technologic basis of these systems in detail, there are unique characteristics of each system that make them more or less suitable for mapping and ablation of AFL.

The EnSite system uses a saline-inflated balloon catheter on which is mounted a wire mesh containing electrodes that are capable of sensing the voltage potential of surrounding atrial endocardium, without actual electrode-tissue contact, from which the computerized mapping system can generate up to 3000 virtual endocardial electrograms and create a propagation map of the AFL. In addition, a low-amplitude high-frequency electrical current emitted from the ablation catheter can be sensed and tracked in 3-D space by the mapping balloon, thus producing a 3-D anatomy by roving the mapping catheter around the right atrial endocardium, on which the propagation map is superimposed. The appropriate ablation target then can be localized and the ablation catheter positioned appropriately and tracked while ablation performed. After ablation, the mapping system can be used to assess for bidirectional CTI conduction block during pacing from the low lateral right atrium and coronary sinus ostium. The

---

Fig. 5. (*A*) A schematic diagram of the expected right atrial activation sequence during pacing in sinus rhythm from the coronary sinus (CS) ostium before (*left panel*) and after (*right panel*) ablation of the CTI. Before ablation the activation pattern during coronary sinus pacing is caudal to cranial in the interatrial septum and low right atrium, with collision of the septal and right atrial wavefronts in the midlateral right atrium. After ablation the activation pattern during coronary sinus pacing still is caudal to cranial in the interatrial septum, but the lateral right atrium now is activated in a strictly cranial to caudal pattern (ie, counterclockwise), indicating complete clockwise conduction block in the CTI. CT, crista terminalis; ER, eustachian ridge; His, His' bundle; IVC, inferior vena cava; SVC, superior vena cava. (*B*) Surface ECG and right atrial endocardial electrograms recorded during pacing in sinus rhythm from the coronary sinus (CS) ostium before (*left panel*) and after (*right panel*) ablation of the CTI. Tracings include surface ECG leads I, aVF, and V1 and endocardial electrograms from the proximal coronary sinus (CSP), His bundle (HIS), tricuspid valve annulus at the 1 o'clock position (HALOP) to the 7 o'clock position (HALOD), and high right atrium (HRA or RFA). Before ablation during coronary sinus pacing, there is collision of the cranial and caudal right atrial wavefronts in the midlateral right atrium (HALO5). After ablation the lateral right atrium is activated in a strictly cranial to caudal pattern (ie, counterclockwise), indicating complete medial to lateral conduction block in the CTI. *Arrows* indicate direction of atrial activation. (*Adapted from* Feld GK, Srivatsa U, Hoppe B. Ablation of isthmus dependent atrial flutters. In: Huang SS, Wood MA, editors. Catheter ablation of cardiac arrhythmias. Philadelphia: Elsevier; 2006. p. 207–8; with permission.)

advantages of the EnSite system include the ability to map the entire AFL activation sequence in one beat, precise anatomic representation of the right atrium (including the CTI and adjacent structures), precise localization of the ablation catheter within the right atrium, and propagation maps of endocardial activation during AFL and pacing after ablation to assess for CTI conduction block. In addition, any ablation catheter system can be used with the EnSite system. The major disadvantage of the EnSite system is the need to use the balloon-mapping catheter, with its large 10-Fr introducer sheath, and the need for full anticoagulation during the mapping procedure.

The CARTO system uses a magnetic sensor in the ablation catheter, a magnetic field generated by a grid placed under the patient, and a reference

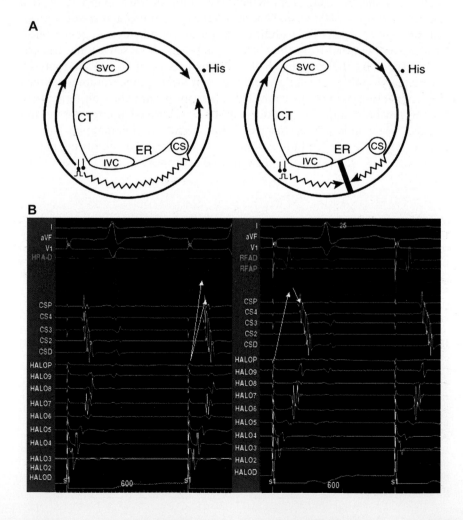

Table 1
Success rates for radiofrequency catheter ablation of atrial flutter

Author/reference	N	Electrode length	% Acute success	Follow-up (months)	% Chronic success
Feld et al [7]	16	4	100	4 ± 2	83
Cosio et al [5]	9	4	100	2–18	56
Kirkorian et al [37]	22	4	86	8 ± 13	84
Fischer et al [36]	80	4	73	20 ± 8	81
Poty et al [46]	12	6/8	100	9 ± 3	92
Schwartzman et al [47]	35	8	100	1–21	92
Chauchemez et al [50]	20	4	100	8 ± 2	80
Tsai et al [43]	50	8	92	10 ± 5	100
Atiga et al [42]	59	4 versus cooled	88	13 ± 4	93
Scavee et al [40]	80	8 versus cooled	80	15	98
Feld et al [31]	169	8 or 10	93	6	97
Calkins et al [51]	150	8	88	6	87
Ventura et al [44]	130	8 versus cooled	100	14 ± 2	98

Acute and chronic success rates are reported as overall results in randomized or comparison studies.

N, number of patients studied; % Acute success, termination of AFL during ablation or demonstration of isthmus block after ablation; % Chronic success, % of patients in whom type 1 AFL did not recur during follow-up.

Adapted from Feld GK, Srivatsa U, Hoppe B. Ablation of isthmus dependent atrial flutters. In: Huang SS, Wood MA, editors. Catheter ablation of cardiac arrhythmias. Philadelphia: Elsevier; 2006. p. 211; with permission.

◀ ───

Fig. 6. (*A*) Schematic diagrams of the expected right atrial activation sequence during pacing in sinus rhythm from the low lateral right atrium before (*left panel*) and after (*right panel*) ablation of the CTI. Before ablation the activation pattern during coronary sinus pacing is caudal to cranial in the right atrial free wall, with collision of the cranial and caudal wavefronts in the mid-septum, with simultaneous activation at the His bundle (HIS) and proximal coronary sinus (CS). After ablation the activation pattern during low lateral right atrial sinus pacing still is caudal to cranial in the right atrial free wall, but the septum now is activated in a strictly cranial to caudal pattern (ie, clockwise), indicating complete lateral to medial conduction block in the CTI. CT, crista terminalis; ER, eustachian ridge; His, His' bundle; IVC, inferior vena cava; SVC, superior vena cava. (*B*) Surface ECG and right atrial endocardial electrograms during pacing in sinus rhythm from the low lateral right atrium before (*left panel*) and after (*right panel*) ablation of the CTI. Tracings include surface ECG leads I, aVF, and V1 and endocardial electrograms from the proximal coronary sinus (CSP), His bundle (HIS), tricuspid valve annulus at the 1 o'clock position (HALOP) to the 7 o'clock position (HALOD), and high right atrium (HRA or RFA). Before ablation during low lateral right atrial pacing, there is collision of the cranial and caudal right atrial wavefronts in the mid-septum (HIS and CSP). After ablation, the septum is activated in a strictly cranial to caudal pattern (ie, clockwise), indicating complete lateral to medial conduction block in the CTI. *Arrows* indicate direction of atrial activation. (*Adapted from* Feld GK, Srivatsa U, Hoppe B. Ablation of isthmus dependent atrial flutters. In: Huang SS, Wood MA, editors. Catheter ablation of cardiac arrhythmias. Philadelphia: Elsevier; 2006. p. 208–9; with permission.)

pad on the skin to track the ablation catheter in 3-D space. The computer system sequentially records anatomic location and electrograms for on-line analysis of activation time and computation of isochronal patterns, which are superimposed on the endocardial geometry (Fig. 7A). A live propagation map also can be produced. The advantages of the CARTO include precise anatomic representation of the right atrium (including the CTI and adjacent structures), precise localization of the ablation catheter within the right atrium, and static activation and propagation maps of endocardial activation that can be constructed during AFL and during pacing after ablation to assess for CTI conduction block (Fig. 7B). The disadvantages of the CARTO system include the need to use the proprietary catheters and ablation generator and the inability to map the entire endocardial activation sequence in one beat.

The 3-D computerized mapping systems, although not required to map and ablate AFL, may be useful particularly in difficult cases, such as those where prior ablation has failed, or in those where complex anatomy may be involved, including idiopathic or postoperative scarring or unoperated or surgically corrected congenital heart disease.

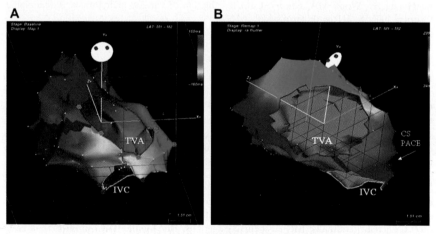

Fig. 7. (*A*) A 3-D electroanatomic (CARTO, Biosense-Webster) map of the right atrium in a patient who had typical AFL before (*A*) and after (*B*) CTI ablation. Note the counterclockwise activation pattern around the tricuspid valve during AFL (*A*), which is based on color scheme indicating activation time from orange (early) to purple (late). (*B*) After ablation of the CTI during pacing from the coronary sinus ostium, there is evidence of medial to lateral isthmus block as indicated by juxtaposition of orange and purple color in the CTI, indicating early and late activation, respectively. A 3-D propagation map also can be produced using the CARTO system, which in some cases allows better visualization of the atrial activation sequence during AFL. CS PACE, pacing from coronary sinus ostium; IVC, inferior vena cava; TVA, tricuspid valve annulus. (*From* Feld GK, Srivatsa U, Hoppe B. Ablation of isthmus dependent atrial flutters. In: Huang SS, Wood MA, editors. Catheter ablation of cardiac arrhythmias. Philadelphia: Elsevier; 2006. p. 213; with permission.)

Alternative energy sources for ablation of type 1 atrial flutter

The development of new energy sources for ablation of cardiac arrhythmias is an ongoing effort because of the disadvantages of radiofrequency energy for ablation, including the risk for coagulum formation, tissue charring, subendocardial steam pops, embolization, failure to achieve transmural ablation, and long procedure and fluoroscopy times required to ablate large areas of myocardium. Many of these disadvantages have been overcome in the case of ablation of type 1 AFL since its first description in 1992. Nonetheless, several clinical and preclinical studies recently have been published on the use of catheter cryoablation and microwave ablation of AFL and other arrhythmias [53–59]. Recent studies demonstrate that catheter cryoablation of type 1 AFL can be achieved with similar results to radiofrequency ablation [53,54,59]. The potential advantages of cryoablation include the lack of pain associated with ablation, the ability to produce a large transmural ablation lesion, and the lack of tissue charring or coagulum formation. Further clinical research is ongoing with respect to the safety and efficacy of catheter cryoablation for fibrillation in the United States (CryoCor, San Diego, California). In addition, early work has begun on the use of a linear microwave ablation catheter system (MedWaves, San Diego, California), with antenna lengths of up to 4 cm [55–58]. These studies show the feasibility of linear microwave ablation for AFL, which may have the advantage of very rapid ablation of the CTI with a single energy application over the entire length of the ablation electrode, less pain associated with ablation, and preservation of the endocardial surface resulting in less risk for thrombus formation [55–58].

Summary

Radiofrequency catheter ablation has become a first-line treatment for type 1 AFL, with nearly uniform acute and chronic success and low complication rates. The most effective approach preferred by most laboratories is combined anatomically and electrophysiologically guided ablation of the CTI, with procedure endpoints of arrhythmia noninducibility and bidirectional CTI conduction block. Currently, the use of a large-tip 8- to 10-mm ablation catheter with a high-output radiofrequency generator (ie, up to 100 W) or a cooled-tip ablation catheter is recommended for optimal success rates. Computerized 3-D activation mapping is an adjunctive method, which, although not mandatory to cure AFL, may have significant advantages in some cases, resulting in overall improved success rates. New alternate energy sources, including cryoablation and microwave ablation, are under investigation with the hope of improving procedure times and success rates further and potentially reducing the risk for complications during AFL ablation.

References

[1] Saoudi N, Cosio F, Waldo A, et al. Classification of atrial flutter and regular atrial tachycardia according to electrophysiologic mechanism and anatomic bases: a statement from a joint expert group from the Working Group of Arrhythmias of the European Society of Cardiology and the North American Society of Pacing and Electrophysiology. J Cardiovasc Electrophysiol 2001;12(7):852–66.

[2] Olshansky B, Okumura K, Hess PG, et al. Demonstration of an area of slow conduction in human atrial flutter. J Am Coll Cardiol 1990;16(7):1639–48.

[3] Lesh MD, Van Hare GF, Epstein LM, et al. Radiofrequency catheter ablation of atrial arrhythmias. Results and mechanisms. Circulation 1994;89(3):1074–89.

[4] Cosio FG, Goicolea A, Lopez-Gil M, et al. Atrial endocardial mapping in the rare form of atrial flutter. Am J Cardiol 1990;66(7):715–20.

[5] Cosio FG, Lopez-Gil M, Goicolea A, et al. Radiofrequency ablation of the inferior vena cava-tricuspid valve isthmus in common atrial flutter. Am J Cardiol 1993;71(8):705–9.

[6] Tai CT, Chen SA, Chiang CE, et al. Electrophysiologic characteristics and radiofrequency catheter ablation in patients with clockwise atrial flutter. J Cardiovasc Electrophysiol 1997;8(1):24–34.

[7] Feld GK, Fleck RP, Chen PS, et al. Radiofrequency catheter ablation for the treatment of human type 1 atrial flutter. Identification of a critical zone in the reentrant circuit by endocardial mapping techniques. Circulation 1992;86(4):1233–40.

[8] Feld GK, Mollerus M, Birgersdotter-Green U, et al. Conduction velocity in the tricuspid valve-inferior vena cava isthmus is slower in patients with type I atrial flutter compared to those without a history of atrial flutter. J Cardiovasc Electrophysiol 1997;8(12):1338–48.

[9] Kinder C, Kall J, Kopp D, et al. Conduction properties of the inferior vena cava-tricuspid annular isthmus in patients with typical atrial flutter. J Cardiovasc Electrophysiol 1997; 8(7):727–37.

[10] Da Costa A, Mourot S, Romeyer-Bouchard C, et al. Anatomic and electrophysiological differences between chronic and paroxysmal forms of common atrial flutter and comparison with controls. Pacing Clin Electrophysiol 2004;27(9):1202–11.

[11] Kalman JM, Olgin JE, Saxon LA, et al. Activation and entrainment mapping defines the tricuspid annulus as the anterior barrier in typical atrial flutter. Circulation 1996;94(3): 398–406.

[12] Olgin JE, Kalman JM, Lesh MD. Conduction barriers in human atrial flutter: correlation of electrophysiology and anatomy. J Cardiovasc Electrophysiol 1996;7(11):1112–26.

[13] Olgin JE, Kalman JM, Fitzpatrick AP, et al. Role of right atrial endocardial structures as barriers to conduction during human type I atrial flutter. Activation and entrainment mapping guided by intracardiac echocardiography. Circulation 1995;92(7):1839–48.

[14] Tai CT, Huang JL, Lee PC, et al. High-resolution mapping around the crista terminalis during typical atrial flutter: new insights into mechanisms. J Cardiovasc Electrophysiol 2004; 15(4):406–14.

[15] Spach MS, Dolber PC, Heidlage JF. Influence of the passive anisotropic properties on directional differences in propagation following modification of the sodium conductance in human atrial muscle. A model of reentry based on anisotropic discontinuous propagation. Circ Res 1988;62(4):811–32.

[16] Spach MS, Miller WT 3rd, Dolber PC, et al. The functional role of structural complexities in the propagation of depolarization in the atrium of the dog. Cardiac conduction disturbances due to discontinuities of effective axial resistivity. Circ Res 1982;50(2):175–91.

[17] Olgin JE, Kalman JM, Saxon LA, et al. Mechanism of initiation of atrial flutter in humans: site of unidirectional block and direction of rotation. J Am Coll Cardiol 1997;29(2):376–84.

[18] Suzuki F, Toshida N, Nawata H, et al. Coronary sinus pacing initiates counterclockwise atrial flutter while pacing from the low lateral right atrium initiates clockwise atrial flutter. Analysis of episodes of direct initiation of atrial flutter. J Electrocardiol 1998;31(4):345–61.

[19] Haissaguerre M, Sanders P, Hocini M, et al. Pulmonary veins in the substrate for atrial fibrillation: the "venous wave" hypothesis. J Am Coll Cardiol 2004;43(12):2290–2.
[20] Sparks PB, Jayaprakash S, Vohra JK, et al. Electrical remodeling of the atria associated with paroxysmal and chronic atrial flutter. Circulation 2000;102(15):1807–13.
[21] Cha Y, Wales A, Wolf P, et al. Electrophysiologic effects of the new class III antiarrhythmic drug dofetilide compared to the class IA antiarrhythmic drug quinidine in experimental canine atrial flutter: role of dispersion of refractoriness in antiarrhythmic efficacy. J Cardiovasc Electrophysiol 1996;7(9):809–27.
[22] Oshikawa N, Watanabe I, Masaki R, et al. Relationship between polarity of the flutter wave in the surface ECG and endocardial atrial activation sequence in patients with typical counterclockwise and clockwise atrial flutter. J Interv Card Electrophysiol 2002;7(3):215–23.
[23] Okumura K, Plumb VJ, Page PL, et al. Atrial activation sequence during atrial flutter in the canine pericarditis model and its effects on the polarity of the flutter wave in the electrocardiogram. J Am Coll Cardiol 1991;17(2):509–18.
[24] Feld GK, Venkatesh N, Singh BN. Pharmacologic conversion and suppression of experimental canine atrial flutter: differing effects of d-sotalol, quinidine, and lidocaine and significance of changes in refractoriness and conduction. Circulation 1986;74(1):197–204.
[25] Feld GK, Nademanee K, Noll E, et al. Oral N-acetylprocainamide compared to quinidine plus digoxin in the chronic suppression of atrial flutter in humans. Cardiovasc Drugs Ther 1989;3(2):191–8.
[26] Feld GK, Venkatesh N, Singh BN. Effects of N-acetylprocainamide and recainam in the pharmacologic conversion and suppression of experimental canine atrial flutter: significance of changes in refractoriness and conduction. J Cardiovasc Pharmacol 1988;11(5):573–80.
[27] Feld GK, Chen PS, Nicod P, et al. Possible atrial proarrhythmic effects of class 1C antiarrhythmic drugs. Am J Cardiol 1990;66(3):378–83.
[28] Kafkas NV, Patsilinakos SP, Mertzanos GA, et al. Conversion efficacy of intravenous ibutilide compared with intravenous amiodarone in patients with recent-onset atrial fibrillation and atrial flutter. Int J Cardiol 2007;118:321–5.
[29] Babaev A, Suma V, Tita C, et al. Recurrence rate of atrial flutter after initial presentation in patients on drug treatment. Am J Cardiol 2003;92(9):1122–4.
[30] Natale A, Newby KH, Pisano E, et al. Prospective randomized comparison of antiarrhythmic therapy versus first-line radiofrequency ablation in patients with atrial flutter. J Am Coll Cardiol 2000;35(7):1898–904.
[31] Feld G, Wharton M, Plumb V, et al. Radiofrequency catheter ablation of type 1 atrial flutter using large-tip 8- or 10-mm electrode catheters and a high-output radiofrequency energy generator: results of a multicenter safety and efficacy study. J Am Coll Cardiol 2004;43(8): 1466–72.
[32] Da Costa A, Thevenin J, Roche F, et al. Results from the Loire-Ardeche-Drome-Isere-Puy-de-Dome (LADIP) trial on atrial flutter, a multicentric prospective randomized study comparing amiodarone and radiofrequency ablation after the first episode of symptomatic atrial flutter. Circulation 2006;114(16):1676–81.
[33] Gilligan DM, Zakaib JS, Fuller I, et al. Long-term outcome of patients after successful radiofrequency ablation for typical atrial flutter. Pacing Clin Electrophysiol 2003;26(1 Pt 1):53–8.
[34] Tai CT, Chen SA, Chiang CE, et al. Long-term outcome of radiofrequency catheter ablation for typical atrial flutter: risk prediction of recurrent arrhythmias. J Cardiovasc Electrophysiol 1998;9(2):115–21.
[35] Scharf C, Veerareddy S, Ozaydin M, et al. Clinical significance of inducible atrial flutter during pulmonary vein isolation in patients with atrial fibrillation. J Am Coll Cardiol 2004;43(11):2057–62.
[36] Fischer B, Haissaguerre M, Garrigues S, et al. Radiofrequency catheter ablation of common atrial flutter in 80 patients. J Am Coll Cardiol 1995;25(6):1365–72.
[37] Kirkorian G, Moncada E, Chevalier P, et al. Radiofrequency ablation of atrial flutter. Efficacy of an anatomically guided approach. Circulation 1994;90(6):2804–14.

[38] Calkins H, Leon AR, Deam AG, et al. Catheter ablation of atrial flutter using radiofrequency energy. Am J Cardiol 1994;73(5):353–6.
[39] Jais P, Haissaguerre M, Shah DC, et al. Successful irrigated-tip catheter ablation of atrial flutter resistant to conventional radiofrequency ablation. Circulation 1998;98(9):835–8.
[40] Scavee C, Jais P, Hsu LF, et al. Prospective randomised comparison of irrigated-tip and large-tip catheter ablation of cavotricuspid isthmus-dependent atrial flutter. Eur Heart J 2004;25(11):963–9.
[41] Calkins H. Catheter ablation of atrial flutter: do outcomes of catheter ablation with "large-tip" versus "cooled-tip" catheters really differ? J Cardiovasc Electrophysiol 2004;15(10):1131–2.
[42] Atiga WL, Worley SJ, Hummel J, et al. Prospective randomized comparison of cooled radiofrequency versus standard radiofrequency energy for ablation of typical atrial flutter. Pacing Clin Electrophysiol 2002;25(8):1172–8.
[43] Tsai CF, Tai CT, Yu WC, et al. Is 8-mm more effective than 4-mm tip electrode catheter for ablation of typical atrial flutter? Circulation 1999;100(7):768–71.
[44] Ventura R, Klemm H, Lutomsky B, et al. Pattern of isthmus conduction recovery using open cooled and solid large-tip catheters for radiofrequency ablation of typical atrial flutter. J Cardiovasc Electrophysiol 2004;15(10):1126–30.
[45] Mangat I, Tschopp DR Jr, Yang Y, et al. Optimizing the detection of bidirectional block across the flutter isthmus for patients with typical isthmus-dependent atrial flutter. Am J Cardiol 2003;91(5):559–64.
[46] Poty H, Saoudi N, Abdel Aziz A, et al. Radiofrequency catheter ablation of type 1 atrial flutter. Prediction of late success by electrophysiological criteria. Circulation 1995;92(6):1389–92.
[47] Schwartzman D, Callans DJ, Gottlieb CD, et al. Conduction block in the inferior vena caval-tricuspid valve isthmus: association with outcome of radiofrequency ablation of type I atrial flutter. J Am Coll Cardiol 1996;28(6):1519–31.
[48] Tada H, Oral H, Sticherling C, et al. Double potentials along the ablation line as a guide to radiofrequency ablation of typical atrial flutter. J Am Coll Cardiol 2001;38(3):750–5.
[49] Tai CT, Haque A, Lin YK, et al. Double potential interval and transisthmus conduction time for prediction of cavotricuspid isthmus block after ablation of typical atrial flutter. J Interv Card Electrophysiol 2002;7(1):77–82.
[50] Cauchemez B, Haissaguerre M, Fischer B, et al. Electrophysiological effects of catheter ablation of inferior vena cava-tricuspid annulus isthmus in common atrial flutter. Circulation 1996;93(2):284–94.
[51] Calkins H, Canby R, Weiss R, et al. Results of catheter ablation of typical atrial flutter. Am J Cardiol 2004;94(4):437–42.
[52] Gronefeld GC, Wegener F, Israel CW, et al. Thromboembolic risk of patients referred for radiofrequency catheter ablation of typical atrial flutter without prior appropriate anticoagulation therapy. Pacing Clin Electrophysiol 2003;26(1 Pt 2):323–7.
[53] Manusama R, Timmermans C, Limon F, et al. Catheter-based cryoablation permanently cures patients with common atrial flutter. Circulation 2004;109(13):1636–9.
[54] Timmermans C, Ayers GM, Crijns HJ, et al. Randomized study comparing radiofrequency ablation with cryoablation for the treatment of atrial flutter with emphasis on pain perception. Circulation 2003;107(9):1250–2.
[55] Adragao P, Parreira L, Morgado F, et al. Microwave ablation of atrial flutter. Pacing Clin Electrophysiol 1999;22(11):1692–5.
[56] Liem LB, Mead RH. Microwave linear ablation of the isthmus between the inferior vena cava and tricuspid annulus. Pacing Clin Electrophysiol 1998;21(11 Pt 1):2079–86.
[57] Iwasa A, Storey J, Yao B, et al. Efficacy of a microwave antenna for ablation of the tricuspid valve–inferior vena cava isthmus in dogs as a treatment for type 1 atrial flutter. J Interv Card Electrophysiol 2004;10(3):191–8.

[58] Chan JY, Fung JW, Yu CM, et al. Preliminary results with percutaneous transcatheter microwave ablation of typical atrial flutter. J Cardiovasc Electrophysiol 2007;18(3):286–9.
[59] Feld GK, Daubert JP, Weiss R, Miles W, et al. for the CAFÉ trial investigators. Acute and chronic efficacy and safety of catheter cryoablation of the cavo-tricuspid isthmus for treatment of atrial flutter. Heart Rhythm 2005;2:S238.

??. ???? ?? ??? ?. ??, ???. ?? ????? ?? ????? ??? ??????? ??? ?????????? ??? ?????? ??????? ?? ???????. ? ?????? ??? ??????? ?? ???. ?
???? ?????. ??????? ?? ????? ?. ????? ??? ???? ??? ?? ???? ??? ?? ?????????? ? ??? ???
?? ?? ????? ??? ?????? ?????????? ??? ????? ?? ??????? ? ?????? ?????? ??? ?? ?? ?????.
? ?????? ???? ??????? ????? ?? ???? ?????? ???.

THE MEDICAL
CLINICS
OF NORTH AMERICA

ELSEVIER
SAUNDERS

Med Clin N Am 92 (2008) 87–99

Postoperative Atrial Fibrillation

Krit Jongnarangsin, MD[a], Hakan Oral, MD[b],*

[a]Division of Cardiovascular Medicine, University of Michigan, Veterans Affairs Ann
Arbor Healthcare System, 2215 Fuller Road, Ann Arbor, MI 48105-2399, USA
[b]Division of Cardiovascular Medicine, University of Michigan, Cardiovascular Center,
Room 2556, 1500 E. Medical Center Drive, Ann Arbor, MI 48109-5853, USA

The incidence of atrial fibrillation (AF) in the general population is estimated to be 0.4% in patients younger than 70 years and 2% to 4% in older
patients [1]. The incidence of AF is higher in patients with cardiovascular
disease. The Cardiovascular Health Study demonstrated that the prevalence
of AF was 9.1%, 4.6%, and 1.6% in patients with clinical, subclinical, and
no cardiovascular disease, respectively [2]. Atrial arrhythmias occur frequently after major cardiothoracic surgery and result in increased morbidity
and length of hospital stay [3–6]. The prevalence of atrial arrhythmias after
cardiac surgery has been reported to range from 10% to 65% [4,7–27]
depending on the type and technique of surgery, patient characteristics,
method of arrhythmia surveillance, and definition of arrhythmia. Postoperative AF may occur in as many as 40% of patients undergoing coronary
artery bypass surgery (CABG) [28–31], in 35% to 40% after valvular surgery [13,28,32], in 60% after combined CABG and valve surgery, and in
11% to 24% after cardiac transplantation [13,33]. In a large, multicenter,
international cohort study, most initial episodes of AF occurred within
the first few (2–5) days after CABG surgery [29].

Pathogenesis

The electrophysiologic mechanisms of AF after cardiac surgery are not
well understood. A pre-existing atrial substrate, such as atrial fibrosis or
dilatation, may predispose to AF [34]. Perioperative factors such as atrial
injury or ischemia, inflammation, an increase in adrenergic tone, catechol-
amines, atrial stretch from volume overload, or electrolyte disturbances

---

* Corresponding author.
E-mail address: oralh@umich.edu (H. Oral).

0025-7125/08/$ - see front matter © 2008 Elsevier Inc. All rights reserved.
doi:10.1016/j.mcna.2007.09.004   *medical.theclinics.com*

may trigger postoperative AF in patients who are susceptible through the dispersion of atrial refractoriness [35,36], nonuniform atrial conduction [37], or increased premature atrial complexes [38].

The expression of proinflammatory cytokines and the activation of oxidases with an increase in oxidative stress have also been implicated in the genesis of postoperative AF [39–46]. Oxidative stress may decrease the atrial effective refractory period and may also promote progressive fibrosis [47]. Consistent with these mechanisms, steroids and statins have been shown to attenuate profibrillatory effects of oxidative stress [48,49].

Clinical implications

Postoperative AF is associated with an increased incidence of postoperative complications and longer length of hospital stay [7,8,13,29,30]. Patients with postoperative AF are more likely to sustain hypotension, pulmonary edema [19], and cerebrovascular accidents [7,8,13,50,51]. The incidence of stroke is significantly higher in patients in whom AF develops after cardiac surgery (3.3% versus 1.4%) [13]. The incidence of a composite outcome including encephalopathy, a decline in Mini-Mental State Examination score, an increase in the National Institutes of Health Stroke Scale score, renal dysfunction, renal failure, pneumonia, mediastinitis or deep sternal wound infection, sepsis, harvest site infection, vascular catheter infection, and genitourinary infection is also higher in patients with postoperative AF (22.6% versus 15.4%) [29]. The cost of care for patients in whom postoperative AF develops is increased by approximately $10,000 per patient [30].

Postoperative AF is also associated with a lower in-hospital and long-term survival. A retrospective cohort study found that patients who experienced AF after CABG surgery had higher in-hospital mortality (odds ratio [OR], 1.7; $P = .0001$) and a decrease in survival at 4 to 5 years (74% versus 87%, $P < .0001$) [30].

Predictors of atrial fibrillation after cardiac surgery

Several clinical factors have been shown to be associated with an increased incidence of AF following cardiac surgery [28,29]. These factors include age, gender, hypertension, a prior history of AF, obesity, chronic obstructive pulmonary disease, left atrial size, and left ventricular ejection fraction [52].

Older age has consistently been shown in multiple studies to be a predictor for postoperative AF. Every 10-year increase in age is associated with a 75% increase in the odds of developing AF, and an age greater than 70 years old alone is considered to be a high risk factor [29]. The increase in postoperative AF in older age is most likely related to degenerative changes in atrial myocardium, dilatation, and nonuniform anisotropic conduction [53].

Men are more likely than women to experience AF after CABG surgery [7–9,21,27]. A previous history of AF also increases the risk of postoperative AF [4,11]. Hypertension is a predictor of AF in the general population as well as after cardiac surgery [7,8]. Higher body mass index has been shown to be an independent predictor for new-onset AF after cardiac surgery [52]. There is a strong correlation between body mass index and left atrial enlargement [54–56]. Patients with chronic obstructive pulmonary disease have been reported to have a 43% increase in the probability of developing postoperative AF [29], most likely owing to an increase in P-wave dispersion and heterogeneity of conduction [57].

Prevention

The incidence of AF after cardiac surgery is high, especially in patients with the multiple risk factors described previously. Although it is often transient, postoperative AF often is associated with increased morbidity and prolonged ICU and hospital stay; therefore, prophylactic therapy should be considered in all patients, particularly those at high risk, who are considered for cardiac surgery. Pharmacologic therapy and cardiac pacing have been evaluated in several trials.

Pharmacologic prophylaxis

β-adrenergic receptor antagonists

β-adrenergic receptor antagonists alone or combined with other antiarrhythmic drugs, such as digitalis or calcium channel blockers, have been commonly used to prevent postoperative AF. Beta-blockers attenuate the effects of beta-adrenergic stimulation, which facilitates vulnerability to AF after cardiac surgery. The efficacy of beta-blockers in reducing the incidence of postoperative AF has been demonstrated in several trials; therefore, beta-blockers should be administered perioperatively in patients without contraindications as the standard therapy to reduce the incidence of AF after CABG [58].

Sotalol

Sotalol, a combined β-receptor and potassium channel–blocking agent, has been shown to decrease postoperative AF by 41% to 93% in comparison with placebo [59–66]. Although sotalol was well tolerated, ventricular arrhythmias were reported in two patients among the six trials [60,61,63–66]. It is not clear whether sotalol provides an incremental antiarrhythmic effect for postoperative AF prophylaxis when compared with regular beta-blockers. Sotalol is considered a class IIb indication for postoperative arrhythmia prevention in the American College of Cardiology/American Heart Association (ACC/AHA) 2004 guidelines for CABG surgery, and low-dose sotalol should be considered in patients who are not candidates for traditional beta-blockers [58].

Amiodarone

Amiodarone is a class III antiarrhythmic agent that inhibits multiple ion channels and α- and β-adrenergic receptors. The efficacy of amiodarone in preventing postoperative AF has been evaluated in multiple randomized trials using various regimens. Overall, it has been shown that amiodarone significantly reduces the incidence of postoperative AF regardless of whether it is administered orally [67–71], intravenously [72–75], or both [76–79]. A meta-analysis of 10 trials confirmed that amiodarone therapy was associated with a significant reduction in the incidence of postoperative AF or atrial flutter (relative risk, 0.64; 95% CI, 0.55 to 0.75) [80].

In the largest double-blind, randomized, controlled trial of prophylactic oral amiodarone for the prevention of arrhythmias (PAPABEAR) [70], postoperative atrial tachyarrhythmias were reduced by 48% in patients who received oral amiodarone (10 mg/kg daily) 6 days before surgery through 6 days after surgery in a comparison with placebo. A reduction in postoperative AF was also observed across subgroups predefined according to age, type of cardiac surgery, and concomitant beta-blocker therapy. Although oral amiodarone has been shown to be effective in postoperative AF prophylaxis, it should be administered several days before surgery. A single-day loading dose of oral amiodarone given 1 day before cardiac surgery has been shown to be ineffective in preventing postoperative AF [81]. An intravenous formulation acts more rapidly than an oral preparation. The Amiodarone Reduction in Coronary Heart (ARCH) trial [73] demonstrated that low-dose intravenous amiodarone (1 g/d for 2 days) administered immediately after cardiac surgery was safe and effective in reducing the incidence of postoperative AF.

The efficacy of amiodarone in preventing postoperative AF was shown to be similar to that of beta-blockers in the meta-analysis of prophylactic therapies against postoperative AF [82]. Side effects of amiodarone therapy were uncommon in clinical trials. Amiodarone was discontinued mainly due to bradycardia. Amiodarone is considered a class IIa indication in the ACC/ AHA 2004 guidelines for CABG surgery. Preoperative administration of amiodarone is an appropriate prophylactic therapy for patients at high risk for postoperative AF who have contraindications to therapy with beta-blockers [58].

Calcium channel antagonists

Prior studies have demonstrated that verapamil does not have a significant effect on the incidence of postoperative AF [15,23,24,83]. A meta-analysis of randomized control trials also confirmed that verapamil does not reduce the probability of developing supraventricular arrhythmias after CABG (OR, 0.91; 95% CI, 0.57–1.46) [84]. Similar to verapamil, diltiazem was not effective in preventing postoperative AF when compared with placebo [85]; therefore, nondihydropyridine calcium channel blockers are considered a class IIa indication primarily for ventricular rate control during

AF. Calcium channel blockers have no role in the prophylaxis of postoperative AF [58].

Digitalis

The efficacy of digitalis for postoperative AF prophylaxis has been previously evaluated in randomized control trials. The results have been conflicting regarding the potential benefits of digitalis for postoperative AF prophylaxis. Two meta-analyses [84,86] showed no significant reduction in the incidence of supraventricular arrhythmias after CABG in patients receiving digitalis in a comparison with controls. Nevertheless, digitalis may be helpful when administered with beta-blockers. Similar to calcium channel blockers, digitalis has a class IIa indication primarily for ventricular rate control. There is no indication for using digitalis for the prevention of postoperative AF.

Magnesium

Hypomagnesemia is common after cardiac surgery and may predispose patients to postoperative arrhythmias. The efficacy of prophylactic magnesium administration on postoperative arrhythmias has been evaluated; however, the results have been variable. A meta-analysis of randomized controlled trials suggested that prophylactic treatment with magnesium reduces postoperative supraventricular arrhythmias by 23% (AF by 29%) [87]. Because of conflicting results, prophylactic magnesium therapy is not routinely recommended; however, serum magnesium levels should be maintained in patients undergoing cardiac surgery [88].

Statins

Statin therapy has been shown to reduce the incidence of postoperative AF after noncardiac thoracic [89] and CABG surgery [90]. Statin therapy was associated with a reduction of postoperative AF regardless of C-reactive protein levels. A recent randomized controlled trial demonstrated that atorvastatin (40 mg/d) starting 7 days before cardiac surgery significantly reduced the incidence of postoperative AF in comparison with placebo (OR, 0.39; 95% CI, 0.18–0.85) [91]. Because the benefits of statins in addition to the prevention of postoperative AF have been well established in patients with coronary artery disease, all patients without contraindications for statin therapy should receive it before CABG surgery.

Corticosteroids

Corticosteroid treatment has been shown to reduce the incidence of postoperative AF after cardiac surgery in previous randomized controlled trials [92,93]. A prospective, double-blind, randomized multicenter study found that intravenous hydrocortisone reduced the relative risk of postoperative AF by 37% when compared with placebo. Corticosteroids may decrease the incidence of postoperative AF by reducing the inflammatory response after surgery. No significant adverse events related to corticosteroid treatment were reported in these trials [92,94].

Atrial pacing

The efficacy of temporary atrial overdrive pacing on postoperative AF prevention has been evaluated in several studies. The algorithm and site of pacing varied among these studies. Although the results of postoperative AF reduction with right atrial pacing are conflicting [95–101], most studies have shown no significant reduction in postoperative AF [96–100]. In contrast, bi-atrial overdrive pacing has been shown to be effective in preventing postoperative AF [99,100,102]. Postoperative atrial pacing at Bachmann's bundle was also evaluated in a prior study [101]. Although pacing at Bachmann's bundle was associated with better thresholds, it did not reduce the incidence of postoperative AF.

Therapy

Although prophylactic therapy can reduce the incidence of postoperative AF, some patients will still experience AF after cardiac surgery. Spontaneous conversion of AF may occur within 2 hours in 15% to 30% of patients and within 24 hours in 25% to 80% of patients. If AF persists or recurs, two therapeutic strategies of rate and rhythm control may be considered.

Rate control

Rate control is a reasonable option in patients who are asymptomatic and hemodynamically stable. A prior study has shown that patients with postoperative AF can be safely discharged home in AF after the ventricular rate has been controlled and anticoagulation initiated [103]. Medications that slow atrioventricular nodal conduction such as beta-blockers, nondihydropyridine calcium channel blockers (verapamil or diltiazem), or digoxin can be used for rate control; however, beta-blockers seem to be the most effective agent for patients with postoperative AF with a rapid ventricular response because of augmented postoperative sympathetic tone. Digoxin alone may control ventricular rate at rest but rarely is adequate when sympathetic tone is high in the postoperative period. Combined therapy may be required to achieve adequate heart rate control. In patients who cannot tolerate beta-blockers or calcium channel blockers, intravenous amiodarone is an alternative option for ventricular rate control [104]. Because amiodarone has sympatholytic and calcium channel blocker action, it is effective in slowing atrioventricular nodal conduction in patients with AF and rapid ventricular response rates.

Rhythm control

Rhythm control is preferred in patients who are highly symptomatic or hemodynamically unstable or when anticoagulation is contraindicated.

Sinus rhythm can be restored by electrical or pharmacologic cardioversion. Direct current cardioversion should be considered in patients who are hemodynamically unstable owing to hypotension or heart failure. In patients with unsuccessful electrical cardioversion or early recurrence of AF, direct current cardioversion may be repeated after administration of antiarrhythmic drugs such as ibutilide [105] or amiodarone. Electrical cardioversion using a rectilinear biphasic waveform is more effective than a monophasic sinusoidal waveform [106].

Pharmacologic conversion can be achieved by class IA (quinidine, procainamide, and disopyramide), class IC (flecainide and propafenone), and class III (amiodarone, sotalol, ibulitide, and dofetilide) agents. Although intravenous administration of class IA and IC agents in patients with AF after CABG surgery results in conversion to sinus rhythm in 40% to 75% of patients within 1 hour [107–110] and in 50% to 90% of patients within 12 hours [16,111–114], class IA agents are not available in the United States and can be proarrhythmic in patients with ischemia or impaired left ventricular systolic function. The efficacy of intravenous class III agents for the acute conversion of postoperative AF seems comparable to that of class IA and IC drugs; however, amiodarone is more preferable than the other antiarrhythmic drugs because it also provides ventricular rate control and is less proarrhythmic, particularly in patients with a reduced ejection fraction.

Anticoagulation

AF is associated with a higher risk of thromboembolic events. There are no specific guidelines for antithrombotic therapy in patients with postoperative AF. Antithrombotic therapy is recommended for all patients with AF that persists more than 48 hours to prevent thromboembolic events [34]. The type and intensity of antithrombotic therapy is based on the risk of thromboembolism. Warfarin with a target international normalized ratio of 2.0 to 3.0 is recommended for patients with prior thromboembolism or more than one moderate risk factor (age > 75 years, hypertension, heart failure, impaired left ventricular systolic function, and diabetes mellitus). Aspirin, 81 to 325 mg daily, is recommended as an alternative to warfarin in low-risk patients or in those with contraindications to warfarin. Routine anticoagulation with heparin to prevent thrombus formation in patients with postoperative AF is generally not advised because of the risk for postoperative bleeding [28]. Although the incidence of large pericardial effusions and cardiac tamponade was found to be higher in patients receiving warfarin [115,116], it still can be administered in the immediate post-CABG period with only a minimal risk for bleeding [116] in the majority of the patients.

Summary

AF is a common arrhythmia that occurs after cardiac surgery. It is associated with an increase in morbidity, length of hospital stay, and mortality.

Patients who are at higher risk of postoperative AF should receive prophylactic treatment. AF usually resolves spontaneously after heart rate is controlled; however, if patients are highly symptomatic or hemodynamically unstable, sinus rhythm should be restored by electrical or pharmacologic cardioversion. Patients with AF of more than 48 hours should receive antithrombotic therapy for thromboembolism prevention.

References

[1] Alpert JS, Petersen P, Godtfredsen J. Atrial fibrillation: natural history, complications, and management. Annu Rev Med 1988;39:41–52.

[2] Furberg CD, Psaty BM, Manolio TA, et al. Prevalence of atrial fibrillation in elderly subjects (the Cardiovascular Health Study). Am J Cardiol 1994;74:236–41.

[3] Hravnak M, Hoffman LA, Saul MI, et al. Predictors and impact of atrial fibrillation after isolated coronary artery bypass grafting. Crit Care Med 2002;30:330–7.

[4] Mathew JP, Parks R, Savino JS, et al. Atrial fibrillation following coronary artery bypass graft surgery: predictors, outcomes, and resource utilization: Multicenter Study of Perioperative Ischemia Research Group. JAMA 1996;276:300–6.

[5] Borzak S, Tisdale JE, Amin NB, et al. Atrial fibrillation after bypass surgery: does the arrhythmia or the characteristics of the patients prolong hospital stay? Chest 1998;113: 1489–91.

[6] Nickerson NJ, Murphy SF, Davila-Roman VG, et al. Obstacles to early discharge after cardiac surgery. Am J Manag Care 1999;5:29–34.

[7] Aranki SF, Shaw DP, Adams DH, et al. Predictors of atrial fibrillation after coronary artery surgery: current trends and impact on hospital resources. Circulation 1996;94:390–7.

[8] Almassi GH, Schowalter T, Nicolosi AC, et al. Atrial fibrillation after cardiac surgery: a major morbid event? Ann Surg 1997;226:501–11 [discussion: 511–3].

[9] Mendes LA, Connelly GP, McKenney PA, et al. Right coronary artery stenosis: an independent predictor of atrial fibrillation after coronary artery bypass surgery. J Am Coll Cardiol 1995;25:198–202.

[10] Crosby LH, Pifalo WB, Woll KR, et al. Risk factors for atrial fibrillation after coronary artery bypass grafting. Am J Cardiol 1990;66:1520–2.

[11] Hashimoto K, Ilstrup DM, Schaff HV. Influence of clinical and hemodynamic variables on risk of supraventricular tachycardia after coronary artery bypass. J Thorac Cardiovasc Surg 1991;101:56–65.

[12] Leitch JW, Thomson D, Baird DK, et al. The importance of age as a predictor of atrial fibrillation and flutter after coronary artery bypass grafting. J Thorac Cardiovasc Surg 1990; 100:338–42.

[13] Creswell LL, Schuessler RB, Rosenbloom M, et al. Hazards of postoperative atrial arrhythmias. Ann Thorac Surg 1993;56:539–49.

[14] Kalman JM, Munawar M, Howes LG, et al. Atrial fibrillation after coronary artery bypass grafting is associated with sympathetic activation. Ann Thorac Surg 1995;60:1709–15.

[15] Ferraris VA, Ferraris SP, Gilliam H, et al. Verapamil prophylaxis for postoperative atrial dysrhythmias: a prospective, randomized, double-blind study using drug level monitoring. Ann Thorac Surg 1987;43:530–3.

[16] Gavaghan TP, Feneley MP, Campbell TJ, et al. Atrial tachyarrhythmias after cardiac surgery: results of disopyramide therapy. Aust N Z J Med 1985;15:27–32.

[17] Caretta Q, Mercanti CA, De Nardo D, et al. Ventricular conduction defects and atrial fibrillation after coronary artery bypass grafting: multivariate analysis of preoperative, intraoperative and postoperative variables. Eur Heart J 1991;12:1107–11.

[18] Frost L, Molgaard H, Christiansen EH, et al. Atrial ectopic activity and atrial fibrillation/flutter after coronary artery bypass surgery: a case-base study controlling for confounding from age, beta-blocker treatment, and time distance from operation. Int J Cardiol 1995;50: 153–62.

[19] Yousif H, Davies G, Oakley CM. Perioperative supraventricular arrhythmias in coronary bypass surgery. Int J Cardiol 1990;26:313–8.

[20] Rubin DA, Nieminski KE, Reed GE, et al. Predictors, prevention, and long-term prognosis of atrial fibrillation after coronary artery bypass graft operations. J Thorac Cardiovasc Surg 1987;94:331–5.

[21] Fuller JA, Adams GG, Buxton B. Atrial fibrillation after coronary artery bypass grafting. Is it a disorder of the elderly? J Thorac Cardiovasc Surg 1989;97:821–5.

[22] Roffman JA, Fieldman A. Digoxin and propranolol in the prophylaxis of supraventricular tachydysrhythmias after coronary artery bypass surgery. Ann Thorac Surg 1981;31:496–501.

[23] Williams DB, Misbach GA, Kruse AP, et al. Oral verapamil for prophylaxis of supraventricular tachycardia after myocardial revascularization: a randomized trial. J Thorac Cardiovasc Surg 1985;90:592–6.

[24] Davison R, Hartz R, Kaplan K, et al. Prophylaxis of supraventricular tachyarrhythmia after coronary bypass surgery with oral verapamil: a randomized, double-blind trial. Ann Thorac Surg 1985;39:336–9.

[25] Tyras DH, Stothert JC Jr, Kaiser GC, et al. Supraventricular tachyarrhythmias after myocardial revascularization: a randomized trial of prophylactic digitalization. J Thorac Cardiovasc Surg 1979;77:310–4.

[26] Ommen SR, Odell JA, Stanton MS. Atrial arrhythmias after cardiothoracic surgery. N Engl J Med 1997;336:1429–34.

[27] Zaman AG, Archbold RA, Helft G, et al. Atrial fibrillation after coronary artery bypass surgery: a model for preoperative risk stratification. Circulation 2000;101:1403–8.

[28] Maisel WH, Rawn JD, Stevenson WG. Atrial fibrillation after cardiac surgery. Ann Intern Med 2001;135:1061–73.

[29] Mathew JP, Fontes ML, Tudor IC, et al. A multicenter risk index for atrial fibrillation after cardiac surgery. JAMA 2004;291:1720–9.

[30] Villareal RP, Hariharan R, Liu BC, et al. Postoperative atrial fibrillation and mortality after coronary artery bypass surgery. J Am Coll Cardiol 2004;43:742–8.

[31] Lauer MS, Eagle KA, Buckley MJ, et al. Atrial fibrillation following coronary artery bypass surgery. Prog Cardiovasc Dis 1989;31:367–78.

[32] Asher CR, Miller DP, Grimm RA, et al. Analysis of risk factors for development of atrial fibrillation early after cardiac valvular surgery. Am J Cardiol 1998;82:892–5.

[33] Pavri BB, O'Nunain SS, Newell JB, et al. Prevalence and prognostic significance of atrial arrhythmias after orthotopic cardiac transplantation. J Am Coll Cardiol 1995;25:1673–80.

[34] Fuster V, Ryden LE, Cannom DS, et al. ACC/AHA/ESC 2006 Guidelines for the Management of Patients with Atrial Fibrillation: a report of the American College of Cardiology/American Heart Association Task Force on Practice Guidelines and the European Society of Cardiology Committee for Practice Guidelines (Writing Committee to Revise the 2001 Guidelines for the Management of Patients With Atrial Fibrillation): developed in collaboration with the European Heart Rhythm Association and the Heart Rhythm Society. Circulation 2006;114:e257–354.

[35] Cox JL. A perspective of postoperative atrial fibrillation in cardiac operations. Ann Thorac Surg 1993;56:405–9.

[36] Sato S, Yamauchi S, Schuessler RB, et al. The effect of augmented atrial hypothermia on atrial refractory period, conduction, and atrial flutter/fibrillation in the canine heart. J Thorac Cardiovasc Surg 1992;104:297–306.

[37] Tsikouris JP, Kluger J, Song J, et al. Changes in P-wave dispersion and P-wave duration after open heart surgery are associated with the peak incidence of atrial fibrillation. Heart Lung 2001;30:466–71.

[38] Frost L, Christiansen EH, Molgaard H, et al. Premature atrial beat eliciting atrial fibrilla-
     tion after coronary artery bypass grafting. J Electrocardiol 1995;28:297–305.
[39] Kim YM, Guzik TJ, Zhang YH, et al. A myocardial Nox2 containing NAD(P)H oxidase
     contributes to oxidative stress in human atrial fibrillation. Circ Res 2005;97:629–36.
[40] Clermont G, Vergely C, Jazayeri S, et al. Systemic free radical activation is a major event
     involved in myocardial oxidative stress related to cardiopulmonary bypass. Anesthesiology
     2002;96:80–7.
[41] Levy JH, Tanaka KA. Inflammatory response to cardiopulmonary bypass. Ann Thorac
     Surg 2003;75:S715–20.
[42] Ochoa JJ, Vilchez MJ, Ibanez S, et al. Oxidative stress is evident in erythrocytes as well as
     plasma in patients undergoing heart surgery involving cardiopulmonary bypass. Free
     Radic Res 2003;37:11–7.
[43] Gaudino M, Andreotti F, Zamparelli R, et al. The -174G/C interleukin-6 polymorphism
     influences postoperative interleukin-6 levels and postoperative atrial fibrillation. Is atrial
     fibrillation an inflammatory complication? Circulation 2003;108(Suppl 1):II195–9.
[44] Mihm MJ, Yu F, Carnes CA, et al. Impaired myofibrillar energetics and oxidative injury
     during human atrial fibrillation. Circulation 2001;104:174–80.
[45] Carnes CA, Chung MK, Nakayama T, et al. Ascorbate attenuates atrial pacing-induced
     peroxynitrite formation and electrical remodeling and decreases the incidence of postoper-
     ative atrial fibrillation. Circ Res 2001;89:E32–8.
[46] Allessie M, Ausma J, Schotten U. Electrical, contractile and structural remodeling during
     atrial fibrillation. Cardiovasc Res 2002;54:230–46.
[47] Griendling KK, Sorescu D, Ushio-Fukai M. NAD(P)H oxidase: role in cardiovascular bi-
     ology and disease. Circ Res 2000;86:494–501.
[48] Shiroshita-Takeshita A, Schram G, Lavoie J, et al. Effect of simvastatin and antioxidant
     vitamins on atrial fibrillation promotion by atrial-tachycardia remodeling in dogs. Circula-
     tion 2004;110:2313–9.
[49] Shiroshita-Takeshita A, Brundel BJ, Lavoie J, et al. Prednisone prevents atrial fibrillation
     promotion by atrial tachycardia remodeling in dogs. Cardiovasc Res 2006;69:865–75.
[50] Reed GL 3rd, Singer DE, Picard EH, et al. Stroke following coronary-artery bypass surgery:
     a case-control estimate of the risk from carotid bruits. N Engl J Med 1988;319:1246–50.
[51] Taylor GJ, Malik SA, Colliver JA, et al. Usefulness of atrial fibrillation as a predictor of
     stroke after isolated coronary artery bypass grafting. Am J Cardiol 1987;60:905–7.
[52] Zacharias A, Schwann TA, Riordan CJ, et al. Obesity and risk of new-onset atrial fibrilla-
     tion after cardiac surgery. Circulation 2005;112:3247–55.
[53] Spach MS, Dolber PC. Relating extracellular potentials and their derivatives to anisotropic
     propagation at a microscopic level in human cardiac muscle: evidence for electrical uncou-
     pling of side-to-side fiber connections with increasing age. Circ Res 1986;58:356–71.
[54] Pritchett AM, Jacobsen SJ, Mahoney DW, et al. Left atrial volume as an index of left atrial
     size: a population-based study. J Am Coll Cardiol 2003;41:1036–43.
[55] Vaziri SM, Larson MG, Lauer MS, et al. Influence of blood pressure on left atrial size: the
     Framingham Heart Study. Hypertension 1995;25:1155–60.
[56] Gerdts E, Oikarinen L, Palmieri V, et al. Correlates of left atrial size in hypertensive patients
     with left ventricular hypertrophy: the Losartan Intervention For Endpoint Reduction in
     Hypertension (LIFE) Study. Hypertension 2002;39:739–43.
[57] Tukek T, Yildiz P, Akkaya V, et al. Factors associated with the development of atrial fibril-
     lation in COPD patients: the role of P-wave dispersion. Ann Noninvasive Electrocardiol
     2002;7:222–7.
[58] Eagle KA, Guyton RA, Davidoff R, et al. ACC/AHA 2004 guideline update for coronary
     artery bypass graft surgery: summary article. A report of the American College of Cardiol-
     ogy/American Heart Association Task Force on Practice Guidelines (Committee to Update
     the 1999 Guidelines for Coronary Artery Bypass Graft Surgery). J Am Coll Cardiol 2004;
     44:e213–310.

[59] Evrard P, Gonzalez M, Jamart J, et al. Prophylaxis of supraventricular and ventricular arrhythmias after coronary artery bypass grafting with low-dose sotalol. Ann Thorac Surg 2000;70:151–6.

[60] Gomes JA, Ip J, Santoni-Rugiu F, et al. Oral d,l sotalol reduces the incidence of postoperative atrial fibrillation in coronary artery bypass surgery patients: a randomized, double-blind, placebo-controlled study. J Am Coll Cardiol 1999;34:334–9.

[61] Jacquet L, Evenepoel M, Marenne F, et al. Hemodynamic effects and safety of sotalol in the prevention of supraventricular arrhythmias after coronary artery bypass surgery. J Cardiothorac Vasc Anesth 1994;8:431–6.

[62] Janssen J, Loomans L, Harink J, et al. Prevention and treatment of supraventricular tachycardia shortly after coronary artery bypass grafting: a randomized open trial. Angiology 1986;37:601–9.

[63] Matsuura K, Takahara Y, Sudo Y, et al. Effect of sotalol in the prevention of atrial fibrillation following coronary artery bypass grafting. Jpn J Thorac Cardiovasc Surg 2001;49: 614–7.

[64] Pfisterer ME, Kloter-Weber UC, Huber M, et al. Prevention of supraventricular tachyarrhythmias after open heart operation by low-dose sotalol: a prospective, double-blind, randomized, placebo-controlled study. Ann Thorac Surg 1997;64:1113–9.

[65] Suttorp MJ, Kingma JH, Peels HO, et al. Effectiveness of sotalol in preventing supraventricular tachyarrhythmias shortly after coronary artery bypass grafting. Am J Cardiol 1991;68:1163–9.

[66] Weber UK, Osswald S, Buser P, et al. Significance of supraventricular tachyarrhythmias after coronary artery bypass graft surgery and their prevention by low-dose sotalol: a prospective double-blind randomized placebo-controlled study. J Cardiovasc Pharmacol Ther 1998;3:209–16.

[67] Giri S, White CM, Dunn AB, et al. Oral amiodarone for prevention of atrial fibrillation after open heart surgery, the Atrial Fibrillation Suppression Trial (AFIST): a randomised placebo-controlled trial. Lancet 2001;357:830–6.

[68] Daoud EG, Strickberger SA, Man KC, et al. Preoperative amiodarone as prophylaxis against atrial fibrillation after heart surgery. N Engl J Med 1997;337:1785–91.

[69] White CM, Giri S, Tsikouris JP, et al. A comparison of two individual amiodarone regimens to placebo in open heart surgery patients. Ann Thorac Surg 2002;74:69–74.

[70] Mitchell LB, Exner DV, Wyse DG, et al. Prophylactic Oral Amiodarone for the Prevention of Arrhythmias that Begin Early After Revascularization, Valve Replacement, or Repair: PAPABEAR. A randomized controlled trial. JAMA 2005;294:3093–100.

[71] Yazigi A, Rahbani P, Zeid HA, et al. Postoperative oral amiodarone as prophylaxis against atrial fibrillation after coronary artery surgery. J Cardiothorac Vasc Anesth 2002;16:603–6.

[72] Lee SH, Chang CM, Lu MJ, et al. Intravenous amiodarone for prevention of atrial fibrillation after coronary artery bypass grafting. Ann Thorac Surg 2000;70:157–61.

[73] Guarnieri T, Nolan S, Gottlieb SO, et al. Intravenous amiodarone for the prevention of atrial fibrillation after open heart surgery: the Amiodarone Reduction in Coronary Heart (ARCH) trial. J Am Coll Cardiol 1999;34:343–7.

[74] Hohnloser SH, Meinertz T, Dammbacher T, et al. Electrocardiographic and antiarrhythmic effects of intravenous amiodarone: results of a prospective, placebo-controlled study. Am Heart J 1991;121:89–95.

[75] Treggiari-Venzi MM, Waeber JL, Perneger TV, et al. Intravenous amiodarone or magnesium sulphate is not cost-beneficial prophylaxis for atrial fibrillation after coronary artery bypass surgery. Br J Anaesth 2000;85:690–5.

[76] White CM, Caron MF, Kalus JS, et al. Intravenous plus oral amiodarone, atrial septal pacing, or both strategies to prevent post-cardiothoracic surgery atrial fibrillation: the Atrial Fibrillation Suppression Trial II (AFIST II). Circulation 2003;108(Suppl 1):II200–6.

[77] Yagdi T, Nalbantgil S, Ayik F, et al. Amiodarone reduces the incidence of atrial fibrillation after coronary artery bypass grafting. J Thorac Cardiovasc Surg 2003;125:1420–5.

[78] Tokmakoglu H, Kandemir O, Gunaydin S, et al. Amiodarone versus digoxin and metopro-lol combination for the prevention of postcoronary bypass atrial fibrillation. Eur J Cardi-othorac Surg 2002;21:401–5.

[79] Butler J, Harriss DR, Sinclair M, et al. Amiodarone prophylaxis for tachycardias after cor-onary artery surgery: a randomised, double blind, placebo controlled trial. Br Heart J 1993; 70:56–60.

[80] Aasbo JD, Lawrence AT, Krishnan K, et al. Amiodarone prophylaxis reduces major car-diovascular morbidity and length of stay after cardiac surgery: a meta-analysis. Ann Intern Med 2005;143:327–36.

[81] Maras D, Boskovic SD, Popovic Z, et al. Single-day loading dose of oral amiodarone for the prevention of new-onset atrial fibrillation after coronary artery bypass surgery. Am Heart J 2001;141:E8.

[82] Crystal E, Connolly SJ, Sleik K, et al. Interventions on prevention of postoperative atrial fibrillation in patients undergoing heart surgery: a meta-analysis. Circulation 2002;106: 75–80.

[83] Smith EE, Shore DF, Monro JL, et al. Oral verapamil fails to prevent supraventricular tachycardia following coronary artery surgery. Int J Cardiol 1985;9:37–44.

[84] Andrews TC, Reimold SC, Berlin JA, et al. Prevention of supraventricular arrhythmias af-ter coronary artery bypass surgery: a meta-analysis of randomized control trials. Circula-tion 1991;84:III236–44.

[85] Babin-Ebell J, Keith PR, Elert O. Efficacy and safety of low-dose propranolol versus diltia-zem in the prophylaxis of supraventricular tachyarrhythmia after coronary artery bypass grafting. Eur J Cardiothorac Surg 1996;10:412–6.

[86] Kowey PR, Taylor JE, Rials SJ, et al. Meta-analysis of the effectiveness of prophylactic drug therapy in preventing supraventricular arrhythmia early after coronary artery bypass grafting. Am J Cardiol 1992;69:963–5.

[87] Shiga T, Wajima Z, Inoue T, et al. Magnesium prophylaxis for arrhythmias after cardiac surgery: a meta-analysis of randomized controlled trials. Am J Med 2004;117:325–33.

[88] Bradley D, Creswell LL, Hogue CW Jr, et al. Pharmacologic prophylaxis: American Col-lege of Chest Physicians guidelines for the prevention and management of postoperative atrial fibrillation after cardiac surgery. Chest 2005;128:39S–47S.

[89] Amar D, Zhang H, Heerdt PM, et al. Statin use is associated with a reduction in atrial fi-brillation after noncardiac thoracic surgery independent of C-reactive protein. Chest 2005;128:3421–7.

[90] Hazelrigg SR, Boley TM, Cetindag IB, et al. The efficacy of supplemental magnesium in reduc-ing atrial fibrillation after coronary artery bypass grafting. Ann Thorac Surg 2004;77:824–30.

[91] Patti G, Chello M, Candura D, et al. Randomized trial of atorvastatin for reduction of postoperative atrial fibrillation in patients undergoing cardiac surgery: results of the ARMYDA-3 (Atorvastatin for Reduction of MYocardial Dysrhythmia After cardiac sur-gery) study. Circulation 2006;114:1455–61.

[92] Prasongsukarn K, Abel JG, Jamieson WR, et al. The effects of steroids on the occurrence of postoperative atrial fibrillation after coronary artery bypass grafting surgery: a prospective randomized trial. J Thorac Cardiovasc Surg 2005;130:93–8.

[93] Halvorsen P, Raeder J, White PF, et al. The effect of dexamethasone on side effects after coronary revascularization procedures. Anesth Analg 2003;96:1578–83.

[94] Halonen J, Halonen P, Jarvinen O, et al. Corticosteroids for the prevention of atrial fibril-lation after cardiac surgery: a randomized controlled trial. JAMA 2007;297:1562–7.

[95] Blommaert D, Gonzalez M, Mucumbitsi J, et al. Effective prevention of atrial fibrillation by continuous atrial overdrive pacing after coronary artery bypass surgery. J Am Coll Cardiol 2000;35:1411–5.

[96] Gerstenfeld EP, Hill MR, French SN, et al. Evaluation of right atrial and biatrial tempo-rary pacing for the prevention of atrial fibrillation after coronary artery bypass surgery. J Am Coll Cardiol 1999;33:1981–8.

[97] Chung MK, Augostini RS, Asher CR, et al. Ineffectiveness and potential proarrhythmia of atrial pacing for atrial fibrillation prevention after coronary artery bypass grafting. Ann Thorac Surg 2000;69:1057–63.

[98] Greenberg MD, Katz NM, Iuliano S, et al. Atrial pacing for the prevention of atrial fibrillation after cardiovascular surgery. J Am Coll Cardiol 2000;35:1416–22.

[99] Fan K, Lee KL, Chiu CS, et al. Effects of biatrial pacing in prevention of postoperative atrial fibrillation after coronary artery bypass surgery. Circulation 2000;102:755–60.

[100] Daoud EG, Dabir R, Archambeau M, et al. Randomized, double-blind trial of simultaneous right and left atrial epicardial pacing for prevention of post-open heart surgery atrial fibrillation. Circulation 2000;102:761–5.

[101] Goette A, Mittag J, Friedl A, et al. Pacing of Bachmann's bundle after coronary artery bypass grafting. Pacing Clin Electrophysiol 2002;25:1072–8.

[102] Levy T, Fotopoulos G, Walker S, et al. Randomized controlled study investigating the effect of biatrial pacing in prevention of atrial fibrillation after coronary artery bypass grafting. Circulation 2000;102:1382–7.

[103] Solomon AJ, Kouretas PC, Hopkins RA, et al. Early discharge of patients with new-onset atrial fibrillation after cardiovascular surgery. Am Heart J 1998;135:557–63.

[104] Clemo HF, Wood MA, Gilligan DM, et al. Intravenous amiodarone for acute heart rate control in the critically ill patient with atrial tachyarrhythmias. Am J Cardiol 1998;81:594–8.

[105] Oral H, Souza JJ, Michaud GF, et al. Facilitating transthoracic cardioversion of atrial fibrillation with ibutilide pretreatment. N Engl J Med 1999;340:1849–54.

[106] Wozakowska-Kaplon B, Janion M, Sielski J, et al. Efficacy of biphasic shock for transthoracic cardioversion of persistent atrial fibrillation: can we predict energy requirements? Pacing Clin Electrophysiol 2004;27:764–8.

[107] Gentili C, Giordano F, Alois A, et al. Efficacy of intravenous propafenone in acute atrial fibrillation complicating open-heart surgery. Am Heart J 1992;123:1225–8.

[108] Geelen P, O'Hara GE, Roy N, et al. Comparison of propafenone versus procainamide for the acute treatment of atrial fibrillation after cardiac surgery. Am J Cardiol 1999;84:345–7, A8–9.

[109] Connolly SJ, Mulji AS, Hoffert DL, et al. Randomized placebo-controlled trial of propafenone for treatment of atrial tachyarrhythmias after cardiac surgery. J Am Coll Cardiol 1987;10:1145–8.

[110] Wafa SS, Ward DE, Parker DJ, et al. Efficacy of flecainide acetate for atrial arrhythmias following coronary artery bypass grafting. Am J Cardiol 1989;63:1058–64.

[111] Delfaut P, Saksena S, Prakash A, et al. Long-term outcome of patients with drug-refractory atrial flutter and fibrillation after single- and dual-site right atrial pacing for arrhythmia prevention. J Am Coll Cardiol 1998;32:1900–8.

[112] Campbell TJ, Morgan JJ. Treatment of atrial arrhythmias after cardiac surgery with intravenous disopyramide. Aust N Z J Med 1980;10:644–9.

[113] Campbell TJ, Gavaghan TP, Morgan JJ. Intravenous sotalol for the treatment of atrial fibrillation and flutter after cardiopulmonary bypass: comparison with disopyramide and digoxin in a randomised trial. Br Heart J 1985;54:86–90.

[114] Gavaghan TP, Koegh AM, Kelly RP, et al. Flecainide compared with a combination of digoxin and disopyramide for acute atrial arrhythmias after cardiopulmonary bypass. Br Heart J 1988;60:497–501.

[115] Malouf JF, Alam S, Gharzeddine W, et al. The role of anticoagulation in the development of pericardial effusion and late tamponade after cardiac surgery. Eur Heart J 1993;14:1451–7.

[116] Weber MA, Hasford J, Taillens C, et al. Low-dose aspirin versus anticoagulants for prevention of coronary graft occlusion. Am J Cardiol 1990;66:1464–8.

THE MEDICAL
CLINICS
OF NORTH AMERICA

Med Clin N Am 92 (2008) 101–120

ELSEVIER
SAUNDERS

Electrical and Pharmacologic Cardioversion for Atrial Fibrillation

Susan S. Kim, MD, Bradley P. Knight, MD*

Clinical Cardiac Electrophysiology, Section of Cardiology, Department of Medicine, University of Chicago Hospitals, University of Chicago, 5758 South Maryland Avenue MC9024, Chicago, IL 60637, USA

Cardioversion is a useful tool in the management of patients who have atrial fibrillation (AF) when rhythm control is appropriate. It is used most frequently for those who are symptomatic or newly diagnosed. Transthoracic electrical cardioversion is the overwhelming method of choice because of its relative simplicity and efficacy. In selected circumstances, pharmacologic cardioversion is preferred. Indications for cardioversion and management of pericardioversion anticoagulation are discussed in this article. Electrical and pharmacologic cardioversion is described in detail. Finally, management strategies are offered for initial failure to convert or immediate recurrence of AF (IRAF).

Patterns of atrial fibrillation

Before discussing the indications for cardioversion, it is useful to define the clinical patterns of the occurrence of AF. Generally speaking, patients who have AF demonstrate one of three clinical patterns: paroxysmal, persistent, or permanent AF (Fig. 1) [1]. Paroxysmal AF consists of self-terminating episodes, each lasting generally less than 7 days in duration, usually less than 24 hours. Persistent AF consists of non–self-terminating episodes, each lasting more than 7 days, whereas permanent AF is defined as a long episode with failed or no attempt at cardioversion.

Given these definitions, cardioversion can be of clinical usefulness in some patients who have paroxysmal AF and in many who have persistent AF. By definition, cardioversion is not used for patients who have permanent AF.

* Corresponding author. University of Chicago, 5758 South Maryland Avenue MC9024, Chicago, IL 60637.
E-mail address: bknight@medicine.bsd.uchicago.edu (B.P. Knight).

0025-7125/08/$ - see front matter © 2008 Elsevier Inc. All rights reserved.
doi:10.1016/j.mcna.2007.08.003
medical.theclinics.com

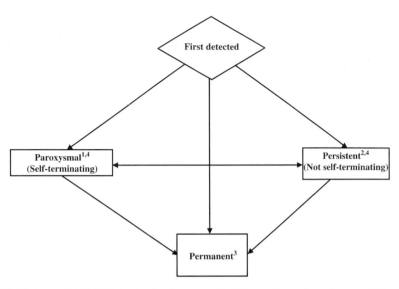

Fig. 1. Patterns of AF. (*1*) Episodes that last generally 7 days or fewer (most less than 24 hours); (*2*) episodes that last usually longer than 7 days; (*3*) cardioversion failed or not attempted; and (*4*) paroxysmal and persistent AF may be recurrent. (*Reprinted from* Fuster V, Ryden LE, Cannom DS, et al. ACC/AHA/ESC 2006 guidelines for the management of patients with atrial fibrillation. Circulation 2006;114(7):e257–354, © 2006; with permission from the American Heart Association).

Indications for cardioversion

Broadly, cardioversion should be considered for two populations of patients: those who are symptomatic with AF and those who present with AF for the first time.

Patients who have symptomatic AF can range from those who have severe enough symptoms—such as severely decompensated heart failure, hypotension, uncontrolled ischemia, or angina—to mandate urgent cardioversion. Other patients who have AF may have less severe, but nevertheless troublesome symptoms, such as palpitations, fatigue, lightheadedness, and exertional dyspnea. Regardless of the degree of severity, any symptoms due to atrial fibrillation warrant consideration of cardioversion as a management option.

Restoration of sinus rhythm is a reasonable goal in patients who have a first-time diagnosis of AF, regardless of symptoms, unless there is some indication that the AF has been present for many years before identification. The purpose of cardioversion even in patients who are asymptomatic or newly diagnosed is potentially to slow the progression of the clinical pattern of AF. There are many lines of evidence that support the principle that "atrial fibrillation begets atrial fibrillation" [2]. Natural history studies show that AF can be a progressive disease: patients who have paroxysmal AF progress to persistent and permanent AF. Even those who have lone paroxysmal AF may progress [3] and the tendency to progress seems to correlate with the duration of the paroxysmal AF episodes [4]. In addition, many clinical trials show that pharmacologic and electrical cardioversion are more likely to succeed in patients who have episodes of shorter duration than in those who have longer-duration episodes [5]. A study comparing short- versus longer-duration episodes of AF in goat hearts demonstrated that with longer-duration episodes, the rate, inducibility, and stability of AF were increased significantly. In addition, a marked shortening of the atrial effective refractory period was seen [2]. These lines of evidence strongly support the principle that AF begets itself; this principle underlies the rationale for cardioverting patients who have newly diagnosed AF.

As evidenced in large-scale, randomized clinical trials, cardioversion and other attempts to maintain sinus rhythm are unlikely to have a meaningful clinical impact on older patients who are asymptomatic. Also, cardioversion is not applied to patients who have permanent AF (discussed previously). Both of these populations of patients, however, should receive therapeutic anticoagulation or antiplatelet therapy as dictated by their risk for a thromboembolic event versus the risks from this therapy [6,7].

An additional population of patients who may benefit from cardioversion is those who have postoperative AF. Postoperative AF occurs most commonly in the first few days after surgery, a time when anticoagulation may be undesirable. Many episodes of postoperative AF resolve spontaneously. Those patients who do not have spontaneous resolution may be cardioverted prior to an AF duration of 48 hours in order to avoid anticoagulation (discussed later).

Pericardioversion anticoagulation

Because AF results in mechanical stasis in the atria, patients who have AF are at risk for developing intracardiac thrombi and subsequent embolization. The risk for a thromboembolic event is particularly high around the time of cardioversion for the following reasons: firstly, if an unstable thrombus is present precardioversion, the recovery of atrial contraction post cardioversion and the force of atrial contraction may cause fragmentation and embolization of the pre-existing thrombus [8,9]. Secondly, in many patients, the recovery of atrial mechanical function can lag behind restoration of normal electrical function [10]. This period of atrial mechanical "stunning" after cardioversion can last up to 4 weeks post cardioversion. Thus, stasis in the atria and the risk for clot formation may endure for several weeks post cardioversion, even with persistent sinus rhythm. As such, the goals of pericardioversion anticoagulation for AF are two-fold: (1) to minimize the likelihood of an unstable thrombus being present at the time of cardioversion and (2) to prevent the formation of new thrombus in the postcardioversion phase. Without anticoagulation, the risk for a thromboembolic event post cardioversion can be as high as 5% [11].

To minimize the likelihood of an unstable thrombus being present at the time of cardioversion, one of two different strategies may be used: (1) empiric anticoagulation for 3 weeks or (2) short-term anticoagulation and transesophageal echocardiography (TEE)-guided cardioversion. Presuming that an unstable thrombus takes approximately 2 weeks to organize and adhere to the atrial wall, under the empiric anticoagulation strategy, patients should be treated for a minimum of 3 weeks with warfarin (target international normalized ratio [INR] 2.5; range 2.0 to 3.0) or enoxaparin before cardioversion [1,9,12]. When using warfarin, it is critical to verify a therapeutic effect with weekly INR levels prior to cardioversion. One retrospective study examined 1435 patients who had AF greater than 48 hours' duration who were receiving warfarin and undergoing direct current cardioversion. In these patients, embolic events were significantly more likely when the INR was 1.5 to 2.4 compared to an INR greater than or equal to 2.5 (0.93% versus 0%, $P = .012$) [13].

Alternatively, patients may be therapeutically anticoagulated with heparin followed by TEE. If no thrombus is seen on TEE, cardioversion is performed. The advantage of TEE-guided cardioversion is a shorter time to cardioversion and, potentially, a shorter total duration of anticoagulation. The validity of TEE-guided cardioversion was demonstrated in a randomized clinical trial involving 1222 patients [14]. Patients who had AF requiring cardioversion were randomized to 24 hours of unfractionated heparin and TEE-guided cardioversion versus empiric anticoagulation for 3 weeks prior to cardioversion. In both strategies, patients were anticoagulated for 4 weeks post cardioversion. After 8 weeks, there was no significant difference in the rate of embolic events (0.8% versus 0.5%, $P = .50$) between the TEE-guided versus warfarin-only groups. There was a significantly decreased rate of hemorrhagic events (2.9% versus 5.5%, $P = .03$) and a shorter time to cardioversion (3.0 versus 30.6 days, $P < .001$) in the TEE-guided versus warfarin-only groups. A smaller, randomized, controlled trial compared low-molecular-weight heparin to unfractionated heparin plus oral anticoagulation [12]. Of the 496 patients in the trial, 431 underwent TEE-guided cardioversion whereas the remaining 65 patients were anticoagulated empirically and cardioverted after 3 weeks. In all strategies, patients underwent 4 weeks of anticoagulation post cardioversion. The use of low-molecular-weight heparin was found noninferior in the empiric-anticoagulation and TEE-guided treatment arms compared to the use of unfractionated heparin plus oral anticoagulation for the primary endpoint of preventing ischemic and embolic events, bleeding complications, and death.

Again, given the delay of up to 4 weeks for recovery of atrial mechanical function post cardioversion, patients should undergo at least 4 weeks of therapeutic anticoagulation post cardioversion [1,9]. Especially in the early postcardioversion period, meticulous attention should be given to anticoagulation status, as most thromboembolic events occur within the first few days post cardioversion (Fig. 2) [15]. In particular, overlapping therapy

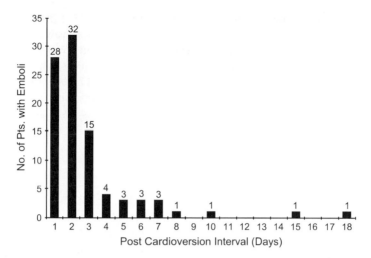

Fig. 2. Interval between cardioversion and thromboembolic events in 92 patients. (*From* Berger M, Schweitzer P. Timing of thromboembolic events after electrical cardioversion of atrial fibrillation or flutter: a retrospective analysis. Am J Cardiol 1998;82(12):1545–7, © Elsevier 1998; with permission).

with heparin (unfractionated or low-molecular-weight) should be administered if the INR is less than 2.0. One analysis that pooled data from 32 studies and included a total of 4621 patients examined the timing of embolic events [15]. Ninety-two (2%) patients had embolic events. Only 11 of the patients were anticoagulated prior to cardioversion. Seventy-five (82%) of the 92 episodes occurred within the first 72 hours post cardioversion (see Fig. 2). Notably, 98% of the embolic events occurred within the first 10 days post cardioversion.

For AF episodes lasting less than 48 hours, the likelihood of thrombus formation and subsequent embolization after cardioversion is low. As such, anticoagulation is not recommended routinely for patients who have episodes of duration less than 48 hours [1]. Neither pre- nor postcardioversion anticoagulation is recommended for these short-duration episodes. One prospective observational study followed 375 patients admitted to the hospital for AF who were identified by symptoms to have an AF episode of less than 48 hours in duration [16]. Patients being treated with anticoagulation using warfarin (INR >1.6) or heparin at the time of presentation were excluded. Two hundred fifty patients converted spontaneously, whereas pharmacologic or electrical conversion was performed in 107 patients. Three patients (0.8% [95% CI, 0.2% to 2.4%]) had a clinical thromboembolic event. Thus, overall, the thromboembolic risk for patients who had short-duration AF seems low.

Determining the true onset of an AF episode can be difficult in the absence of electrocardiographic documentation (eg, telemetry or 12-lead

ECG). Symptoms generally are unreliable as a marker of the presence of absence of AF. One study in patients who had pacemakers showed that more
than 90% of atrial tachyarrhythmia events documented by the pacemaker
were not perceived by the patients, even in those patients who otherwise
were believed symptomatic with their arrhythmias [17]. As such, in the
absence of electrocardiographic evidence of the true onset of an episode of
AF, it is most prudent to assume that the episode has been going on for
more than 48 hours.

Cardioversion

Most patients who require cardioversion undergo transthoracic electrical
cardioversion rather than an attempt at pharmacologic conversion, because
of its shorter overall procedure duration and high rate of success (as high as
over 90%) [18]. Although at least deep sedation is required for transthoracic
electrical cardioversion, if short-acting agents are used, patients may be
discharged within hours after recovery from anesthesia. Antiarrhythmic
medications play two primary roles in cardioversion for AF: (1) used alone,
they are effective in timely termination of symptomatic AF of short duration, and (2) used together with electrical cardioversion, they help facilitate
achieving persistent sinus rhythm in two distinct populations of patients: (1)
those who have IRAF (successful conversion to sinus rhythm [even just one
beat] followed by recurrence of AF within minutes) and (2) those who truly
fail cardioversion with no achievement of sinus rhythm at all.

Electrical cardioversion: biphasic waveforms superior
to monophasic waveforms

The success of cardioversion and defibrillation depends on the delivery of
adequate current flow through the heart [19]. At the same time, excessive
current delivery can lead to myocardial damage, leading to ST-segments
changes, enzyme release, depression of myocardial function, and reduced
mean arterial pressures [20,21].

The two major determinants of current delivery through an external defibrillator are energy selection and the shock waveform used. When Bernard
Lown reported the first series of AF cardioversions using an external defibrillator in 1963 [22], he was using what is termed, monophasic damped
sinusoidal (MDS) waveform, or the "Lown waveform," for energy delivery
(Fig. 3) [23]. This waveform, displayed as current amplitude over time, is
characterized by an initial high peak followed by an exponential decay of
the current to zero. The MDS waveform remained the dominant waveform
in external defibrillators until biphasic waveforms emerged. Under pressure
to reduce the size of implantable defibrillator generators, device manu-
factures developed biphasic waveforms, which demonstrated a significant
decrease in defibrillation energy requirements for ventricular fibrillation

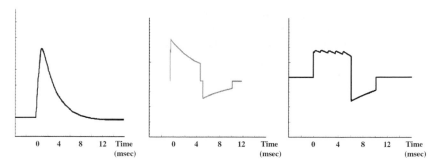

Fig. 3. Shock waveforms: (*left*) MDS waveform; (*middle*) BTE waveform; (*right*) RBW. The vertical axis represents current amplitude. (*From* Mittal S, Stein KM, Markowitz SM, et al. An update on electrical cardioversion of atrial fibrillation. Card Electrophysiol Rev 2003;7(3):285–9, © 2003 Springer; with kind permission from Springer Science and Business Media).

[24,25]. Given their superiority in implantable defibrillators, biphasic waveforms then were tried in external defibrillators. Currently, two types of biphasic waveforms are used in most commercially available external defibrillators: biphasic truncated exponential (BTE) waveforms and rectilinear biphasic waveforms (RBW) (see Fig. 3). Both biphasic waveforms are characterized by lower peak current amplitudes (compared to monophasic waveform energies of similar clinical efficacy) and a second phase with a negative or inverted polarity. The lower peak current amplitudes may be associated with less myocardial injury than higher peak current shocks [26].

Biphasic waveforms are proved to convert AF at much lower energies and at higher rates than the MDS waveform. One study compared the RBW waveform to the MDS waveform [18]. Here, 165 patients who had AF were randomized to monophasic shocks using a dose escalation of 100, 200, 300, and 360 J or biphasic shocks using 70, 120, 150, and 170 J. With the first shock, the RBW was significantly more successful than the MDS shock, with a 60/88 (68%) versus 16/77 (21%) ($P < .0001$) conversion rate. There still was a significantly higher success rate in the biphasic versus monophasic shock group after the highest energy shock (83/88 [94%] versus 61/77 [79%], $P = .005$). At all comparable energy levels and across all impedances, peak currents in the biphasic shocks measured at approximately 50% of the peak current amplitude seen with monophasic shocks.

Two randomized studies compared the BTE waveform with the MDS waveform for AF cardioversion. In the first study, 57 patients were randomized to cardioversion with 150 J, then 360 J with a MDS defibrillator versus 150 J followed by another 150 J with a BTE defibrillator. With the first shock (each at 150 J), the cardioversion success rate was 16/27 (59%) versus 26/30 (86%) in the MDS and BTE groups, respectively [27]. Cumulative success rates after the second shock and after crossover were not significantly different between the two groups (88% versus 93% and 92% versus 96%, respectively). In the second study, 203 patients were randomized to an

MDS versus a BTE waveform with delivery of 100 J, 150 J, or 200 J, then maximum output (360 J and 200 J, respectively) shocks [28]. At each of the first three energy levels, the cumulative cardioversion success rate was significantly higher in the BTE group versus the MDS group: for example, at 200 J, the success rate was 86/96 (90%) versus 57/107 (53%) ($P < .0001$). At the highest energies, there was no statistically significant difference in outcome between groups: 87/96 (91%) versus 91/107 (85%) ($P = .29$). Also, at equal energy levels, the BTE waveform was associated with significantly less dermal injury than the MDS waveform.

Finally, biphasic external defibrillators are more efficacious in patients who have AF resistant to monphasic cardioversion [29]. Fifty-six patients who had AF and who had failed at least one 360-J monophasic shock were randomized to progressive 150-J, 200-J, and 360-J BTE shocks or one 360-J monophasic shock. Sinus rhythm was restored in 17 of 28 (61%) patients who had biphasic versus 5 of 28 (18%) who had monophasic shocks ($P = .001$). With crossover allowed after failed shocks, 78% of patients who had a failed monophasic shock were cardioverted successfully with a biphasic shock, whereas only 27% of those patients who had failed biphasic shocks converted with the high-energy monophasic shock.

Currently, the preponderance of evidence favors the use of biphasic external defibrillators for AF cardioversion because of their categorically lower energy requirements and greater efficacy compared to monophasic defibrillators.

Electrical cardioversion: practical considerations

Anesthesia
Patients undergoing elective cardioversion should receive at least deep sedation, as high-energy shock can cause significant discomfort. Short-acting agents, such as midazolam, fentanyl, and propofol, are desirable given their rapid onset and short half-life. In some cases, general anesthesia may be indicated. Anesthesia and cardioversion should be performed in the post-absorptive state. Even when urgent cardioversion is required, as in cases of hypotension, severe decompensated heart failure, angina, or ischemia, attempts should be made to sedate patients as circumstances allow.

Pad or paddle positioning and size
A handful of studies have examined the effect of electrode (pad or paddle) positioning, anterior-posterior (AP) versus anterior-lateral (AL), on cardioversion success. One study randomized 301 patients who had AF to AP or AL pad positioning. The AP position was associated with a significantly higher rate of successful cardioversion and lower cumulative energy requirement (Fig. 4) [30]. Two subsequent studies show no effect of pad placement on cardioversion success in AF [31,32]. The second of the two studies also showed that an increased pad size (13 cm versus the standard 8.5 cm) did not improve the likelihood of cardioversion [32].

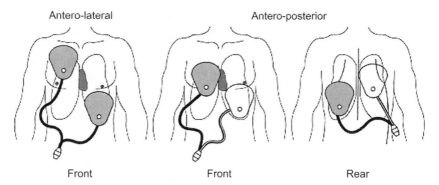

Fig. 4. Electrode positions: anterolateral, ventricular apex-right infraclavicular area paddle position; (modified) antero-posterior, right sternal body at the third intercostal space-angle of the left scapula paddle position; front, front view; rear, rear view. (*Reproduced from* Botto GL, Politi A, Bonini W, et al. External cardioversion of atrial fibrillation: role of paddle position on technical efficacy and energy requirements. Heart 1999;82:726–30; with permission from the BMJ Publishing Group).

Shock delivery

To avoid shock delivery during the vulnerable phase of the cardiac cycle ("shock on T") and subsequent ventricular fibrillation, shocks should be delivered in a synchronized fashion. In the synchronized mode, intrinsic R waves are sensed and shock delivery is timed to minimize the risk of delivery during the vulnerable period. This is in contrast to the defibrillation mode where shocks are delivered in an asynchronous or random fashion without regard to the cardiac cycle. This mode is appropriate for ventricular fibrillation or very rapid ventricular tachycardia where synchronized delivery is not possible and immediate shock is desired.

Energy selection

Energy level is related directly to current amplitude, and adequate current delivery determines successful cardioversion. As such, one choice may be to start with the highest energy for every cardioversion (360 J with monophasic defibrillators and 200 J or even 360 J in some biphasic defibrillators). The advantage is a high probability of successful cardioversion and, thus, a shorter duration of sedation. The disadvantage of higher energy shocks, especially with monophasic defibrillators, mostly is with thermal injury to the skin [28,33]. Any potential myocardial damage, from even high-energy cardioversion, rarely is of clinical consequence.

Because current is related inversely to impedance, increased transthoracic impedance can diminish current delivery to myocardium. In one study, increased transthoracic impedance was found significantly and independently associated with lower rates of successful cardioversion [18]. Incomplete pad or paddle contact also may increase transthoracic impedance. Adequate contact medium (usually gel or paste) and firm pad or paddle contact should be assured. Other factors that increase transthoracic impedance include obesity, emphysema, and asthma. In patients who have these conditions, selection of a high level of energy is appropriate. Delivering shocks during the expiratory phase of the respiratory cycle also may decrease transthoracic impedance.

Patients who have AF of longer duration have lower rates of successful cardioversion [18,30]. They also may have more success with higher energy shocks.

Lower-energy shocks are appropriate when patients are smaller in size or have AF of shorter duration. Also, patients with atrial flutter may successfully convert with low energies (as low as 100 J monophasic or 50 J biphasic defibrillators) for successful cardioversion. Even with lower energy shocks, patients can experience significant discomfort and still should undergo at least deep sedation.

Patients who have implanted devices

Under the proper circumstances, patients who have implanted devices (permanent pacemakers or implantable cardioverter-defibrillators [ICDs]) can undergo external cardioversion with minimal risk to their devices and to themselves. Potential risks at the time of shock include alteration of programmed data or, if electricity is conducted down an implanted lead, endocardial injury with transient or permanent exit block. These risks are maximized when pads or paddles are placed, one over the pulse generator and one at the apex of the heart. AP positioning seems to lower these risks [1]. Pre- and post cardioversion, devices should be interrogated with complete lead testing and device reprogramming as needed.

In patients who have ICDs, cardioversion may be achieved with a commanded internal shock delivered through the device. Device-mediated cardioversion has the advantage of avoiding potential damage to the implanted system. A disadvantage is that each shock contributes to significant decrease in battery life—up to approximately 1 month for each maximum-energy shock. Internal shocks can cause significant discomfort, so patients still should receive at least deep sedation. For patients who have atrial flutter, device-delivered antitachycardia pacing should be attempted; because it is painless, sedation is not needed.

Electrical cardioversion: internal via intracardiac catheters

Thus far, the discussion of electrical cardioversion primarily has been about external transthoracic cardioversion. Prior to the development of biphasic defibrillators, AF cardioversion failure rates were significantly higher. In that setting, internal cardioversion was established as next-line therapy for patients who had failed external cardioversion. The technique eventually evolved to placement of intracardiac catheters in the right atrium, coronary sinus, and left pulmonary artery, through which low-energy shocks were delivered [34]. This treatment option may be useful in patients for whom all other cardioversion techniques have failed (discussed later).

Electrical cardioversion: outcomes

The three potential outcomes after electrical cardioversion are (1) restoration of sinus rhythm that persists, (2) restoration of sinus rhythm (at least one sinus beat) followed by IRAF, or (3) failed cardioversion with no evidence of sinus rhythm. Results from many studies show that patients who have IRAF can achieve rates of long-term freedom from AF [35,36] comparable to those patients who have persistent sinus rhythm post cardioversion. The rates of long-term freedom from AF are significantly worse, however, in patients who have true failed cardioversion who ultimately achieve sinus rhythm. Thus, it is critical to distinguish between patients who have IRAF (those patients who have even just one sinus beat after cardioversion) and those who have true failed cardioversion. Because patients who have IRAF can achieve favorable long-term outcomes, aggressive measures should be taken to facilitate persistent postcardioversion sinus rhythm.

Immediate recurrence of atrial fibrillation

IRAF is defined as AF recurring within the first few minutes after cardioversion. One study suggests that if AF recurs within the first 24 hours post cardioversion, it will occur within the first few minutes after cardioversion [37]. Even when only one beat of sinus rhythm is seen, the subsequent AF is considered IRAF as opposed to true failed cardioversion. The incidence of IRAF ranges from 5% to 25% [38].

The distinction between IRAF and true failed cardioversion is important as the two populations have different long-term outcomes [36]: patients who have IRAF who ultimately achieve persistent sinus rhythm post cardioversion (usually pharmacologically facilitated) have better rates of long-term freedom from AF than patients who have true failed cardioversion who subsequently achieve sinus rhythm.

IRAF seems to be triggered by very early coupled premature atrial beats (PABs). In one study of patients undergoing internal cardioversion for AF, IRAF was noted in 13% (5/38) of patients. IRAF in these patients always was seen to reinitiate with noncatheter-induced PABs. PAB coupling intervals that led to IRAF were significantly shorter than those not leading to IRAF [35]. Pretreatment with atropine or flecainide facilitated cardioversion without IRAF in three patients whereas repeat shock alone was successful for two patients. In another study, this time in patients undergoing catheter ablation for AF, PABs triggering IRAF also were significantly shorter than PABs not triggering AF [39]. In this study, 20% of IRAF episodes were documented as initiated by pulmonary vein activity. In every one of these cases, the pulmonary vein activity took the form of a rapid pulmonary vein tachycardia. In a third study, also in patients undergoing catheter ablation for AF, again, coupling intervals for IRAF-initiating PABs were significantly shorter than those not initiating IRAF. IRAF was seen more frequently in patients who had AF lasting less than 1 month in duration than in those who had longer episodes. Long-term, patients who had IRAF had similar freedom from AF as those who did not have IRAF [40].

The increased incidence of IRAF in patients who have shorter-duration episodes of AF also was seen in another study [38]. Patients who had implantable atrial defibrillators and patients undergoing external transthoracic cardioversion were studied. In patients who received cardioversion within 1 hour of the onset of AF, IRAF occurred at a rate of 56% compared to those whose AF endured more than 24 hours, where the rate of IRAF was 12%. This finding suggests a possible lower limit of AF duration below which cardioversion may be less likely to lead to persistent sinus rhythm.

Patients who have IRAF successfully have achieved persistent postcardioversion sinus rhythm or suppression of IRAF in many studies using a variety of antiarrhythmic medications. An early demonstration of successful pharmacologic suppression of IRAF was published in 1967 with the use of quinidine [41]. Fifty patients received oral quinidine (1200 mg) 1 day prior to cardioversion. Successful cardioversion was achieved in 92% versus 64% ($P < .01$) of quinidine versus control patients, predominantly because of the prevention of IRAF. Another Vaughan-Williams class IA agent, procainamide, has no effect on the rate of successful cardioversion compared to placebo [42].

In another study, 50 patients were randomized to propafenone (750 mg per day) or placebo for 2 days prior to cardioversion. Propafenone patients had a significantly lower likelihood of IRAF and, thus, a higher overall likelihood of persistent sinus rhythm post cardioversion compared to patients receiving placebo (0% versus 17% IRAF, 84% versus 65% sinus rhythm at 48 hours) [43]. A subsequent study showed that the addition of verapamil to propafenone was superior to propafenone, alone, in suppressing IRAF [44].

Sotalol and amiodarone suppress IRAF effectively. Sotalol suppressed IRAF effectively in patients undergoing internal cardioversion [45]. Amiodarone was studied in 27 patients who had either IRAF (group A) or a failed cardioversion (group B) [36]. All patients received oral amiodarone loading (600 mg per day for 4 weeks) followed by 200 mg per day for 4 weeks if sinus rhythm was ultimately achieved. Five out of eleven (46%) of group A patients converted during loading whereas only 1 of 16 (6%) group B patients did. After electrical cardioversion, the total number of group A patients in sinus rhythm was 10 of 11 (91%) versus 7 of 16 (44%) in group B. At 1-month follow-up, all 10 of 11 (91%) of group A patients versus only 5 of 16 (33%) of group B patients remained in sinus rhythm. This study, although small, demonstrated a significant outcome difference between patients who had IRAF post cardioversion versus those who had failed cardioversion. These findings suggest that in patients who have IRAF, restoration of persistent sinus rhythm should be pursued aggressively.

Another study demonstrated favorable outcomes in pharmacologically facilitated cardioversion in patients who had IRAF, this time using intravenous verapamil or ibutilide. These medications have been shown to attenuate the shortening of the atrial refractory period seen in post-AF patients; that is, they prolong the atrial refractory period [46]. Subsequently, both medications were studied in patients who had IRAF [47]. Verapamil (0.15 mg/kg at 2 mg/min) was assigned randomly to 11 patients versus ibutilide (1 mg) over 10 minutes in nine patients. IRAF occurred in 73% of verapamil patients and in only 22% of ibutilide patients ($P < .05$). After crossover, ibutilide continued to have a higher rate of IRAF suppression than verapamil. These findings correlated with ibutilide's much greater effect on the atrial refractory period compared to verapamil's in the earlier study [46].

Verapamil was used alone in one uncontrolled study of 19 patients who had IRAF after each of three cardioversions [48]. Each patient received 10 mg intravenously followed by a fourth cardioversion attempt. IRAF was suppressed in 9 of 19 (47%) of patients whereas sinus rhythm duration prior to IRAF was increased in those patients who did experience IRAF.

For patients undergoing transthoracic cardioversion, same-day options for pharmacologic suppression of IRAF include intravenous verapamil and ibutilide, with higher success rates seen with ibutilide. Because ibutilide is contraindicated in patients who have depressed left ventricular systolic function, intravenous verapamil (in the absence of decompenstaed heart failure) or outpatient loading with amiodarone should be used.

Failed cardioversion

Even in the era of biphasic defibrillation, up to 10% or more of patients may have true failed cardioversion, that is, no evidence of any sinus activity after cardioversion. Certainly the use of monophasic rather than biphasic waveforms is associated with higher failure rates [18,27,28]. Longer duration of episodes and increased transthoracic impedance also are associated with higher cardioversion failure rates [18,30]. In contrast, younger age and smaller left atrial size are found independently associated with successful cardioversion [5,49].

When conventional external cardioversion fails, the following tactics may be effective: (1) Repeat shock at highest energy. Because success of cardioversion is probabilistic, a failed attempt at maximum output does not imply that it never will work. Although most biphasic defibrillators deliver a maximum of 200 J, some biphasic defibrillators can deliver up to 360 J; (2) Reposition the pads or paddles. If the electrodes are in the AL position, reposition them to the AP position: right sternal body at the third intercostal space and angle of the left scapula (see Fig. 4) [30]. The goal is to direct the energy vector optimally through the atria; (3) Apply manual pressure on the anterior pad at the time of shock delivery. With the pads in the AP position, while ensuring electrical insulation, apply mechanical pressure to the anterior pad to decrease the distance (thus, the impedance) between the two pads; (4) Deliver the shock during the expiration. In theory, this may decrease transthoracic impedance; (5) Consider pharmacologic facilitation of cardioversion (discussed later); (6) Try the "double-paddle" technique. In one study, patients who had AF and who had failed 360-J monophasic cardio-version were loaded with amiodarone orally. If repeat 360-J monophasic cardioversion failed again, the patients underwent the double-paddle tech-nique: two monophasic defibrillators were used with two sets of paddles for each patient; each defibrillator was set for a synchronous shock at the maxiumum output of 360 J; they then were discharged simultaneously; thirteen of 15 patients were converted successfully [50]; and (7) Consider internal cardioversion.

In addition to facilitating persistent sinus rhythm for patients who have IRAF (discussed previously), antiarrhythmic medications effectively can facilitate successful cardioversion for patients who have true failure to cardiovert (ie, no evidence of any sinus activity).

Amiodarone and ibutilide show the strongest success in pharmacologic facilitation of cardioversion after true failed cardioversion. Although some data exist showing decreased IRAF when using propafenone, verapamil, and quinidine, it is less clear whether or not they increase the likelihood of cardioversion in patients who have had true cardioversion failure.

Amiodarone, used pre- and post cardioversion, increases the rate of successful cardioversion in patients undergoing initial cardioversion [51] and in patients who have failed cardioversion in the past [36,52]. In patients who have failed past cardioversion, success rates were 7/16 (44%) with 4 weeks of amiodarone (600 mg per day by mouth) and 32/49 (65%) with amiodarone (6.0-g load by mouth) given prior to cardioversion.

Ibutilide clearly is shown to facilitate successful cardioversion in patients who have failed direct current cardioversion [53]. In one study, 100 patients who had long-duration AF (mean 117 ± 201 days) and a high prevalence of structural heart disease (89%) were randomized to undergo transthoracic electrical cardioversion with or without pretreatment with ibutilide (1 mg). Remarkably, conversion to sinus rhythm occurred in 50 of 50 (100%) of patients pretreated with ibutilide compared to 36 of 50 (72%) of patients who did not have pretreatment. Additionally, all 14 patients in the untreated group were cardioverted successfully after ibutilide pretreatment. Sustained polymorphic ventricular tachycardia occurred in 2 of 64 patients treated with ibutilide; both patients had ejection fractions less than or equal to 20%.

Thus, amiodarone and ibutilide facilitate cardioversion effectively in patients who have true failed cardioversion. Conveniently, ibutilide can be administered over a short timeframe for same-day treatment. Ibutilide, however, should not be used in patients who have low ejection fractions. In patients who have ejection fractions less than or equal to 30%, oral load-ing with amiodarone is the preferred option.

Electrical cardioversion: complications

The risks and complications of cardioversion fall largely into three categories: (1) risks associated with sedation, (2) thromboembolic events

(<1% with appropriate anticoagulation) [12,14], and (3) postcardioversion arrhythmias. Overall, the risk for electrical cardioversion in patients who are selected properly is low [1,54].

Pharmacologic cardioversion: general considerations

As discussed previously, because of the relative simplicity and high efficacy, most cardioversions are performed electrically. Pharmacologic cardioversion is used primarily in two settings: (1) for short-duration AF in highly symptomatic patients who have little or no structural heart disease and (2) as adjunct therapy to facilitate electrical cardioversion in patients who have failed cardioversion or have IRAF. In rare instances, such as to avoid anesthesia, pharmacologic cardioversion also may be indicated.

The principles of pericardioversion anticoagulation apply whether or not cardioversion is performed electrically or pharmacologically. That is, if patients' AF episodes have persisted for more than 48 hours or for unknown duration, those patients should undergo therapeutic anticoagulation for 3 weeks or TEE with heparin administration prior to initiation of any antiarrhythmic medication, even those with low efficacy. In particular, amiodarone frequently is used in patients who have AF. Because amiodarone has the potential to convert the AF to sinus rhythm, pericardioversion anticoagulation principles should be applied.

Pharmacologic cardioversion: short-duration atrial fibrillation

In patients who have little comorbid disease and short-duration AF, antiarrhythmic agents show no significant difference in long-term cardioversion outcomes compared to placebo. Class IC agents, however, show a faster time to cardioversion and, thus, may be useful in terminating short-duration episodes of AF more rapidly for patients who are highly symptomatic [55,56]. This finding underlies the "pill-in-the-pocket" approach to management of symptomatic, short-duration AF in patients who have little to no structural heart disease. One study examined 268 patients who had little structural heart disease and who had presented to an emergency department for symptomatic AF [57]. On discharge from the hospital, patients were instructed in out-of-hospital self-administration of flecainide or propafenone after the onset of symptoms. Patients weighing more than 70 kg received flecainide (300 mg) or propafenone (600 mg); those weighing less than 70 kg in weight received flecainide (200 mg) or propafenone (450 mg). This approach was successful in 94% of episodes (534/569) with time to resolution of symptoms at 113 ± 93 minutes. In 139 of 165 patients, the medication was effective for all arrhythmic episodes. Also, the number of monthly emergency room visits and hospitalizations decreased significantly after the initiation of this management strategy. Overall, 12 of 268 patients (7%) experienced adverse effects, including nausea, asthenia, and vertigo. One episode of atrial flutter with 1:1 AV conduction occurred. Given its overall safety and efficacy, the pill-in-the-pocket strategy can be useful in a select population of patients who have AF.

Pharmacologic cardioversion: longer-duration atrial fibrillation

In patients who have structural heart disease and longer-duration AF, pharmacologic cardioversion demonstrates only modest success (20%–30%) [53,58]. As such, electrical cardioversion is used more commonly. Antiarrhythmic medications provide useful adjunct therapy for postcardioversion patients experiencing IRAF or those who have true cardioversion failure (discussed previously).

Atrial flutter

Generally, the principles discussed previously are valid for atrial flutter, except as specifically noted. In particular, anticoagulation for patients who have atrial flutter should be handled just as it would be for patients who have AF.

Summary

In summary, cardioversion is a useful option in managing patients who have AF. It is useful especially for patients who are symptomatic or newly diagnosed or for some patients who have postoperative AF. To minimize the presence of thrombus at the time of cardioversion, patients who have AF of more than 48 hours' duration should receive therapeutic anticoagulation for 3 weeks prior (full-dose low-molecular-weight heparin or warfarin— INR target 2.5, range 2.0–3.0) or TEE accompanied by heparin prior to cardioversion. To minimize the formation of thrombus post cardioversion in patients who have AF duration for more than 48 hours, therapeutic anticoagulation should be continued for 4 weeks, keeping in mind that the greatest risk for systemic embolization is in the first few days post cardioversion. Electrical, pharmacologic, or a combined approach to cardioversion can be taken. In the majority of cases, transthoracic electrical cardioversion is indicated, given its simplicity and high efficacy, especially in the era of biphasic-waveform defibrillators. Pharmacologic cardioversion with class IC agents may be useful for early conversion to sinus rhythm in patients who have minimal structural heart disease and short-duration, symptomatic AF. Antiarrhythmic agents also are useful in the setting of two distinct postcardioversion outcomes: (1) IRAF: recurrence within minutes post cardioversion after even just one sinus beat and (2) true failed cardioversion (no sinus beats seen). Patients who have IRAF and who achieve persistent sinus rhythm may have good rates of long-term freedom from AF and should be treated aggressively with pharmacologically facilitated cardioversion.

Ibutilide, amiodarone, and verapamil along with propafenone and quinidine are effective. For patients who have true failed cardioversion, ibutilide and amiodarone are effective. Given its short administration period and strong clinical efficacy, ibutilide is an excellent agent for facilitated cardioversion except in patients who have ejection fractions less than or equal to 30%. Because of the potential for cardioversion, regardless of indication or level of efficacy, antiarrhythmic medications should be given only with proper application of the principles of pericardioversion anticoagulation.

References

[1] Fuster V, Ryden LE, Cannom DS, et al. ACC/AHA/ESC 2006 Guidelines for the Management of Patients with Atrial Fibrillation: a report of the American College of Cardiology/American Heart Association Task Force on Practice Guidelines and the European Society of Cardiology Committee for Practice Guidelines (Writing Committee to Revise the 2001 Guidelines for the Management of Patients With Atrial Fibrillation): developed in collaboration with the European Heart Rhythm Association and the Heart Rhythm Society. Circulation 2006;114(7):E257–354.

[2] Wijffels MCEF, Kirchhof CJHJ, Dorland R, et al. Atrial fibrillation begets atrial fibrillation. Circulation 1995;92:1954–68.

[3] Kopecky SL, Gersh BJ, McGoon MD, et al. The natural history of lone atrial fibrillation: a population based study over three decades. N Engl J Med 1987;317:669–74.

[4] Godtfredsen J. Atrial fibrillation: etiology, course and prognosis: a follow-up study of 1212 cases. Copenhagen (Denmark): Munksgaard; 1975.

[5] Van Gelder IC, Crijns HJ, Van Gilst WH, et al. Prediction of uneventful cardioversion and maintenance of sinus rhythm from direct-current electrical cardioversion of chronic atrial fibrillation and flutter. Am J Cardiol 1991;68(1):41–6.

[6] The Atrial Fibrillation Follow-up Investigation of Rhythm Management (AFFIRM) Investigators. A comparison of rate control and rhythm control in patients with atrial fibrillation. N Engl J Med 2002;347:1825–33.

[7] Van Gelder IC, Hagens VE, Bosker HA, et al. Rate Control versus Electrical Cardioversion for Persistent Atrial Fibrillation Study Group. A comparison of rate control and rhythm control in patients with recurrent persistent atrial fibrillation. N Engl J Med 2002;347(23): 1834–40.

[8] O'Neill PG, Puleo PR, Bolli R, et al. Return of atrial mechanical function following electrical conversion of atrial dysrhythmias. Am Heart J 1990;120(2):353–9.

[9] Laupacis A, Albers G, Dalen J, et al. Antithrombotic therapy in atrial fibrillation. Chest 1998;114(5 Suppl):579S–89S.

[10] Manning WJ, Leeman DE, Gotch PJ, et al. Pulsed Doppler evaluation of atrial mechanical function after electrical cardioversion of atrial fibrillation. J Am Coll Cardiol 1989;13(3): 617–23.

[11] Bjerkelund C, Orning O. The efficacy of anticoagulant therapy in preventing embolism related to DC electrical conversion of atrial fibrillation. Am J Cardiol 1969;23:208–16.

[12] Stellbrink C, Nixdorff U, Hofmann T, et al. ACE (Anticoagulation in Cardioversion using Enoxaparin) Study Group. Safety and efficacy of enoxaparin compared with unfractionated heparin and oral anticoagulants for prevention of thromboembolic complications in cardioversion of nonvalvular atrial fibrillation: the Anticoagulation in Cardioversion using Enoxaparin (ACE) trial. Circulation 2004;109(8):997–1003.

[13] Gallagher MM, Hennessy BJ, Edvardsson N, et al. Embolic complications of direct current cardioversion of atrial arrhythmias: association with low intensity of anticoagulation at the time of cardioversion. J Am Coll Cardiol 2002;40(5).926–33.

[14] Klein AL, Grimm RA, Murray RD, et al. Assessment of Cardioversion Using Transesophageal Echocardiography Investigators. Use of transesophageal echocardiography to guide cardioversion in patients with atrial fibrillation. N Engl J Med 2001;344(19):1411–20.

[15] Berger M, Schweitzer P. Timing of thromboembolic events after electrical cardioversion of atrial fibrillation or flutter: a retrospective analysis. Am J Cardiol 1998;82(12):1545–7, A8.

[16] Weigner MJ, Caulfield TA, Danias PG, et al. Risk for clinical thromboembolism associated with conversion to sinus rhythm in patients with atrial fibrillation lasting less than 48 hours. Ann Intern Med 1997;126(8):615–20.

[17] Strickberger SA, Ip J, Saksena S, et al. Relationship between atrial tachyarrhythmias and symptoms. Heart Rhythm 2005;2(2):125–31.

[18] Mittal S, Ayati S, Stein KM, et al. Transthoracic cardioversion of atrial fibrillation: comparison of rectilinear biphasic versus damped sine wave monophasic shocks. Circulation 2000; 101(11):1282–7.

[19] Zhou X, Daubert JP, Wolf PD, et al. Epicardial mapping of ventricular defibrillation with monophasic and biphasic shocks in dogs. Circ Res 1993;72(1):145–60.

[20] Dahl CF, Ewy GA, Warner ED, et al. Myocardial necrosis from direct current countershock: effect of paddle electrode size and time interval between discharges. Circulation 1974;50: 956–61.

[21] Joglar JA, Kessler DJ, Welch PJ, et al. Effects of repeated electrical defibrillations on cardiac troponin I levels. Am J Cardiol 1999;83:270–2, A6.

[22] Lown B, Perlroth MG, Kaidbey S, et al. "Cardioversion" of atrial fibrillation. A report on the treatment of 65 episodes in 50 patients. N Engl J Med 1963;269:325–31.

[23] Mittal S, Stein KM, Markowitz SM, et al. An update on electrical cardioversion of atrial fibrillation. Card Electrophysiol Rev 2003;7(3):285–9.

[24] Winkle RA, Mead H, Ruder MA, et al. Improved low energy defibrillation efficacy in man with the use of a biphasic truncated exponential waveform. Am Heart J 1989;117:122–7.

[25] Kroll M, Anderson K, Supino C, et al. Decline in defibrillation thresholds. Pacing Clin Electrophysiol 1993;16(1 pt 2):213–7.

[26] Bardy GH, Marchlinski FE, Sharma AD, et al. Multicenter comparison of truncated biphasic shocks and standard damped sine wave monophasic shocks for transthoracic ventricular defibrillation. Transthoracic Investigators. Circulation 1996;94(10):2507–14.

[27] Ricard P, Levy S, Boccara G, et al. External cardioversion of atrial fibrillation: comparison of biphasic vs. monophasic waveform shocks. Europace 2001;3(2):96–9.

[28] Page RL, Kerber RE, Russell JK, et al. BiCard Investigators. Biphasic versus monophasic shock waveform for conversion of atrial fibrillation: the results of an international randomized, double-blind multicenter trial. J Am Coll Cardiol 2002;39(12):1956–63.

[29] Khaykin Y, Newman D, Kowalewski M, et al. Biphasic versus monophasic cardioversion in shock-resistant atrial fibrillation. J Cardiovasc Electrophysiol 2003;14(8):868–72.

[30] Botto GL, Politi A, Bonini W, et al. External cardioversion of atrial fibrillation: role of paddle position on technical efficacy and energy requirements. Heart 1999;82:726–30.

[31] Brazdzionyte J, Babarskiene RM, Stanaitiene G. Anterior-posterior versus anterior-lateral electrode position for biphasic cardioversion of atrial fibrillation. Medicina (Kaunas) 2006;42(12):994–8.

[32] Kerber RE, Jensen SR, Grayzel J, et al. Elective cardioversion: influence of paddle-electrode location and size on success rates and energy requirements. N Engl J Med 1981;305:658–62.

[33] Ambler JJ, Deakin CD. A randomised controlled trial of the effect of biphasic or monophasic waveform on the incidence and severity of cutaneous burns following external direct current cardioversion. Resuscitation 2006;71(3):293–300.

[34] Levy S. Internal defibrillation: where we have been and where we should be going? J Interv Card Electrophysiol 2005;13(Suppl 1):61–6.

[35] Timmermans C, Rodriguez LM, Smeets JL, et al. Immediate reinitiation of atrial fibrillation following internal atrial defibrillation. J Cardiovasc Electrophysiol 1998;9(2):122–8.

[36] Van Noord T, Van Gelder IC, Schoonderwoerd BA, et al. Immediate reinitiation of atrial fibrillation after electrical cardioversion predicts subsequent pharmacologic and electrical conversion to sinus rhythm and amiodarone. Am J Cardiol 2000;86(12):1384–5, A5.

[37] Tieleman RG, Van Gelder IC, Crijns HJ, et al. Early recurrences of atrial fibrillation after electrical cardioversion: a result of fibrillation-induced electrical remodeling of the atria? J Am Coll Cardiol 1998;31(1):167–73.

[38] Oral H, Ozaydin M, Sticherling C, et al. Effect of atrial fibrillation duration on probability of immediate recurrence after transthoracic cardioversion. J Cardiovasc Electrophysiol 2003; 14(2):182–5.

[39] Chugh A, Ozaydin M, Scharf C, et al. Mechanism of immediate recurrences of atrial fibrillation after restoration of sinus rhythm. Pacing Clin Electrophysiol 2004;27(1): 77–82.

[40] Husser D, Bollmann A, Kang S, et al. Determinants and prognostic significance of immediate atrial fibrillation recurrence following cardioversion in patients undergoing pulmonary vein isolation. Pacing Clin Electrophysiol 2005;28(2):119–25.

[41] Rossi M, Lown B. The use of quinidine in cardioversion. Am J Cardiol 1967;19(2):234–8.

[42] Jacobs LO, Andrews TC, Pederson DN, et al. Effect of intravenous procainamide on direct-current cardioversion of atrial fibrillation. Am J Cardiol 1998;82(2):241–2.

[43] Bianconi L, Mennuni M, Lukic V, et al. Effects of oral propafenone administration before electrical cardioversion of chronic atrial fibrillation: a placebo-controlled study. J Am Coll Cardiol 1996;28(3):700–6.

[44] De Simone A, Stabile G, Vitale DF, et al. Pretreatment with verapamil in patients with persistent or chronic atrial fibrillation who underwent electrical cardioversion. J Am Coll Cardiol 1999;34(3):810–4.

[45] Tse HF, Lau CP, Ayers GM. Incidence and modes of onset of early reinitiation of atrial fibrillation after successful internal cardioversion, and its prevention by intravenous sotalol. Heart 1999;82(3):319–24.

[46] Sticherling C, Hsu W, Tada H, et al. Effects of verapamil and ibutilide on atrial fibrillation and postfibrillation atrial refractoriness. J Cardiovasc Electrophysiol 2002;13(2):151–7.

[47] Sticherling C, Ozaydin M, Tada H, et al. Comparison of verapamil and ibutilide for the suppression of immediate recurrences of atrial fibrillation after transthoracic cardioversion. J Cardiovasc Pharmacol Ther 2002;7(3):155–60.

[48] Daoud EG, Hummel JD, Augostini R, et al. Effect of verapamil on immediate recurrence of atrial fibrillation. J Cardiovasc Electrophysiol 2000;11(11):1231–7.

[49] Frick M, Frykman V, Jensen-Urstad M, et al. Factors predicting success rate and recurrence of atrial fibrillation after first electrical cardioversion in patients with persistent atrial fibrillation. Clin Cardiol 2001;24(3):238–44.

[50] Kabukcu M, Demircioglu F, Yanik E, et al. Simultaneous double external DC shock technique for refractory atrial fibrillation in concomitant heart disease. Jpn Heart J 2004;45(6): 929–36.

[51] Manios EG, Mavrakis HE, Kanoupakis EM, et al. Effects of amiodarone and diltiazem on persistent atrial fibrillation conversion and recurrence rates: a randomized controlled study. Cardiovasc Drugs Ther 2003;17(1):31–9.

[52] Opolski G, Stanislawska J, Gorecki A, et al. Amiodarone in restoration and maintenance of sinus rhythm in patients with chronic atrial fibrillation after unsuccessful direct-current cardioversion. Clin Cardiol 1997;20(4):337–40.

[53] Oral H, Souza JJ, Michaud GF, et al. Facilitating transthoracic cardioversion of atrial fibrillation with ibutilide pretreatment. N Engl J Med 1999;340(24):1849–54.

[54] Ditchey RV, Karliner JS. Safety of electrical cardioversion in patients without digitalis toxicity. Ann Intern Med 1981;95(6):676–9.

[55] Capucci A, Lenzi T, Boriani G, et al. Effectiveness of loading oral flecainide for converting recent-onset atrial fibrillation to sinus rhythm in patients without organic heart disease or with only systemic hypertension. Am J Cardiol 1992;70:69–72.

[56] Crijns HJ, van Wijk LM, van Gilst WH, et al. Acute conversion of atrial fibrillation to sinus rhythm: clinical efficacy of flecainide acetate. Comparison of two regimens. Eur Heart J 1988; 9(6):634–8.

[57] Alboni P, Botto GL, Baldi N, et al. Outpatient treatment of recent-onset atrial fibrillation with the "pill-in-the-pocket" approach. N Engl J Med 2004;351(23):2384–91.

[58] Singh S, Zoble RG, Yellen L, et al. Efficacy and safety of oral dofetilide in converting to and maintaining sinus rhythm in patients with chronic atrial fibrillation or atrial flutter the symptomatic atrial fibrillation investigative research on dofetilide (SAFIRE-D) study. Circulation 2000;102:2385–90.

ELSEVIER
SAUNDERS

THE MEDICAL
CLINICS
OF NORTH AMERICA

Med Clin N Am 92 (2008) 121–141

Drug Therapy for Atrial Fibrillation

Simone Musco, MD[a], Emily L. Conway, MD[a],
Peter R. Kowey, MD[a,b,*]

[a]Division of Cardiovascular Diseases, Main Line Heart Center, 556 Medical Office,
Building East, 100 Lancaster Avenue, Wynnewood, PA 19096, USA
[b]Thomas Jefferson University, 1020 Walnut Street,
Philadelphia, PA 19107, USA

Atrial fibrillation (AF) is the most frequently diagnosed arrhythmia, affecting an estimated 2.3 million people in the United States. Prevalence increases with age, occurring in 3.8% of people age 60 and older and in up to 9% of people over age 80 [1].

One of the fundamental considerations in the management of AF is whether or not to attempt to restore sinus rhythm or to allow AF to continue while controlling the ventricular rates. The decision depends on the severity of symptoms, associated heart disease, age, and other comorbidities that may limit therapeutic options.

AF can be classified as paroxysmal, persistent, or permanent. Paroxysmal AF terminates spontaneously, with episodes typically lasting less than 24 hours but possibly lasting up to 7 days. Persistent AF requires cardioversion (pharmacologic or electrical) to terminate, and episodes last greater than 7 days. Permanent AF describes continuous AF that has failed cardioversion or where cardioversion never has been attempted. Recurrent AF describes two or more episodes of paroxysmal or persistent AF.

Determining how symptomatic patients are from AF can be difficult. Symptoms of palpitations, dyspnea, lightheadedness, or syncope generally are related to rapid, irregular ventricular rates. By slowing the heart rate with atrioventricular (AV) nodal blocking agents, these symptoms may abate. Some patients may notice a subtle decline in exercise tolerance or complain of generalized fatigue despite adequate rate control resulting from loss of atrial mechanical function. Patients who have hypertension, left ventricular hypertrophy, impaired diastolic relaxation, and restrictive cardiomyopathy are particularly sensitive to the loss of AV synchrony and the resultant decrease

---

* Corresponding author. Division of Cardiovascular diseases, Main Line Heart Center, 556 Medical Office, Building East, 100 Lancaster Avenue, Wynnewood, PA 19096.
E-mail address: koweyp@mlhs.org (P.R. Kowey).

0025-7125/08/$ - see front matter © 2008 Elsevier Inc. All rights reserved.
doi:10.1016/j.mcna.2007.08.002
medical.theclinics.com

in diastolic filling. Patients who clearly are symptomatic from AF may benefit from an attempt to control rhythm. In asymptomatic patients who have no appreciable decline in functional status in AF, rate control may be sufficient.

Rhythm versus rate control

Multiple prospective randomized studies have examined the issue of rhythm versus rate control. The two largest trials, Atrial Fibrillation Follow-up Investigation of Rhythm Management (AFFIRM) and Rate Control Versus Electrical Cardioversion for Persistent Atrial Fibrillation (RACE), failed to show any benefit in the rhythm control arm [2,3]. The AFFIRM trial enrolled more than 4000 patients who had paroxysmal and persistent AF. Patients were randomized to receive rate control or antiar-rhythmic drug therapy. All patients initially were anticoagulated, but patients in the rhythm control group who had remained in sinus rhythm for at least 3 months could stop warfarin. There was no significant difference in the primary endpoint of overall mortality, with a trend toward increased risk in the rhythm control group (5-year mortality, 24% versus 21%). A trend toward higher risk for ischemic stroke was seen in the rhythm control group, however, mainly in patients who were not receiving adequate anticoagulation. This emphasizes the need for indefinite anticoagulation for rate and rhythm control methods in high-risk patients, as asymptomatic recurrences of AF predispose to thromboembolic events.

The RACE trial randomized 522 patients who had persistent AF, despite previous electrical cardioversion, into rate control or rhythm control groups. All patients were anticoagulated. The study protocol allowed patients in the rhythm control group who had maintained sinus rhythm for 1 month the option of discontinuing warfarin therapy. The primary end-point was a composite of death from cardiovascular causes, heart failure, thromboembolic complications, bleeding, implantation of a pacemaker, or severe adverse reactions to drugs. After a mean of 2.3 years of follow-up, the trial found rate control was not inferior to rhythm control for the pre-vention of death or morbidity. Only 39% of the rhythm control group was in sinus rhythm compared with 10% of the rate control group. Within the rhythm control group, hypertension and female gender were associated with a higher risk for an event. Higher rates of thromboembolic events occurred in the rhythm control group, with the majority of the events asso-ciated with subtherapeutic anticoagulation. Cessation of anticoagulation also was associated with a higher risk for thromboembolic events.

To address the issue of whether or not patients had any difference in ex-ercise tolerance with rate versus rhythm control, a substudy of the AFFIRM trial performed serial 6-minute walk tests on 245 study patients [4]. Walk distances improved in both groups over time, with slightly longer distances observed in the rhythm control group. It was unclear whether or not the difference in walk distances was clinically significant.

The results from the AFFIRM and RACE trials are most applicable to elderly patients (mean ages of study patients were 70 and 68, respectively) who have few or no symptoms from AF, for whom anticoagulation and a strategy of rate control may be most appropriate. For younger, symptomatic patients who do not have underlying heart disease, restoration of sinus rhythm still must be considered a valid approach.

Rate control agents

The goal of rate control is to control the resting heart rate and the heart rate during exercise while avoiding excessive bradycardia. Persistent tachycardia may lead to development of cardiomyopathy, which usually is reversible with adequate rate control. Although criteria for adequate rate control vary among trials, typical goals for ventricular rates range from 60 to 80 beats per minute at rest and between 90 and 115 beats per minute during exercise [5]. Given that rates may be well controlled at rest but may increase significantly during exercise, it is useful to record heart rates during exercise stress testing or by 24-hour ambulatory EKG monitoring.

Ventricular rate during AF is a factor of the refractoriness of the AV node, sympathetic and parasympathetic tone, and intrinsic conduction. Agents that prolong the refractory period of the AV node effectively control ventricular rate. β-Blockers, calcium channel blockers, and digoxin all slow conduction through the AV node and may be used alone or in combination for rate control.

β-Blockers are the most effective monotherapy for rate control, especially in high adrenergic states. In the AFFIRM trial, 70% of patients on β-blockers achieved adequate rate control (as defined previously) compared with 54% of patients on calcium channel blockers [2]. In the acute setting, intravenous beta-blockade with esmolol, metoprolol, propanolol, or atenolol has a rapid onset. Esmolol may be given as a continuous intravenous infusion. Caution is advised when starting β-blockers in patients who have heart failure or hypotension. In hemodynamically stable patients, oral beta-blockade is safe and effective for controlling ventricular rates. Sotalol, a β-blocker with Vaughan-Williams class III antiarrhythmic properties that suppresses AF, is associated with slower ventricular rates with AF recurrences.

Calcium channel blockers (nondihydropyridines) may be preferred in patients who have preserved left ventricular systolic function and severe chronic obstructive pulmonary disease. Verapamil and diltiazem are equally effective in controlling ventricular rates. Given intravenously, calcium channel blockers have a rapid onset of action (2–7 minutes). To maintain effectiveness, a continuous drip usually is given because of the drugs' short half-lives.

Digoxin, once considered first-line treatment for rate control in the acute management of AF, is less effective than β-blockers or calcium channel blockers. Intravenous digoxin requires 60 minutes to take effect, whereas its peak effect may not be seen for 6 hours. Digoxin is not shown more effective than placebo in converting AF to sinus rhythm. Digoxin may be used in patients who cannot tolerate β-blockers or calcium channel blockers because of heart failure or hypotension. Digoxin is less effective in settings of high sympathetic tone and does not slow heart rates during exercise. In sedentary patients who do not exercise, digoxin alone may be sufficient to control rates at rest [5]. Often, patients require combination therapy to achieve sufficient rate control.

Rhythm control: pharmacologic cardioversion

Once the decision is made to proceed with restoration of sinus rhythm, it can be pursued pharmacologically or electrically. The duration of AF is an important factor. Patients who have recent-onset AF (less than 48 hours) have a high rate of spontaneous conversion, up to 60% at 24 hours [6]. Pharmacologic or electrical cardioversion in this setting allows faster restoration of sinus rhythm, with resolution of symptoms and shorter lengths of stay. Success rates for direct current electrical cardioversion range from 75% to 93%. Administration of antiarrhythmic drugs before electrical cardioversion increases long-term success rates. Achievement of sinus rhythm with pharmacologic cardioversion alone varies by agent, averaging approximately 50% after 1 to 5 hours [7]. Biphasic electrical cardioversion may be more effective than pharmacologic cardioversion but requires pain control (general anesthesia or conscious sedation) and a 6- to 8-hour fasting period.

Once an episode of AF is present for more than 7 days, electrical cardioversion is preferred. Spontaneous conversion rates are much lower after 1 week, and pharmacologic therapy also is less effective. With either method, adequate anticoagulation must be achieved before cardioversion and for a period of 4 weeks after, as the risks for thromboembolic events are similar.

Maintenance of sinus rhythm

For patients who have recurrent paroxysmal or persistent AF, the choice of agent for long-term antiarrhythmic therapy must be individualized. The benefit of maintaining sinus rhythm must be balanced with the side-effect profile of the antiarrhythmic drug. Even after successful cardioversion, recurrence of AF is high in untreated patients, with relapse rates of 71% to 84% at 1 year [8]. Using a rhythm control strategy, recurrence is reduced by 30% to 50% [8].

Amiodarone is the most effective drug for preventing recurrence of AF [8–10]. In the Sotalol Amiodarone Atrial Fibrillation Efficacy Trial (SAFE-T), 665 patients who had persistent AF were randomized to receive amiodarone, sotalol, or placebo and followed for 1 to 4.5 years. Recurrence rates at 1 year were 48% with amiodarone, 68% with sotalol, and 87% in the placebo group. A higher incidence of minor bleeding episodes was seen in the amiodarone group, likely because of interaction with warfarin levels [11]. The Canadian Trial of Atrial Fibrillation (CTAF) found similar results among 403 patients assigned to amiodarone, sotalol, or propafenone. After a mean follow-up period of 16 months, the recurrence rate for the amiodarone group was 35%, compared with 63% in the sotalol or propafenone group. However, 18% of patients in the amiodarone group withdrew because of adverse events compared with 11% in the sotalol or propafenone group [9]. In a post hoc analysis of the Veterans Affairs Congestive Heart Failure: Survival Trial of Antiarrhythmic Therapy (CHF-STAT), amiodarone facilitated conversion to and maintenance of sinus rhythm in patients who had left ventricular systolic dysfunction. Furthermore, the subset of patients who were maintained in sinus rhythm had lower overall mortality. Amiodarone was not linked to worsening of heart failure [12]. Despite its effectiveness over other agents, the lengthy list of potential adverse effects associated with amiodarone use makes it a second-line agent in patients who do not have contraindications to other antiarrhythmic drugs. Major side effects of amiodarone include potentially fatal pulmonary toxicity, thyroid dysfunction, hepatic toxicity, optic neuropathy, peripheral neuropathy, gastrointestinal upset, skin discoloration, and, rarely, torsades de pointes.

In patients who have no evidence of structural heart disease, class IC agents are first-line therapy for maintaining sinus rhythm, based on the guidelines recently issued by the American College of Cardiology, American Heart Association, and European Society of Cardiology [5]. Propafenone and flecainide generally are well tolerated, show similar effectiveness, and have a low risk for toxicity [13]. The Rythmol Atrial Fibrillation Trial (RAFT), a randomized control trial of 523 patients, tested sustained-release propafenone in three doses (225 mg, 325 mg, and 425 mg). At the end of the 39-week follow-up period, recurrence rate of AF was 69% in the placebo group compared with 52%, 42%, and 30% in the propafenone groups (225 mg, 325 mg, and 425 mg, respectively). Similar results were found in the European Rythmol/Rytmonorm Atrial Fibrillation Trial (ERAFT) of similar design [14]. There were significantly higher withdrawals because of adverse events in the 425-mg group than any other group [15]. Propafenone may cause gastrointestinal symptoms, such as nausea, and should be avoided in patients who have severe obstructive lung disease. Flecainide may cause mild neurologic side effects. Side effects of both agents may include hypotension and bradycardia after conversion to sinus rhythm. Class IC agents also may convert AF into a slow atrial flutter. The slow flutter rate may conduct 1:1, causing rapid ventricular conduction with a wide complex QRS, which may be mistaken for ventricular tachycardia. To prevent rapid ventricular rates, an agent to slow AV nodal conduction, such as a β-blocker or calcium channel blocker, may be coadministered with propafenone or flecainide. Because of the negative inotropic effect and proarrhythmic potential of class IC drugs, they should be avoided in patients who have heart failure or ischemic heart disease.

Sotalol, although not a useful agent for cardioverting AF to sinus rhythm, can be used to maintain sinus rhythm. Sotalol is a nonselective β-blocker, in addition to its class III potassium channel-blocking effects. Sotalol has the added benefit of slowing AV nodal conduction should AF recur, which may decrease symptoms during AF episodes. In the SAFE-T and CTAF studies, recurrence rates of AF with sotalol were significantly lower compared with placebo, although higher than with amiodarone [9,11]. Sotalol prolongs the QT interval and has a risk for torsades de pointes. Sotalol should not be used in patients who have significant left ventricular hypertrophy or heart failure.

Dofetilide is a class III antiarrhythmic drug that selectively inhibits the delayed rectifier potassium current and increases the atrial and ventricular effective refractory period, thus prolonging repolarization. Plasma concentrations peak 2 to 3 hours after oral dosing. The corrected QT interval (QTc) lengthens in a linear, dose-dependent fashion. Unlike class IC agents, dofetilide has no negative inotropic effects. The safety of dofetilide in heart failure has been studied by the Danish Investigations of Arrhythmia and Mortality ON Dofetilide (DIAMOND) study group in two large randomized control trials, DIAMOND-CHF and DIAMOND-AF [16,17]. DIAMOND-CHF enrolled 1518 patients who had severe symptomatic left ventricular dysfunction randomized to dofetilide or placebo. The primary endpoint was all-cause mortality. After a median of 18 months' follow-up, there was no difference in survival in the two groups (41% versus 42%). DIAMOND-AF was a substudy of 506 heart failure patients who had baseline AF or flutter. Over the course of the study, 44% in the dofetilide group converted to sinus rhythm by 1 year compared with 14% in the placebo group. At 1 year, patients receiving dofetilide had a 79% probability of maintaining sinus rhythm versus 42% in the placebo arm.

Because of its QTc prolonging effect, dofetilide use carries a risk for torsades de pointes. In the DIAMOND-CHF study, the incidence of torsades de pointes was 3.3%, with 76% of cases occurring within 3 days of initiation of dofetilide. During the study, dose reduction based on creatinine clearance decreased the incidence of torsades de pointes [16]. The risk for torsades de pointes can be minimized by adjusting the dose for renal function, along with instituting a 72-hour in-hospital monitoring period on initiation of dofetilide.

The Symptomatic Atrial Fibrillation Investigative Research on Dofetilide (SAFIRE-D) tested safety and efficacy of dofetilide in a group of 325 patients who had persistent AF. The trial reported a 58% efficacy for maintaining sinus rhythm at 1 year (versus 25% with placebo) along with a much lower incidence of torsades de pointes (0.8%) compared with DIAMOND-AF. Dofetilide dosing in this study was reduced for impaired renal function and for prolongation of the QTc over 15% of baseline [18]. Similar results were reported in the European and Australian Multicenter Evaluative Research on Atrial Fibrillation and Dofetilide (EMERALD) study [19].

Because of the complexity of dosing regimens, the United States Food and Drug Administration (FDA) has restricted prescription of dofetilide to registered hospitals, physicians, pharmacists, and nurses who have completed specific training in the use of the drug.

Selection of a specific antiarrhythmic agent usually is determined by the presence or absence of underlying cardiac disease (Fig. 1). Class IC antiarrhythmic drugs are contraindicated in patients who have marked left ventricular hypertrophy, coronary artery disease, or congestive heart failure because of the risk for ventricular arrhythmias. In patients who do not have structural heart disease, flecainide, propafenone, or sotalol is preferred because of their effectiveness and low risk for toxicity. Among class III drugs, dofetilide and sotalol are associated with QT prolongation and torsades de pointes and should be avoided in the presence of marked left ventricular hypertrophy. In patients who have congestive heart failure, only amiodarone and dofetilide are safe for use.

Outpatient versus inpatient initiation of therapy

For paroxysmal AF, inpatient versus outpatient initiation of antiarrhythmic drug therapy is an important consideration. For symptomatic patients, the "pill-in-the-pocket" approach uses self-administration of a single dose of a drug shortly after the start of palpitations. The goal of this method is to terminate an episode and prevent recurrence while decreasing the need for emergency room visits, hospitalizations, and direct current cardioversions. This approach has been studied in patients who do not have structural heart disease, primarily with flecainide and propafenone [20]. After oral administration, an effect usually is seen in 3 to 4 hours [21].

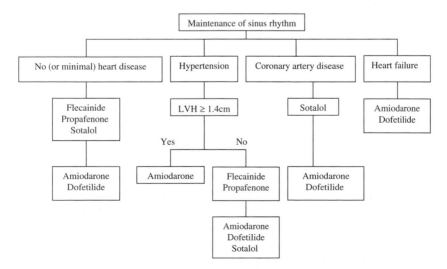

Fig. 1. Algorithm for antiarrhythmic drugs selection for maintenance of sinus rhythm.

Certain class III agents may be started as outpatient treatment in certain patient populations under careful observation. Sotalol may be initiated as outpatient treatment in patients who have little or no heart disease, if the baseline QT interval is less than 450 milliseconds, the electrolytes are normal, and there are no predisposing factors to development of torsades de pointes [5]. Amiodarone has low proarrhythmic potential and may be prescribed without an inpatient evaluation in patients who do not have severe conduction disease. Dofetilide, by FDA mandate, requires inpatient monitoring for initiation.

Patients maintained on antiarrhythmic drugs need close follow-up [22]. Those on class III agents should have renal function, potassium, and magnesium levels checked periodically. An EKG should be performed every 6 months to measure the QT interval. Echocardiograms and stress testing should be checked at appropriate intervals for ischemic disease in patients on class IC antiarrhythmics. Amiodarone use mandates semiannual monitoring of thyroid, liver, and pulmonary function and yearly ocular examinations.

Future pharmacologic therapy

The marginal efficacy and safety of commercially available drugs has stimulated the development of new compounds in two major directions: (1) modification of existing drugs and (2) designing drugs with new targets. Table 1 is a list of investigational compounds and their putative mechanism of action [23,24]. Although much interest has been generated by the modification of current class III agents, the discovery and characterization of novel ion channels believed to participate in onset and perpetuation of AF has provided a new way forward in drug development. Much of the research has focused on blocking potassium channels but several new ideas are being explored.

The next paragraphs review the current evidence that supports the potential usefulness of these novel compounds.

Amiodarone analogs

Dronedarone

Dronedarone is an amiodarone-like compound that lacks the iodine moiety that may be responsible for the pulmonary, thyroid, hepatic, and ocular toxicity of amiodarone. Like amiodarone, dronedarone has complex antiarrhythmic properties that span all classes of the Vaughan-Williams classification. Dronedarone inhibits potassium currents I_{Na}, I_{Kr}, and I_{KAch} and L-type calcium current; has α- and β-adrenergic blocking properties; and prolongs the action potential duration in atria and ventricles with no significant reverse-use dependence. Dronedarone and amiodarone have similar electrophysiologic properties in animal models, but their pharmacokinetic profiles differ

Table 1
Investigational antiarrhythmic drug in development

Modification of existing compound	Novel mechanism of action
Amiodarone analogs	Serotonin type 4 antagonists
Dronedarone (I_{Kr} I_{Ks} β1 I_{Ca} I_{to} I_{Na})	Piboserod
Celivarone (I_{Kr} I_{Ks} β1 I_{Ca} I_{to} I_{Na})	RS100302
ATI-2042 (I_{Kr} I_{Ks} β1 I_{Ca} I_{to} I_{Na})	SB203186
ATI-2001 (I_{Kr} I_{Ks} β1 I_{Ca} I_{to} I_{Na})	Atrial selective repolarization delaying agents
GYKI-16638 (I_{Kr} I_{KI} I_{Na})	AZD 7009 (I_{Kr} I_{Na} I_{Kur})
KB 130015 (I_{KAch} I_{Na} I_{Ca} I_{KATP})	AVE 0118 (I_{Kur} I_{to})
Conventional class III agents	AVE 1231 (I_{Kur} I_{to})
Azimilide (I_{Kr} I_{Ks})	Vernakalant (I_{Kur} I_{to} I_{Na} I_{Ach})
Tedisamil (I_{Kr} I_{to} I_{KATP} I_{Kur} I_{Na})	Almokalant (I_{Kur} I_{to} I_{Na} I_{Ach})
Bertosamil (I_{Kr} I_{to} I_{KATP} I_{Kur} I_{Na})	Terikalant (I_{Kur} I_{to} I_{Na} I_{Ach})
SB-237376 (I_{Kr})	Nifekalant (I_{Kur} I_{to} I_{Na} I_{Ach})
NIP-142 (I_{Kur} I_{KAch})	S-9947 (I_{Kur})
L-768673 (I_{Ks})	S-20951 (I_{Kur})
HMR-1556 (I_{Ks})	Miscellaneous compounds
HMR-1402($I_{Ks.}$ I_{ATP})	ZP-123 (GAP 486)
Miscellaneous compounds	AAP 10 (connexin modulator)
Ersentilide (I_{Kr} β)	GsMtx4 (stretch receptor)
Trecetilide (I_{Kr} β)	
CP060S (I_{Na} I_{Ca})	
KB-R7943 (I_{Na} I_{Ca})	
Cariporide (I_{Na} I_{H})	
JTV-519 (I_{Na} I_{Kr} I_{Ca})	

The drugs are classified by mechanism of action.

Abbreviations: β, β-adrenergic antagonist; I_{Ca}, inward calcium current; I_{Kach}, Ach-sensitive inward potassium current; I_{KATP}, ATP-sensitive inward potassium current; I_{KI}, inward potassium rectifier; I_{Kr}, rapid component of the delayed rectifier potassium inward current; I_{KS}, slow component of the delayed rectifier potassium inward current; I_{Kur}, ultra rapid component of the delayed rectifier potassium inward current; I_{Na}, inward sodium current; I_{to}, transient outward potassium current.

Data from Goldstein RN, Stambler BS. New antiarrhythmic drugs for prevention of atrial fibrillation. Prog Cardiovasc Dis 2005;48(3):193–208; and Pecini R, Elming H, Pedersen OD, et al. New antiarrhythmic agents for atrial fibrillation and atrial flutter. Expert Opin Emerg Drugs 2005;10(2):311–22.

significantly. Dronedarone has a 24-hour half-life and far less tissue accumulation [25,26].

The Dronedarone Atrial Fibrillation Study After Electrical Cardioversion (DAFNE) trial was designed to determine the most appropriate dose of dronedarone for prevention of AF after cardioversion. After 6-months' follow-up, 800 mg daily was deemed the optimal dose [27]. Thyroid, pulmonary, ocular, hepatic toxicity, or proarrhythmic effects were not seen at any of the study doses.

In the European Trial in Atrial Fibrillation or Flutter Patients Receiving Dronedarone for the Maintenance of Sinus Rhythm (EURIDIS) and its sister trial, the American-Australian-African Trial with Dronedarone in Atrial Fibrillation or Flutter Patients for the Maintenance of Sinus Rhythm

(ADONIS), dronedarone administered at a dose of 400 mg twice daily was effective in preventing symptomatic and asymptomatic recurrences of AF or atrial flutter, the primary endpoint of the trials. A secondary endpoint of both trials, mean ventricular rate during AF atrial flutter at first recorded recurrence, also was reduced significantly. The incidence of adverse events in both trials was similar in the dronedarone and placebo groups [28].

In the phase III study, Efficacy and Safety of Dronedarone for the Control of Ventricular Rate (ERATO), dronedarone was tested in patients who had symptomatic permanent AF for its effect on heart rate. Dronedarone significantly reduced average resting and maximal exercise heart rates compared with placebo [29].

The Antiarrhythmic Trial with Dronedarone in Moderate to Severe Congestive Heart Failure Evaluating Morbidity Decrease (ANDROMEDA) was a double-blind, placebo-controlled study evaluating the tolerability of dronedarone in high-risk patients who had congestive heart failure and ventricular dysfunction. The primary endpoint of the trial was death or hospitalization for heart failure The study was ended prematurely after an interim safety analysis showed an excess risk for death in patients on active treatment [30].

Because ANDROMEDA raised concerns over the safety of dronedarone in the heart failure population, further studies are needed. The ongoing trial, A Trial With Dronedarone to Prevent Hospitalization or Death in Patients With Atrial Fibrillation (ATHENA), will examine further the safety and efficacy of dronedarone in a larger study group [31]. Inclusion of patients who have ejection fractions of less than 40% will help elucidate the role of dronedarone in a more ill patient population.

Celivarone

Celivarone (SSR149744C) is a new noniodinated benzofuran derivative structurally related to amiodarone and dronedarone. Like its parent compounds, celivarone inhibits several potassium currents: I_{Kr}, I_{Ks}, I_{KAch}, $I_{Kv1.5}$, and the L-type calcium current. Studies in canine models show relative atrial selectivity [32]. Two clinical trials currently are evaluating the role of celivarone in conversion and maintenance of AF.

The Maintenance of Sinus Rhythm in Patients with Recent Atrial Fibrillation/Flutter (MAIA) trial, a placebo controlled double-blind study, is comparing the efficacy and safety of celivarone in a range of dosages to amiodarone for maintenance of sinus rhythm after electrical, pharmacologic, or spontaneous conversion of AF or atrial flutter [33].

The Double Blind Placebo Controlled Dose Ranging Study of the Efficacy and Safety of ssr149744c 300 or 600 mg for the Conversion of Atrial Fibrillation/Flutter (CORYFEE) trial will assess the efficacy of celivarone in converting AF or flutter to sinus rhythm at the time of planned electrical cardioversion [34].

ATI-2001 and related compounds

ATI-2001 is a synthetic amiodarone analog shown to retain the electro-physiologic properties of amiodarone in regards to ventricular tachyar-rhythmia initiation, perpetuation, and termination in guinea pigs isolated hearts [35]. In the same animal model, ATI-2001 was significantly more potent than amiodarone in its atrial and AV nodal electrophysiologic prop-erties [36]. A recent study, however, showed that the half-life of ATI-2001 in human plasma is only 12 minutes, making the drug more suitable for acute termination of arrhythmias than for long-term management [37]. Of the ATI-2001 congeners, ATI-2042 may have more favorable pharmacokinetic properties and currently is in phase 2 development [38].

Traditional class III agents

Azimilide

Azimilide is a selective once-daily class III antiarrhythmic agent that prolongs action, potential duration,and refractory periods in both atria and lacks reverse-use dependence [39]. The optimal dose, as determined in the Azimilide Supraventricular Arrhythmia Program (ASAP), was 125 mg daily [40]. Unfortunately, after 180 days' follow-up, only 50% of patients enrolled maintained sinus rhythm.

The Azimilide Postinfarct Survival Evaluation (ALIVE), a large random-ized trial of high-risk patients, as defined by low ejection fraction and recent myocardial infarction, showed no difference in all-cause mortality. The azimilide group, however, had fewer occurrences of AF and higher mainte-nance of sinus rhythm at 1 year [41].

Three other studies have evaluated the role of azimilide in the treatment of symptomatic supraventricular arrhythmias [42]. The North American Azimilide Cardioversion Maintenance Trial (A-COMET) I investigated the role of azimilide compared with placebo for maintenance of sinus rhythm after electrical cardioversion of patients who had symptomatic AF. There was no significant difference between placebo and azimilide [43].

The A-COMET II Trial, conducted in Europe, compared azimilide (125 mg daily) to sotalol (160 mg twice daily) or placebo in patients under-going electrical cardioversion. Although azimilide was superior to placebo, it was inferior to sotalol with regard to efficacy and safety [44]. The Azimilide Supraventricular Tachyarrhythmia Reduction (A-STAR) trial also tested 125 mg of azimilide daily versus placebo in patients who had symptomatic paroxysmal AF and structural heart disease. The primary endpoint was the time to the first symptomatic recurrence. No statistically significant difference was seen in the study groups [45].

Although in these trials azimilide generally was well tolerated, early-onset, reversible neutropenia has been reported in 0.2% and torsades de pointes in 0.9% of patients [46]. Based on its modest efficacy and these safety issues, it is unlikely that azimilide will be available for the treatment of AF.

Tedisamil

Tedisamil is a class III antiarrhythmic agent that blocks multiple potassium channels and slows sinus rate. Tedisamil prolongs action potential duration more strongly in the atria than in the ventricles [47]. Tedisamil also possesses significant antianginal and anti-ischemic properties.

In a study of 175 patients, tedisamil was shown to be superior to placebo in acutely terminating AF or atrial flutter [48]. The study, however, showed significant lengthening of the QTc and a 4% risk for ventricular tachycardia during the administration of the drug at its higher dose. Larger-scale studies are in progress to assess the safety and efficacy of tedisamil, although the initial report of torsades de pointes may make it a less desirable compound for widespread clinical use. Bertosamil, a structural analog of tedisamil, has similar pharmacologic properties. It has been studied in vitro but no clinical trials to date have been performed to validate its safety and efficacy.

Atrial repolarization delaying agents

Vernakalant

Vernakalant (RSD1235) is a sodium and potassium channel blocker with atrial selectivity [49,50]. The drug is demonstrated as safe in a variety of doses in healthy volunteers [51]. Initial studies showed vernakalant superior to placebo in the acute termination of recent-onset AF, with a 61% conversion rate [52]. The preliminary results of two-phase III studies recently were reported [53]. In the Atrial Arrhythmia Conversion Trials (ACTs) 1 and 3, vernakalant was superior to placebo in converting AF to sinus rhythm, but only in patients who had recent onset AF. No cases of torsades de pointes were reported.

ACT 4 recently was started to gather additional efficacy and safety data to supplement ACT 1 and ACT 3 pivotal trial results [54]. The ongoing study, ACT 2, is evaluating vernakalant for prevention of recurrence of AF and conversion of atrial arrhythmia to sinus rhythm in subjects after valvular or coronary artery bypass graft surgery [55,56].

AVE0118

AVE0118 selectively blocks I_{Kur}, I_{to}, and I_{KACh} in atrial tissue in several preclinical models [57,58]. In animal models, AVE0118 successfully converted 63% of persistent AF and increased the fibrillation wavelength significantly. Unlike dofetilide and ibutilide, AVE0118 did not have any appreciable effect on QT duration. Although preliminary studies of AVE0118 in animal models show promise, safety and efficacy in humans not yet are established.

AZD7009

AZD7009 is a mixed ion channel blocker (I_{Kr}, I_{Na}, and I_{Kur}) that prolongs atrial repolarization [59]. Animal models showed that AZD7009 effectively terminated all sustained episodes of induced AF and atrial flutter and prevented 95% of recurrences. Although QTc interval prolongation was noted, torsades de pointes were not induced [60].

A phase II clinical trial designed to assess the efficacy and safety of intravenous AZD7009 in conversion of AF currently is in progress [61].

Serotonin antagonists

The serotonin type 4 receptors are found in the atria but not in the ventricles. Stimulation of serotonin type 4 receptors of atrial human cells in vitro produces positive chronotropic effects and induces arrhythmias [62,63]. Efficacy of RS-100302, a selective serotonin type 4 antagonist, was tested in a pig model of AF and atrial flutter [64]. In experimental conditions, the agent terminated atrial flutter in 75% of the animals and AF in 88% of the animals and prevented reinduction of sustained tachycardia in all animals.

At this time, there are not any positive clinical trial data with serotonin type 4 antagonists.

Adjuvant therapy for maintenance of sinus rhythm

RAAS

Angiotensin-converting enzyme inhibitors
Remodeling of atrial tissue may contribute to the initiation and perpetuation of AF, especially in the heart failure population (Table 2). Recent studies show that blockade of RAAS prevents left atrial dilatation and atrial fibrosis, slows atrial conduction velocity, and reduces inflammation [65,66]. Several human and animal models show that the inhibition of the RAAS

Table 2
Drugs used as adjuvant therapy of atrial fibrillation and their proposed mechanism of action

Drugs	Proposed mechanism of action
ACE-I	Blockade of the RAAS
ARB	Inhibition of atrial remodeling
Aldosterone	Inhibition of atrial fibrosis
	Anti-inflammatory effect
Omega-3 fatty acids	Unclear, may be direct antiarrhythmic effect
Steroids	Anti-inflammatory effect
Statins	Anti-inflammatory effect

may help prevent AF [67]. A substudy of the Trandolapril Cardiac Evaluation (TRACE) trial analyzed patients who had sinus rhythm at the time of randomization. After a 2 to 4 years of follow-up, significantly more patients in the placebo group developed AF compared with the trandolapril group [68]. Similarly, a retrospective analysis conducted by a single center participating in the Studies of Left Ventricular Dysfunction (SOLVD) revealed that treatment with enalapril markedly reduced the risk for developing AF in patients who had heart failure [69]. In a longitudinal cohort study that included hypertensive patients treated with antiogensin-converting enzyme inhibitors (ACE-Is) or calcium channel blockers, ACE-Is were associated with a lower incidence of developing AF [70]. This favorable effect of ACE-Is is supported further by meta-analyses of published data [71,72]. The addition of enalapril to amiodarone increases the chances of maintaining sinus rhythm after cardioversion compared with amiodarone alone [73]. A study currently in progress will test the hypothesis that angiotensin-converting enzyme inhibition with ramipril or aldosterone receptor antagonism with spironolactone will decrease the incidence of AF in patients undergoing cardiothoracic surgery [74].

Angiotensin receptor blockers

Clinical and experimental data support the notion that angiotensin receptor blockers (ARBs) have similar effects as ACE-Is in affecting atrial structural remodeling and reducing atrial arrhythmias [75,76]. A retrospective analysis of two large randomized clinical trials, Valsartan Heart Failure Trial (Val-HeFT) and Losartan Intervention for Endpoint Reduction in Hypertension (LIFE), demonstrates that valsartan and losartan significantly reduced new-onset AF compared with the control groups, respectively, placebo and atenolol [77,78]. These findings were confirmed further in a prospective trial of hypertensive patients who had paroxysmal AF randomized to losartan or amlodipine, both in combination with amiodarone [79]. Also, treatment with irbesartan and amiodarone was found more effective than amiodarone alone in preventing recurrence of AF after electrical cardioversion [80].

Conversely, the Candesartan in the Prevention of Relapsing Atrial Fibrillation (CAPRAF) trial did not show significant difference in maintenance of sinus rhythm after electrical cardioversion in patients treated with candesartan or placebo [81].

Larger prospective trials are needed to test the efficacy of ARBs in adjunctive treatment of AF. The results of ongoing prospective trials, such as Angiotensin II-Antagonist in Paroxysmal Atrial Fibrillation (ANTIPAF) trial [82] and the Gruppo Italiano per lo Studio della Sopravvivenza nell'Infarto Miocardico (GISSI)–Atrial Fibrillation Trial [83], are awaited eagerly.

Aldosterone antagonists

Although to date no clinical trial has evaluated the effect of aldosterone blockade in AF, in vitro experimental data suggest a beneficial effect. Spironolactone and its major metabolite, canrenoic acid, successfully inactivated the potassium channels, HERG, hKv1.5, Kv4.3, and Kv7.1+mink, that generate the human I_{Kur}, I_{to} and I_{Ks} currents when transfected in murine cell lines [84,85]. Prospective clinical trials testing the efficacy of aldosterone antagonists are awaited.

Miscellaneous agents

Anti-inflammatory agents: steroids and statins

A largely unexplored field is the relationship between inflammation and AF. This seems of particular importance in postoperative states and in cases of myopericarditis. Some experimental models point to a role for steroids as anti-inflammatory agents. The use of prednisone at high doses in a canine model suppresses the expression of markers of inflammation and the onset and perpetuation of atrial flutter and AF [86].

A recently published trial of patients undergoing coronary bypass graft surgery with or without aortic valve replacement found that perioperative use of corticosteroids decreased the incidence of post operative AF [87]. The trial corroborated earlier findings from smaller studies [88,89], but because of their adverse effects, more evidence is needed before the routine use of corticosteroids can be recommended.

Statins exhibit anti-inflammatory properties. Given the theory that AF is linked to inflammation, studies have begun to examine whether or not statins decrease the occurrence of AF [90,91]. In a small study of persistent AF, the use of statins was associated with a significant decrease in the risk for arrhythmia recurrence after successful cardioversion [92]. In an observational study in a large outpatient cardiology practice, statin therapy seemed protective against the development of AF [93]. Statins are effective in preventing AF after lung, esophageal, and coronary bypass surgery [94,95].

The Atorvastatin Therapy for the Prevention of Atrial Fibrillation (SToP-AF) trial is a prospective randomized placebo controlled study that will test whether or not atorvastatin (80 mg daily) can reduce the recurrence rate of AF after elective electrical cardioversion compared with standard therapy [96].

Omega-3 fatty acids

Incorporation of dietary omega-3 fatty acids into rabbit atrial tissue reduces stretch-induced susceptibility to AF [97]. In a study of patients who had paroxysmal atrial tachycardia and an implanted permanent pacemaker, daily intake of omega-3 fatty (1g) acids reduced the number of episodes and total burden of atrial arrhythmia significantly [98]. Additionally, a recent trial randomized patients undergoing elective coronary bypass surgery to omega-3 fatty acids (2 g daily) or placebo [99]. Patients receiving omega-3 fatty acid had a significantly lower incidence of postoperative AF and a shorter hospital stay than those receiving placebo.

The Rotterdam study prospectively examined the relationship between dietary fish intake, long-chain omega-3 fatty acid supplementation, and the incidence of AF. After a mean follow-up of 6.4 years, neither omega-3 fatty acid nor dietary fish intake was linked to a lower incidence of AF [100].

Given conflicting results in the current literature, large randomized control trials are needed to delineate better what effect, if any, omega-3 fatty acids have on AF. These trials are in progress.

Summary

Many options are available for the treatment of AF. The results of large clinical trials, such as AFFIRM and RACE, suggest that controlling ventricular rates during AF is a valid approach. For symptomatic patients, sinus rhythm can be restored and maintained using pharmacologic or ablative therapy. Table 3 lists the antiarrhythmic drugs currently available for use in patients who have AF. In addition to these drugs, several agents that target remodeling and inflammation can be used for prevention of AF or as adjunctive therapy. New and promising pharmacologic agents

Table 3
Currently available drugs for treatment of atrial fibrillation according to the Vaughan-Williams classification, their mechanism of action, and their main adverse effects

Drug	Mechanism of action	Main adverse effect
Class I		
Ia—quinidine	Sodium channel blockade, delays phase 0 of action potential	Torsades de pointes, diarrhea, dyspepsia, hypotension
Ic—flecainide	Sodium channel blockade, strongly delays phase 0 of action potential	Ventricular tachycardia, congestive heart failure, increased AV conduction
Ic—propafenone	Sodium channel blockade, strongly delays phase 0 of action potential	Ventricular tachycardia, congestive heart failure, increased AV conduction
Class III		
Amiodarone	Multichannel blockade	Thyroid toxicity, pulmonary toxicity, hepatic toxicity, dyspepsia, QT prolongation, torsades de pointes (rare), hypotension, bradycardia
Sotalol	Potassium channel blockade (mainly I_{Kr}), β-receptor blockade	Torsades de pointes, congestive heart failure, bronchospasm
Dofetilide	Potassium channel blockade (mainly I_{Kr})	QT prolongation, torsades de pointes
Ibutilide	Potassium channel blockade (mainly I_{Kr}), activation of a slow, delayed I_{Na} current that occurs early during repolarization	QT prolongation, torsades de pointes

are under investigation. All of these approaches will increase the ability to control the increasing prevalence of AF, especially in the growing aging population.

References

[1] Go A, Hylek E, Phillips K, et al. Prevalence of diagnosed atrial fibrillation in adults: national implications for rhythm management and stroke prevention: the anticoagulation and risk factors in atrial fibrillation study. JAMA 2001;285:2370–5.

[2] Wyse DG, Waldo JP, DiMarco JM, et al. The AFFIRM Investigators. A comparison of rate control and rhythm control in patients with atrial fibrillation. N Engl J Med 2002; 347:1825–33.

[3] Van Gelder I, Hagens V, Bosker H, et al. A comparison of rate control and rhythm control in patients with recurrent persistent atrial fibrillation. N Engl J Med 2002;347:1834–40.

[4] Chung MK, Shemanski L, Sherman DG, et al. Functional status in rate–versus rhythm control strategies for atrial fibrillation. J Am Coll Cardiol 2005;46:1891–9.

[5] Fuster V, Ryden LE, Cannom DS, et al. ACC/AHA/ESC 2006 guidelines for the management of patients with atrial fibrillation. J Am Coll Cardiol 2006;48(4):e149–246.

[6] Naccarelli GV, Wolbrette DL, Bhatta L, et al. A review of clinical trials assessing the efficacy and safety of newer antiarrhythmic drugs in atrial fibrillation. J Interv Card Electrophysiol 2003;9:215–22.

[7] Nattel S, Lionel HO. Controversies in atrial fibrillation. Lancet 2006;367:262–72.

[8] Lafuente-Lafuente C, Mouly S, Longas-Tejero MA, et al. Antiarrhythmic drugs for maintaining sinus rhythm after cardioversion of atrial fibrillation. Arch Intern Med 2006;166:719–28.

[9] Naccarelli GV, Wolbrette DL, Khan M, et al. Old and new antiarrhythmic drugs for converting and maintaining siuns rhythm in atrial fibrillation: comparative efficacy and results of trials. Am J Cardiol 2003;91(Suppl):15D–26D.

[10] Roy D, Talajic M, Dorian P, et al. Amiodarone to prevent recurrence of atrial fibrillation. N Engl J Med 2000;342:913–20.

[11] Singh BN, Singh SN, Reda DJ, et al. Amiodarone versus sotalol for atrial fibrillation. N Engl J Med 2005;352:1861–72.

[12] Deedwania PC, Singh BN, Ellenbogen K, et al. Spontaneous conversion and maintenance of sinus rhythm by amiodarone in patients with heart failure and atrial fibrillation. Circulation 1998;98:2574–9.

[13] Chimenti M, Cullen MT, Casadei G. Safety of long-term flecainide and propafenone in the management of patients with symptomatic paroxysmal atrial fibrillation: report from the Flecainide and Propafenone Italian Study Investigators. Am J Cardiol 1996;77(3):60A–75A.

[14] Meinertz T, Lip GY, Lombardi F, et al. Efficacy and safety of propafenone sustained release in the prophylaxis of symptomatic paroxysmal atrial fibrillation (The European Rythmol/Rytmonorm Atrial Fibrillation Trial [ERAFT] Study). Am J Cardiol 2002; 90(12):1300–6.

[15] Pritchett ELC, Page RL, Carlson M, et al. Efficacy and safety of sustained-release propafenone (Propafenone SR) for patients with atrial fibrillation. Am J Cardiol 2003;92:941–6.

[16] Torp-Pederson C, Mooler M, Block-Thomsen PE, et al. Dofetilide in patients with congestive heart failure and left ventricular dysfunction. N Engl J Med 1999;341:857–65.

[17] Pedersen OD, Bagger H, Keller N, et al. Efficacy of Dofetilide in the treatment of atrial fibrillation-flutter in patients with reduced left ventricular function. Circulation 2001;104: 292–6.

[18] Singh S, Zoble RG, Yellen L, et al. Efficacy and safety of oral dofetilide in converting to and maintaining sinus rhythm in patients with chronic atrial fibrillation or atrial flutter. Circulation 2000;102:2385–90.

[19] Greenbaum RA, Campbell TJ, Channer KS, et al. Conversion of atrial fibrillation and maintenance of sinus rhythm by dofetilide. The EMERALD (European and Australian Multicenter Evaluative Research on Atrial Fibrillation Dofetilide) Study [abstract]. Circulation 1998;98:1633.

[20] Alboni P, Botto GL, Baldi N, et al. Outpatient treatment of recent-onset atrial fibrillation with the "Pill-in-the-Pocket" approach. N Engl J Med 2004;351:2384–91.

[21] Boriani G, Diemberger I, Biffi M, et al. Pharmacological cardioversion of atrial fibrillation: current management and treatment options. Drugs 2004;64(24):2741–62.

[22] Reiffel JA. Maintenance of normal sinus rhythm with antiarrhythmic drugs. In: Kowey P, Naccarelli G, editors. Atrial fibrillation. New York: Marcel Dekker; 2005. p. 195–217.

[23] Goldstein RN, Stambler BS. New antiarrhythmic drugs for prevention of atrial fibrillation. Prog Cardiovasc Dis 2005;48(3):193–208.

[24] Pecini R, Elming H, Pedersen OD, et al. New antiarrhythmic agents for atrial fibrillation and atrial flutter. Expert Opin Emerg Drugs 2005;10(2):311–22.

[25] Sun W, Sarma JS, Singh BN. Electrophysiological effects of dronedarone (SR33589), a noniodinated benzofuran derivative, in the rabbit heart: comparison with amiodarone. Circulation 1999;100(22):2276–81.

[26] Sun W, Sarma JS, Singh BN. Chronic and acute effects of dronedarone on the action potential of rabbit atrial muscle preparations: comparison with amiodarone. J Cardiovasc Pharmacol 2002;39(5):677–84.

[27] Touboul P, Brugada J, Capucci A, et al. Dronedarone for prevention of atrial fibrillation: a dose-ranging study. Eur Heart J 2003;24(16):1481–7.

[28] Hohnloser SH. EURIDIS and ADONIS: maintenance of sinus rhythm with dronedarone in patients with atrial fibrillation or flutter. Hot Line II: acute coronary syndromes/medical treatment II. Presented at the European Society of Cardiology Congress 2004. Munich (Germany), August 28–September 1, 2004.

[29] Davy JM, on behalf of the ERATO Investigators. Dronedarone demonstrates additional rate control on top of standard pharmacotherapies in the treatment of atrial fibrillation. American Heart Association, Scientific sessions 2005, session number APS.52.4, presentation 2737.

[30] Sanofi-Aventis. Discontinuation of one of the studies (ANDROMEDA) with dronedarone. 17 January 2003. Press release.

[31] Available at: http://www.clinicaltrials.gov Trial identifier NCT00174785.

[32] Gautier P, Guillemare E, Djandjighian L, et al. In vivo and in vitro characterization of the novel antiarrhythmic agent SSR149744C: electrophysiological, anti-adrenergic, and anti-angiotensin II effects. J Cardiovasc Pharmacol 2004;44(2):244–57.

[33] Available at: http://www.clinicaltrials.gov. Trial identifier NCT00233441.

[34] Available at: http://www.clinicaltrials.gov. Trial identifier NCT00232310.

[35] Raatikainen MJ, Napolitano CA, Druzgala P, et al. Electrophysiological effects of a novel, short-acting and potent ester derivative of amiodarone, ATI-2001, in guinea pig isolated heart. J Pharmacol Exp Ther 1996;277(3):1454–63.

[36] Raatikainen MJ, Morey TE, Druzgala P, et al. Potent and reversible effects of ATI-2001 on atrial and atrioventricular nodal electrophysiological properties in guinea pig isolated perfused heart. J Pharmacol Exp Ther 2000;295(2):779–85.

[37] Juhasz A, Bodor N. Cardiovascular studies on different classes of soft drugs. Pharmazie 2000;55(3):228–38.

[38] Morey TE, Seubert CN, Raatikainen MJ, et al. Structure-activity relationships and electrophysiological effects of short-acting amiodarone homologs in guinea pig isolated heart. J Pharmacol Exp Ther 2001;297(1):260–6.

[39] Salata JJ, Brooks R. Pharmacology of Azimilide Dihydrochloride (NE-10064). Cardiovasc Drug Rev 1997;15:137–56.

[40] Pritchett EL, Page RL, Connolly SJ, et al. Antiarrhythmic effects of azimilide in atrial fibrillation: efficacy and dose-response. Azimilide Supraventricular Arrhythmia Program 3 (SVA-3) Investigators. J Am Coll Cardiol 2000;36(3):794–802.

[41] Camm AJ, Pratt CM, Schwartz PJ, et al. AzimiLide post Infarct surVival Evaluation (ALIVE) Investigators. Mortality in patients after a recent myocardial infarction: a randomized, placebo-controlled trial of azimilide using heart rate variability for risk stratification. Circulation 2004;109(8):990–6.
[42] Page RL. A-STAR and A-COMET trials (Azimilide in atrial fibrillation) [abstract]. Europace 2002;3:A-2.
[43] Pritchett EL, Kowey P, Connolly S, et al. Antiarrhythmic efficacy of azimilide in patients with atrial fibrillation. Maintenance of sinus rhythm after conversion to sinus rhythm. Am Heart J 2006;151(5):1043–9.
[44] Lombardi F, Borggrefe M, Ruzyllo W, et al. Azimilide vs. placebo and sotalol for persistent atrial fibrillation: the A-COMET-II (Azimilide-CardiOversion MaintEnance Trial-II) trial. Eur Heart J 2006;27(18):2224–31.
[45] Kerr CR, Connolly SJ, Kowey P, et al. Efficacy of azimilide for the maintenance of sinus rhythm in patients with paroxysmal atrial fibrillation in the presence and absence of structural heart disease. Am J Cardiol 2006;98(2):215–8.
[46] Connolly SJ, Schnell DJ, Page RL, et al. Dose-response relations of azimilide in the management of symptomatic, recurrent, atrial fibrillation. Am J Cardiol 2001;88:974–9.
[47] Ravens U, Amos GJ, Li Q, et al. Effects of the antiarrhythmic agent tedisamil. Exp Clin Cardiol 1997;2:231–6.
[48] Hohnloser SH, Dorian P, Straub M, et al. Safety and efficacy of intravenously administered tedisamil for rapid conversion of recent-onset atrial fibrillation or atrial flutter. J Am Coll Cardiol 2004;44(1):99–104.
[49] Beatch GN, Shinagawa K, Johnson B, et al. RSD1235 selectively prolongs atrial refractoriness and terminates AF in dogs with electrically remodeled atria [abstract]. Pacing Clin Electrophysiol 2002;25:698.
[50] Beatch GN, Lin S-P, Hesketh JC, et al. Electrophysiological mechanism of RSD1235, a new atrial fibrillation converting drug [abstract]. Circulation 2003;108:IV85.
[51] Ezrin AM, Grant SM, Bell G, et al. A dose-ranging study of RSD1235, a novel antiarrhythmic agent, in healthy volunteers [abstract]. Pharmacologist 2002;44(Suppl 1):A15.
[52] Roy D, Rowe BH, Stiell IG, et al, CRAFT Investigators. A randomized, controlled trial of RSD1235, a novel anti-arrhythmic agent, in the treatment of recent onset atrial fibrillation. J Am Coll Cardiol 2004;44(12):2355–61.
[53] Available at: http://www.cardiome.com/RSD1235Intravenous.php.
[54] Available at: http://www.cardiome.com/VernakalantIntravenous.php.
[55] Available at: http://www.clinicaltrials.gov Trial identifier: NCT00267930.
[56] Available at: http://www.clinicaltrials.gov Trial identifier: NCT00125320.
[57] Wirth KJ, Paehler T, Rosenstein B, et al. Atrial effects of the novel K(+)-channel-blocker AVE0118 in anesthetized pigs. Cardiovasc Res 2003;60(2):298–306.
[58] Blaauw Y, Gogelein H, Tieleman RG, et al. "Early" class III drugs for the treatment of atrial fibrillation: efficacy and atrial selectivity of AVE0118 in remodeled atria of the goat. Circulation 2004;110(13):1717–24.
[59] Goldstein RN, Khrestian C, Carlsson L, et al. Azd7009: a new antiarrhythmic drug with predominant effects on the atria effectively terminates and prevents reinduction of atrial fibrillation and flutter in the sterile pericarditis model. J Cardiovasc Electrophysiol 2004;15(12):1444–50.
[60] Wu Y, Carlsson L, Liu T, et al. Assessment of the proarrhythmic potential of the novel antiarrhythmic agent AZD7009 and dofetilide in experimental models of torsades de pointes. J Cardiovasc Electrophysiol 2005;16(8):898–904.
[61] Available at: http://www.clinicaltrials.gov. Trial identifier: NCT00255281.
[62] Kaumann AJ, Sanders L, Brown AM, et al. A 5-HT receptor in human atrium. Br J Pharmacol 1990;100:879–85.

[63] Grammer JB, Zeng X, Bosch RF, et al. Atrial L-type Ca2+-channel, beta-adrenorecptor, and 5-hydroxytryptamine type 4 receptor mRNAs in human atrial fibrillation. Basic Res Cardiol 2001;96(1):82–90.

[64] Rahme MM, Cotter B, Leistad E, et al. Electrophysiological and antiarrhythmic effects of the atrial selective 5-HT(4) receptor antagonist RS-100302 in experimental atrial flutter and fibrillation. Circulation 1999;100(19):2010–7.

[65] Xiao XD, Fuchs S, Campbell DJ, et al. Mice with cardiac-restricted ACE have atrial enlargement, cardiac arrhythmias and sudden death. Am J Pathol 2004;165:1019–32.

[66] Boss CJ, Lip GY. Targeting the renin-angiotensin-aldosterone system in atrial fibrillation: from pathophysiology to clinical trials. J Hum Hypertens 2005;19:855–9.

[67] Shi Y, Tardif JC, Nattel S. Enalapril effects on atrial remodeling and atrial fibrillation in experimental congestive heart failure. Cardiovasc Res 2002;54:456–61.

[68] Pedersen OD, Bagger H, Kober L, et al. Trandolapril reduces the incidence of atrial fibrillation after acute myocardial infarction in patients with left ventricular dysfunction. Circulation 1999;100(4):376–80.

[69] Vermes E, Tardif JC, Bourassa MG, et al. Enalapril decreases the incidence of atrial fibrillation in patients with left ventricular dysfunction: insight from the Studies Of Left Ventricular Dysfunction (SOLVD) trials. Circulation 2003;107(23):2926–31.

[70] L'Allier PL, Ducharme A, Keller PF, et al. Angiotensin-converting enzyme inhibition in hypertensive patients is associated with a reduction in the occurrence of atrial fibrillation. J Am Coll Cardiol 2004;44(1):159–64.

[71] Anand K, Mooss AN, Hee TT, et al. Meta-analysis: inhibition of renin-angiotensin system prevents new-onset atrial fibrillation. Am Heart J 2006;152(2):217–22.

[72] Healey JS, Baranchuk A, Crystal E, et al. Prevention of atrial fibrillation with angiotensin-converting enzyme inhibitors and angiotensin receptor blockers: a meta-analysis. J Am Coll Cardiol 2005;45:1832–9.

[73] Ueng KC, Tsai TP, Yu WC, et al. Use of enalapril to facilitate sinus rhythm maintenance after external cardioversion of long-standing persistent atrial fibrillation. Results of a prospective and controlled study. Eur Heart J 2003;24(23):2090–8.

[74] Available at: http://www.clinicaltrials.gov/ct/show/NCT00141778?order=1.

[75] Nakashima H, Kumagai K, Urata H, et al. Angiotensin II antagonist prevents electrical remodeling in atrial fibrillation. Circulation 2000;101(22):2612–7.

[76] Kumagai K, Nakashima H, Urata H, et al. Effects of angiotensin II type 1 receptor antagonist on electrical and structural remodeling in atrial fibrillation. J Am Coll Cardiol 2003; 41(12):2197–204.

[77] Maggioni AP, Latini R, Carson PE, et al. Val-HeFT Investigators. Valsartan reduces the incidence of atrial fibrillation in patients with heart failure: results from the Valsartan Heart Failure Trial (Val-HeFT). Am Heart J 2005;149(3):548–57.

[78] Wachtell K, Lehto M, Gerdts E, et al. Angiotensin II receptor blockade reduces new-onset atrial fibrillation and subsequent stroke compared to atenolol: the Losartan Intervention For End Point Reduction in Hypertension (LIFE) study. J Am Coll Cardiol 2005;45(5): 712–9.

[79] Fogari R, Mugellini A, Destro M, et al. Losartan and prevention of atrial fibrillation recurrence in hypertensive patients. J Cardiovasc Pharmacol 2006;47(1):46–50.

[80] Madrid AH, Bueno MG, Rebollo JM, et al. Use of irbesartan to maintain sinus rhythm in patients with long-lasting persistent atrial fibrillation: a prospective and randomized study. Circulation 2002;106(3):331–6.

[81] Tveit A, Grundvold I, Olufsen M, et al. Candesartan in the prevention of relapsing atrial fibrillation. Int J Cardiol 2007;120(1):85–91.

[82] Available at: http://www.clinicaltrials.gov/ct/show/NCT00098137?order=1.

[83] Disertori M, Latini R, Maggioni AP, et al. Rationale and design of the GISSI-Atrial Fibrillation Trial: a randomized, prospective, multicentre study on the use of valsartan,

an angiotensin II AT1-receptor blocker, in the prevention of atrial fibrillation recurrence. J Cardiovasc Med (Hagerstown) 2006;7(1):29–38.

[84] Caballero R, Moreno I, Gonzalez T, et al. Spironolactone and its main metabolite, canrenoic acid, block human ether-a-go-go-related gene channels. Circulation 2003;107(6): 889–95.

[85] Gomez R, Nunez L, Caballero R, et al. Spironolactone and its main metabolite canrenoic acid block hKv1.5, Kv4.3 and Kv7.1 + minK channels. Br J Pharmacol 2005;146(1): 146–61.

[86] Goldstein RN, Kyungmoo R, Van Wagoner DR, et al. Prevention of postoperative atrial fibrillation and flutter using steroids [abstract]. Pacing Clin Electrophysiol 2003;26:1068.

[87] Halonen J, Halonen P, Jarvinen O, et al. Corticosteroids for the prevention of atrial fibrillation after cardiac surgery. JAMA 2007;297:1562–7.

[88] Prasongsukarn K, Abel JG, Jamieson WR, et al. The effects of steroids on the occurrence of postoperative atrial fibrillation after coronary artery bypass grafting surgery: a prospective randomized trial. J Thorac Cardiovasc Surg 2005;130(1):93–8.

[89] Halvorsen P, Raeder J, White PF, et al. The effect of dexamethasone on side effects after coronary revascularization procedures. Anesth Analg 2003;96(6):1578–83.

[90] Kumagai K, Nakashima H, Saku K. The HMG-CoA reductase inhibitor atorvastatin prevents atrial fibrillation by inhibiting inflammation in a canine sterile pericarditis model. Cardiovasc Res 2004;62(1):105–11.

[91] Shiroshita-Takeshita A, Schram G, Lavoie J, et al. Effect of simvastatin and antioxidant vitamins on atrial fibrillation promotion by atrial-tachycardia remodeling in dogs. Circulation 2004;110(16):2313–9.

[92] Siu CW, Lau CP, Tse HF. Prevention of atrial fibrillation recurrence by statin therapy in patients with lone atrial fibrillation after successful cardioversion. Am J Cardiol 2003; 92(11):1343–5.

[93] Young-Xu Y, Jabbour S, Goldberg R, et al. Usefulness of statin drugs in protecting against atrial fibrillation in patients with coronary artery disease. Am J Cardiol 2003;92(12): 1379–83.

[94] Amar D, Zhang H, Heerdt PM, et al. Statin use is associated with a reduction in atrial fibrillation after noncardiac thoracic surgery independent of C-reactive protein. Chest 2005;128(5):3421–7.

[95] Marin F, Pascual DA, Roldan V, et al. Statins and postoperative risk of atrial fibrillation following coronary artery bypass grafting. Am J Cardiol 2006;97(1):55–60.

[96] Available at: http://www.clinicaltrials.gov/ct/show/NCT00252967?order=1.

[97] Ninio DM, Murphy KJ, Howe PR, et al. Dietary fish oil protects against stretch-induced vulnerability to atrial fibrillation in a rabbit model. J Cardiovasc Electrophysiol 2005; 16(11):1189–94.

[98] Biscione F, Totteri A, De Vita A, et al. Effect of omega-3 fatty acids on the prevention of atrial arrhythmias. Ital Heart J 2005;6(1):53–9.

[99] Calo L, Bianconi L, Colivicchi F, et al. N-3 Fatty acids for the prevention of atrial fibrillation after coronary artery bypass surgery: a randomized, controlled trial. J Am Coll Cardiol 2005;45(10):1723–8.

[100] Brouwer IA, Heeringa J, Geleijnse JM, et al. Intake of very long-chain n-3 fatty acids from fish and incidence of atrial fibrillation. The Rotterdam Study. Am Heart J 2006;151(4): 857–62.

ELSEVIER
SAUNDERS

THE MEDICAL
CLINICS
OF NORTH AMERICA

Med Clin N Am 92 (2008) 143–159

Anticoagulation: Stroke Prevention in Patients with Atrial Fibrillation

Albert L. Waldo, MD*

*Department of Medicine, Division of Cardiovascular Medicine, Case Western Reserve
University/University Hospitals of Cleveland Case Medical Center, Cleveland, OH, USA*

Epidemiology of stroke risk

It is well recognized that during atrial fibrillation (AF), clots may form in the left atrium. This, in turn, may lead to embolization of the clot, with resulting ischemic stroke or systemic embolism. Also, the presence of AF confers a fivefold increased risk for stroke [1]. Moreover, the prevalence of stroke in patients who have AF increases with increasing age. Below age 60, it is less than 0.5%. Then, beginning with the seventh decade, the prevalence of AF doubles with each decade, so that it is 2% to 3% for patients in their 60s, 5% to 6% in their 70s, and 8% to 10% in their 80s [1]. The population attributable risk also increases with age, such that by the 70s, it is 16.5%, and by the 80s, it is just over 30%. [1]. Thus, it is of little surprise that AF is the most common and important cause of stroke resulting from any cause.

Stroke risk stratification schemes for patients who have atrial fibrillation

The risk for stroke is not the same for all patients who have AF. Based on a series of studies, the widely recognized risk factors for stroke are prior stroke or transient ischemic attack (TIA), hypertension, age 75 years or older, heart failure and poor left ventricular function, and diabetes [2,3]. Other recognized stroke risk factors include mechanical prosthetic valve, mitral stenosis, coronary artery disease, age 65 to 74 years, thyrotoxicosis, and female gender [4]. All these are factored in when considering indications for

Supported in part by Grant R01 HL38408 from the United States Public Health Service, National Institutes of Health, National Heart, Lung and Blood Institute, Bethesda, Maryland, and Grant BRTT/WCI TECH 05-066 from the Ohio Wright Center of Innovations, a Third Frontier program from The State of Ohio, Columbus, OH.

* Division of Cardiology, MS LKS 5038, University Hospitals of Cleveland, 11100 Euclid Avenue, Cleveland, OH 44106-5038.

E-mail address: albert.waldo@case.edu

oral anticoagulation. As incorporated into the American College of Cardiology/American Heart Association/European Society of Cardiology (ACC/AHA/ESC) 2006 revised Guidelines for the Management of Patients with Atrial Fibrillation (discussed later), not all stroke risk factors have the same degree of association with stroke in patients who have AF [4].

There arc several stroke risk stratification schemes for patients who have AF. One that has gained great favor is the CHADS$_2$ scheme [5]. Based on analysis of 1773 patients in the National Registry of Atrial Fibrillation, it uses most, but not all, of the accepted stroke risk factors to assess individual patient risk. The "C" stands for recent congestive heart failure, the "H" for hypertension, the "A" for age 75 or older, the "D" for diabetes, and the "S" for prior stroke or TIA. Each category gets one point except stroke or TIA, which gets 2 because of its high association with subsequent stroke. The adjusted stroke rate per 100 patient years increases as the CHADS$_2$ score increases (Fig. 1).

The Framingham risk score [6] uses five steps to predict the 5-year risk of stroke in AF (Fig. 2). The steps consider age, gender, systolic blood pressure, diabetes, and prior stroke or TIA and assign points depending on these factors. The points from steps 1 through 5 are added. Then the predicted 5-year stroke risk is determined for each individual in the absence of anticoagulation therapy from a table. This may be helpful in weighing available therapeutic options and even helping patients understand the need for anticoagulation therapy in the first place.

Warfarin therapy provides effective prophylaxis against stroke

Many clinical trials have demonstrated warfarin's remarkable efficacy in reducing stroke risk in patients who have AF. As demonstrated

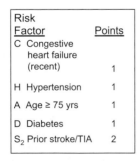
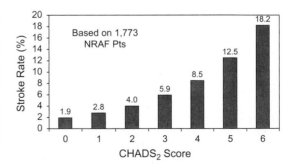

Fig. 1. Key AF stroke risk factors: CHADS2 risk stratification scheme. NRAF, National Registry of Atrial Fibrillation. (*Data from* Gage BF, Waterman AD, Shannon W, et al. Validation of clinical classification schemes for predicting stroke: results from a national registry of atrial fibrillation. JAMA 2001;285:2864–70.)

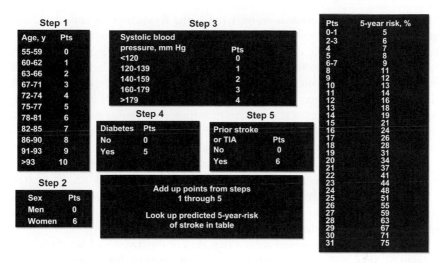

Fig. 2. Framingham risk score for predicting the 5-year risk of stroke in patients who have AF. (*Data from* Wang TJ, Massaro JM, Levy D, et al. A risk score for predicting stroke or death in individuals with new-onset atrial fibrillation in the community: the Framingham Heart Study. JAMA 2003;290:1049–105.)

overwhelmingly more than a decade ago in a meta-analysis of five random-ized, controlled clinical trials comparing warfarin and placebo in patients who had AF (the Copenhagen Atrial Fibrillation Aspirin and Anticoagula-tion (AFASAK) trial [7], the Stroke Prevention in Atrial Fibrillation [SPAF] trial [8], the Boston Area Anticoagulation Trial for Atrial Fibrillation (BAATAF) [9], the Canadian Atrial Fibrillation Anticoagulation (CAFA) trial [10], and the Stroke Prevention in Nonrheumatic Atrial Fibrillation (SPINAF) trial [11]), an intention-to-treat analysis showed that there was a 68% risk reduction in stroke for patients taking warfarin compared with patients taking placebo ($P < .001$) [3]. An on-treatment analysis of these same trials demonstrated an 83% risk reduction in stroke for patients taking warfarin compared with placebo [12]. These and subsequent data established warfarin's therapeutic range as an international normalized ratio (INR) between 2 and 3, with a target INR of 2.5 to provide efficacy and safety.

Despite warfarin's well-demonstrated efficacy as prophylaxis against stroke in patients who have AF, many problems have an impact on its use. They include a narrow therapeutic range (INR 2–3), an unpredictable and patient-specific dose response, delayed onset and offset of action, need for anticoagulation monitoring, slow reversibility when that may be necessary, and many drug-drug and drug-food interactions that affect the INR levels [13]. Interactions with warfarin are common. Among the many interactions with drugs, virtually all the anti-inflammatory drugs interact with warfarin, as do most antibiotics, many diuretics, phenytoin, predni-sone, thyroid hormone replacement, tamoxifen, alcohol, and statins, to list a few [13]. Many foods do as well, including foods high in vitamin K (eg, green, leafy vegetables; kiwi; etc.), high-dose vitamin C, vitamin E, cranberries, and licorice, amongst others [13]. It is important to emphasize warfarin's narrow therapeutic range, because once the INR falls below 2, there is a steep rise in the odds ratio for stroke (eg, an INR of 1.7 doubles this risk) (Fig. 3) [14]. When the INR rises above 3, it does not enhance the efficacy, but it does increase the risk for bleeding, with major hemorrhage and intracranial hemorrhage the two greatest concerns. The incidence of intracranial hemorrhage is flat [15,16], varying between 0.3 and 0.6 per 100 person years, with an INR ranging from less than 1.5 until the INR gets over 3.5 (see Fig. 3), and is remarkably flat until patients' age is 85 or greater. There is no difference with regard to occurrence of intracerebral hemorrhage or subdural hematoma [16]. These data help to understand the therapeutic range and target for the INR.

In view of the recognized difficulties in administration of warfarin, the United States Food and Drug Administration recently has approved safety labeling revisions to advise about the need for individualization of warfarin therapy to minimize the risk for bleeding [13]. The most serious risks of anticoagulant therapy with warfarin are hemorrhage in any tissue or organ and, less frequently (incidence < 0.1%), necrosis or gangrene of skin or other tissues. The risk for bleeding is highest during treatment initiation and with higher doses. Risk factors include a high intensity of anticoagulation (INR ≥ 4), age 65 or greater, high variability of INRs, history of gastrointestinal bleeding, hypertension, cerebrovascular disease, serious heart

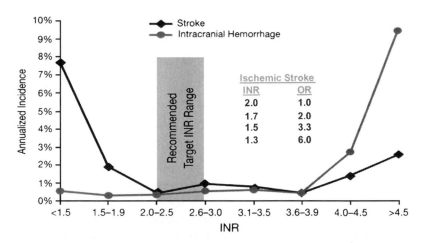

Fig. 3. Annualized incidence of stroke or intracranial hemorrhage according to INR. Also included is the odds ratio (OR) for ischemic stroke in patients who have AF based on their INR. (*Data from* Hylek E, Skates S, Sheehan M, et al. An analysis of the lowest effective intensity of prophylactic anticoagulation for patients with nonrheumatic atrial fibrillation. N Engl J Med 1996;335:540–6; and Hylek EM, Go AS, Chang Y, et al. Effect of intensity of oral anticoagulation on stroke severity and mortality in atrial fibrillation. N Engl J Med 2003;349:1019–26.)

disease, anemia, malignancy, trauma, renal insufficiency, concomitant drugs, and long duration of warfarin therapy. This safety relabeling appropriately emphasizes the need for individualization of treatment with warfarin because of a low therapeutic index and potential effects from interaction with other drugs or dietary vitamin K intake. Regular monitoring of the INR, usually at least monthly, is recommended for all patients. Those at high risk for bleeding may benefit from more frequent monitoring, careful dose adjustments to achieve the desired INR, and, when possible, shorter duration of therapy. To minimize the risk for bleeding, patients should be advised to avoid initiating or discontinuing other medications, including salicylates, and should be wary of other over-the-counter medications and herbal products. Maintenance of a balanced diet with a consistent amount of vitamin K is advised. Drastic changes in diet (eg, eating large amounts of green leafy vegetables) and consumption of cranberry juice or its products should be avoided.

Despite the recognized indications for warfarin use and its clear efficacy in stroke prevention, warfarin therapy remains underused [17]. Most studies indicate usage between 40% and 60% in patients who have AF and risk factors for stroke. Additionally, although the risk for stroke notably increases with increasing age, the use of warfarin decreases as patients get older [17]. It is the elderly who use warfarin the least. In this group, a principle reason seems to be fear of an intracranial hemorrhage. Although decisions of whether or not to use warfarin must be made on a case-by-case basis, the risks for potential intracranial hemorrhage or major bleeding usually are outweighed significantly by the risks for stroke or systemic embolus, such that most of the time, warfarin therapy is warranted [18,19].

Aspirin is significantly less effective as prophylaxis against stroke

Use of aspirin as prophylaxis against stroke in patients who have AF and stroke risks is controversial. Meta-analysis of studies comparing aspirin with placebo suggest a relative risk reduction of approximately 22% with use of aspirin [20]. This largely is driven, however, by data from one clinical trial, the SPAF I study (Fig. 4). Only the SPAF I data indicate that aspirin is significantly better than placebo. It is worth examining those data closely (see Fig. 4) [21]. SPAF I was a National Institutes of Health–sponsored trial that randomized patients to AF to warfarin, aspirin, or placebo (group I) or to aspirin versus placebo for those patients who had a relative or absolute contraindication to warfarin (group II). In group I, of 206 patients in the aspirin arm, there was only one event, whereas in 211 patients in the placebo arm, there were 18 events, giving aspirin a risk reduction of 94% ($P < .001$). No other data have come close to confirming these results, suggesting that they are outliers. Moreover, in group II patients, of 346 patients in the aspirin arm, there were 25 events, and of 357 patients in the placebo arm,

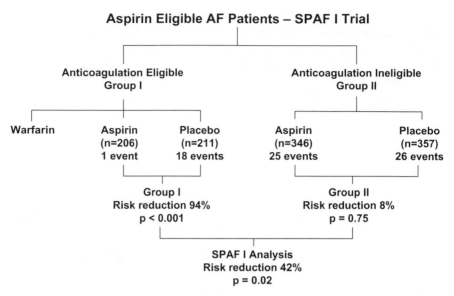

Fig. 4. Analysis of the data from the SPAF I trial in patients taking aspirin compared with placebo. (*Data from* The SPAF Investigators. A differential effect of aspirin on prevention of
stroke in atrial fibrillation. J Stroke Cerebrovasc Dis 1993;3:181–8.)

there were 26 events, giving aspirin a relative risk reduction of 8% ($P = .75$).
The aspirin versus placebo data from groups I and II were pooled, such that
the relative risk reduction using aspirin was 42% ($P = .02$). The confidence
intervals of the pooled data are wide, however, because of the disparate nature
of the data reported. Thus, this relative risk reduction should be considered
unreliable.

There are other data that suggest aspirin is less effective than desirable.
Aspirin never has been shown to affect mortality in patients who have
AF, as opposed to warfarin, which has [22]. In addition, the SPAF III trial
[23] evaluated the benefit of an adjusted dose of warfarin (INR 2–3; target
2.5) versus low-intensity, fixed-dose warfarin (INR 1.2–1.5) plus aspirin in
patients who had AF at high risk for stroke (ie, patients who had one or
more of the following risk factors: female gender and age 75 years; impaired
left ventricular function; systolic blood pressure greater than 160 mm Hg, or
prior thromboembolism) [24]. It was reasoned that warfarin was more effective than aspirin as prophylaxis against stroke, but there was concern about
excess and serious bleeding in patients receiving warfarin. It was hoped that
if aspirin (324 mg daily) was combined with a fixed but low dose of warfarin
to achieve an INR between 1.2 and 1.5, the combined beneficial effects of
aspirin and warfarin would provide effective stroke prevention but avoid
the bleeding risks associated with adjusted-dose warfarin administered to
achieve an INR between 2 and 3. But, the trial was stopped early (after
a mean follow-up of 1.1 years) because the event rate in patients on the

combination therapy was 7.9% per year versus an event rate on adjusted-dose warfarin of 1.9% per year ($P = .001$) (Fig. 5) [23]. Moreover, there was no significant difference in the major bleeding rate or the intracranial hemorrhage rate between the two groups. There was slightly more major bleeding and intracranial hemorrhage in the aspirin plus fixed low-dose warfarin group compared with the adjusted-dose warfarin group (see Fig. 5). And in the adjusted-dose warfarin group, the annual event rate of stroke began to increase as soon as the INR fell below 2; whereas in the combination aspirin fixed low-dose warfarin group, the incidence of stroke decreased as the INR approached 2 (Fig. 6). Additionally, in SPAF III, there was a low stroke risk patient cohort (patients who had AF who did not have any high risk factors for stroke) who were in a nonrandomized, aspirin-only arm of this trial. In these latter patients, just a history of hypertension conferred a 3.6% risk for stroke or systemic embolism per year [24].

There are more data indicating the problems with aspirin therapy compared with warfarin therapy. Hylek and colleagues [14] studied a cohort of 13,559 patients who had nonvalvular AF who suffered 596 ischemic strokes. Thirty-two percent were on warfarin, 27% were on aspirin therapy, and 42% had neither warfarin nor aspirin therapy. They compared the severity of neurologic deficit at discharge and the early and 30-day mortality rates in patients who had a stroke while receiving warfarin (with an INR ≥ 2 or an INR < 2), aspirin, or no antithrombotic therapy. For patients taking aspirin or taking warfarin but who had an INR of less than 2, there was a 2.6- to 3-fold increase in the severity of the stroke, including early (in-hospital) fatality or stroke resulting in total dependence, compared with

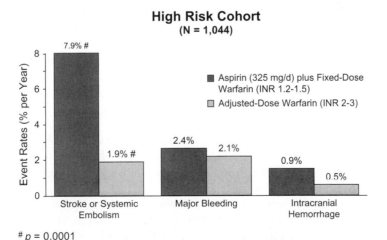

Fig. 5. Analysis of the SPAF III data in the high-risk patient cohort. (*Data from* Israel CW, Gronefeld G, Ehrlich JR, et al. Long-term risk of recurrent atrial fibrillation as documented by an implantable monitoring device: implications for optimal patient care. J Am Coll Cardiol 2004;43:47–52.)

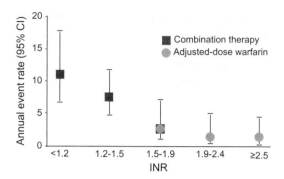

Fig. 6. SPAF III relative risk for stroke or systemic embolism in adjusted-dose warfarin and combination therapy cohorts. Event rates for ischemic stroke for systemic embolism based on the INR in SPAF III patients in the combination therapy (square) and adjusted-dose warfarin therapy (circle) groups. (*Data from* The SPAF Investigators. Adjusted-dose warfarin versus low-intensity, fixed dose warfarin plus aspirin for high-risk patients with atria fibrillation: Stroke Prevention in Atrial Fibrillation III randomized clinical trial. Lancet 1996;348:633–8.)

patients who had an INR of greater than or equal to 2. Similarly, the 30-day mortality rate was approximately 2.5 times greater in patients taking aspirin or who had an INR less than 2 if taking warfarin compared with patients who had an INR greater than or equal to 2. In short, these data demonstrated that warfarin with an INR greater than or equal to 2 not only reduced the frequency of ischemic stroke but also reduced the severity and risk for death from stroke compared with aspirin.

A useful way to think about risks versus benefits of prophylaxis with warfarin or aspirin comes from the data of van Walraven and colleagues [25]. Their meta-analysis concludes that treating 1000 patients who have AF for 1 year with warfarin instead of aspirin would prevent 23 ischemic strokes but cause nine additional major bleeds, including two hemorrhagic strokes. Thus, in patients who have AF and stroke risk factors, the risk for stroke or systemic embolism is significant. Nevertheless, it is apparent that the risks for bleeding also must be taken into account. In most patients, however, the risk for stroke outweighs the risk for bleeding, such that in patients who have AF and are at high risk for stroke, warfarin therapy should be administered. For patients who have AF and are not at high risk for stroke or systemic embolism, although the Guidelines for the Management of Atrial Fibrillation (discussed later) offer aspirin or warfarin as options for therapy [4], administration of warfarin seems to make the most sense unless it is contraindicated. In sum, in patients at risk for stroke resulting from AF, anticoagulation with warfarin (INR 2–3; target 2.5) reduces stroke rate and mortality and morbidity associated with stroke if the latter should occur. Aspirin has considerably less, if not just minimal, effect on stroke rate and severity, and no demonstrated effect on mortality associated with stroke in patients at risk for stroke resulting from AF.

American Heart Association/American College of Cardiology/European Society of Cardiology 2006 guidelines on risk factors for stroke and stroke prevention in atrial fibrillation

The ACC/AHA/ESC 2006 revised Guidelines for the Management of Patients with Atrial Fibrillation [4] have divided risk factors for stroke into three groups (Table 1). High-risk factors include prior stroke, TIA, or thromboembolism; mitral stenosis; or presence of a prosthetic mechanical heart valve. Moderate risk factors include age greater than 75 years, hypertension, heart failure, left ventricular ejection fraction less than or equal to 0.35, or diabetes mellitus. There is a third category that might be called low risk but is formally labeled less validated or weaker risk factors. These include female gender, age 65 to 74 years, coronary artery disease, and thyrotoxicosis.

In the presence of these risk factors, the following recommendations for antithrombotic therapy have been made (see Table 1) [4]. For patients who have any high risk factor for stroke, oral anticoagulation with warfarin therapy (range 2–3; target 2.5) is recommended. For patients who have two or more moderate stroke risk factors, similarly, oral anticoagulation with warfarin is recommended. For patients who have one moderate risk factor, aspirin (81 or 324 mg) or oral anticoagulation with warfarin is recommended. For patients who have less validated or weaker risk factors, aspirin (81 or 324 mg) or oral anticoagulation is recommended. For patients less than 60 years of age, aspirin (81 or 324 mg) or no therapy is recommended. For patients who have no risk factors who are 60 to 65 years of age, aspirin

Table 1
American Heart Association/American College of Cardiology/European Society of Cardiology 2006 revised guidelines for antithrombotic therapy based on stroke risk

Less validated or weaker risk factors	Moderate risk factors	High risk factors
Rx: ASA or OAC	Rx: 1 risk factor—ASA or OAC; ≥2 risk factors—OAC	Rx: OAC
Female gender	Age > 75 years	Prior stroke, TIA, or embolism
Age 65 to 74 years	Hypertension	Mitral stenosis
Coronary artery disease	Heart failure	Mechanical heart valve
Thyrotoxicosis	LVEF ≤ 0.35	
	Diabetes mellitus	

Abbreviations: ASA, aspirin; LVEF, left ventricular ejection fraction; OAC, oral anticoagulation with warfarin; RF, stroke risk factor; Rx, therapy.

Data from Fuster V, Ryden LE, Cannom DS, et al. ACC/AHA/ESC 2006 Guidelines for the management of patients with atrial fibrillation: a report of the American College of Cardiology/American Heart Association Task Force on Practice Guidelines and the European Society of Cardiology Committee for Practice Guidelines (Writing Committee to revise the 2001 guidelines for the management of patients with atrial fibrillation). J Am Coll Cardiol 2006;48:854–906.

(81 or 324 mg) or oral anticoagulation with warfarin is recommended. There is no difference in the indications for antithrombotic therapy between persistent, permanent, or paroxysmal AF.

Other considerations

Although these guidelines were thought out carefully, there are some concerns. As discussed previously, data supporting the use of aspirin in patients who have stroke risk factors are wanting. The guidelines suggest that in patients over age 75 who have risk factors for stroke and in whom there is concern for bleeding, administering warfarin to achieve an INR of 1.6 to 2.5 with a target of 2 should be considered if there is no history of prior stroke [4]. As the Hylek and colleagues [15] data show, however (discussed previously), lowering the INR below 2 does not decrease the incidence of intracranial hemorrhage. It reduces the efficacy of warfarin therapy, however, such that the odds ratio for stroke goes up dramatically (see Fig. 3). Thus, think carefully about applying this recommendation (IIc) of the guidelines.

Managing anticoagulation interruptions is important. In general, the average weekly risk for stroke in the absence of oral anticoagulation is low but not zero. The highest risk is believed to be in patients who have mechanical heart valves or prior stroke [4]. In those patients in whom there is a need to stop the oral anticoagulation for a procedure, bridging the interruption with unfractionated heparin or low-molecular-weight heparin therapy is recommended [4]. Thus, heparin or low-molecular-weight heparin therapy would be administered in lieu of warfarin through the day before the procedure, when it, too, must be stopped. Then, warfarin or bridging with heparin usually is reinstated at a safe time after the procedure.

Cardioversion

The question of adequate anticoagulation to prevent stroke in association with cardioversion has been standardized for while and has not changed with the 2006 revised ACC/AHA/ESC guidelines (Box 1) [4]. It is based on data and on consensus. If AF is known to have been present for less than 48 hours, cardioversion may proceed without any anticoagulation. If AF has been present 48 or more hours, however, cardioversion seems to raise the risk for embolism, with a 1% to 5% risk of emboli occurring within hours to weeks after cardioversion in the absence of anticoagulation. But anticoagulation well before and after cardioversion greatly reduces this risk. Therefore, if AF has been present for 2 or more days or for an unknown period of time, the guidelines state that the INR should be between 2 and 3 for 3 consecutive weeks before cardioversion and for at least 4 weeks after restoring and maintaining normal sinus rhythm.

Box 1. Elective cardioversion of atrial fibrillation anticoagulation —standards for use of anticoagulation in connection with cardioversion of atrial fibrillation

- Cardioversion seems to raise the risk for embolism:
  AC well before and after greatly reduces risk
  For use of AC, risk factors for stroke in AF do not apply
- Standard guidelines for electrical or drug cardioversion:
  INR 2 to 3 for weeks before cardioversion and INR 2 to 3 for 4
  weeks after normal sinus rhythm (continue warfarin beyond
  4 weeks if stroke risk factors present)
  If AF<2 days' duration, may proceed without AC
  If perform transesophageal echocardiography and
  No thrombus—AC just before and 4 weeks after
  cardioversion
  Thrombus present—AC with INR 2–3 for 3 weeks and
  reevaluate

Abbreviation: AC, anticoagulation.

Data from Fuster V, Ryden LE, Cannom DS, et al. ACC/AHA/ESC 2006 guidelines for the management of patients with atrial fibrillation: a report of the American College of Cardiology/American Heart Association Task Force on Practice Guidelines and the European Society of Cardiology Committee for Practice Guidelines (Writing Committee to revise the 2001 guidelines for the management of patients with atrial fibrillation). J Am Coll Cardiol 2006;48:854–906.

If AF is present for 2 or more days in the absence of warfarin therapy with an INR in the therapeutic range, and if one wants to perform a cardioversion, there are two options. One option is to perform a transesophageal echocardiogram in the presence of therapeutic heparin administration. If no thrombus is present, anticoagulation with heparin (unfractionated or low molecular weight) is continued through the cardioversion and as a bridge to achieving a therapeutic INR on warfarin, at which time the heparin is stopped. The warfarin is continued, maintaining an INR in the therapeutic range for at least 1 month after the successful cardioversion. Then if there is an indication for chronic warfarin therapy, it is continued. If there is no such indication, the warfarin is stopped. If there is a thrombus present at the time of the precardioversion transesophageal echocardiography, however, anticoagulation with an INR between 2 and 3 for 3 consecutive weeks is recommended, followed by reevaluation. The second option simply is to anticoagulate the patient orally with warfarin, and, after achieving an INR in the therapeutic range for 3 consecutive weeks, perform the cardioversion. Again, if there is no indication for long-term warfarin therapy, it may be stopped after 1 month. Otherwise, it is continued long term. The ACUTE study [26] demonstrates that there is no important difference between either approach (transesophageal echocardiography with heparin before cardioversion or 3 consecutive weeks of an INR in the therapeutic range on warfarin) in terms of morbidity and mortality.

Risk factors for stroke in AF do not apply to these rules. Thus, if patients have no risk factor for stroke and ordinarily would not need warfarin long term, patients still should be anticoagulated before cardioversion if AF has been present for 48 or more hours or an unknown duration. The main reason for this is that there is an approximately 25% incidence of atrial stunning (absence of atrial contraction) after cardioversion for patients who have had AF for 48 or more hours [27]. The stunning may last up to 1 month, although most often it lasts only for hours or days after restoration of sinus rhythm [27]. It is during this period of stunning when it is believed the milieu that predisposes to left atrial clots still is present, such that clots may form in the left atrium during sinus rhythm. For patients who do not have a need for long-term anticoagulation, ordinarily the anticoagulation would be stopped after 1 month of therapy.

Issues in long-term use of oral anticoagulation

What about continuation of warfarin therapy for patients who have AF and risk factors for stroke who achieve and seem to maintain sinus rhythm? Data from the Atrial Fibrillation Follow-Up Investigation of Rhythm Management (AFFIRM) [28,29] and the Comparison of Rate Control and Rhythm Control in Patients With Recurrent Persistent Atrial Fibrillation (RACE) [30] trials are most instructive in this regard. In the AFFIRM trial, if a patient achieved sinus rhythm and maintained it for at least 1 month, warfarin therapy could be stopped. This was worrisome because of the known tendency for AF to recur but was requested by the study sites because they believed it would have a negative impact on patient recruitment to the study. The result was that patients in the rhythm control arm did well initially, with more than 90% of patients taking warfarin in the first 4 months after randomization. But by the end of year 1, this dropped to just under 80%, and by years 2 to 5, only approximately 70% were taking warfarin in the rhythm control arm. In the rate control arm, where failure to use warfarin was a protocol violation, more than 90% of patients were taking warfarin through year 4, although by year 5, only approximately 85% were taking warfarin. At the end of the AFFIRM trial, when the relationship of ischemic stroke, INR, and the presence of AF in the rate versus rhythm control arms were examined (Table 2), the incidence of ischemic stroke was not significantly different between the rhythm and rate control arms ($P = .79$). However, 57% of the patients in the rhythm control arm who had a stroke were not taking warfarin. Although documented only partly in this trial, it is likely that these patients had recurrence of AF and that much of it was asymptomatic [31,32]; another 22% of patients who had a stroke in the rhythm control arm had an INR of less than 2,

Table 2
The relationship between ischemic stroke, international normalization ratio, and presence or absence of atrial fibrillation

	Rate control, n (%)	Rhythm control, n (%)
Ischemic stroke	77 (5.5)[a]	80 (7.1)[a]
INR $\geq$ 2	23 (31)	16 (21)
INR < 2	27 (36)	17 (22)
Not taking warfarin	25 (33)	44 (57)
AF at time of event	42 (69)	25 (37)

[a] Event rates derived from Kaplan-Meier analysis ($P = .79$).

Data from Wyse DG, Waldo AL, DiMarco JP, et al. A comparison of rate control and rhythm control in patients with recurrent persistent atrial fibrillation. N Engl J Med 2002;347:1825–33.

again emphasizing the importance of maintaining the INR in the therapeutic range. Additionally, in the rate control arm, 33% of patients who had a stroke were not taking warfarin, a protocol violation. This emphasizes the difficulty of keeping patients on warfarin therapy even though there is a clear indication for its use. Moreover, 36% of patients who had a stroke in the rate control arm also had an INR of less than 2, again emphasizing the importance of maintaining the INR in the therapeutic range. Similar data were reported in the RACE trial [30].

In patients who have AF, it is estimated that 10% to 30% of all AF cases are totally asymptomatic and that up to 70% of patients who have symptomatic AF also have symptomatic episodes [31]. The risk for stroke in symptomatic and asymptomatic AF is similar, such that asymptomatic AF requires not only ventricular rate control but also adherence to anticoagulation guidelines. In addition, Israel and colleagues [32] examined the incidence of asymptomatic AF in patients who had a history of AF who also had an implanted pacemaker with excellent stored memory capacity and the ability to detect atrial arrhythmias. In 38% of patients who had a history of AF and had AF recurrences, the AF was asymptomatic and of more than 48 hours' duration, and 16% who developed asymptomatic AF of more than 48 hours' duration did so even after documentation of freedom from AF for 3 months. The implication is that success rates of maintaining continuous sinus rhythm in patients who have a history of AF often are grossly overestimated. And for patients who have AF and risk factors for stroke, the data suggest they should receive warfarin therapy indefinitely, even when sinus rhythm seems to have been restored and maintained.

Long-term anticoagulation after radiofrequency ablation of atrial fibrillation

What to do about long-term anticoagulation for patients who undergo apparently successful ablation to cure AF has yet to be determined. The hope is that these patients truly would be cured, such that the need for anti-coagulation to prevent stroke resulting from AF no longer is present. There is an uncertain but real incidence of asymptomatic AF recurrence in these patients, however, both early and late after the ablation [33]. A difficulty in assessing long-term warfarin need in these patients is the absence of long-term data to give perspective, not only on the incidence of recurrence of AF beyond the 2- to 3-month "blanking period," when AF recurrence may not indicate failure of the procedure, but also on the incidence of stroke in the absence of anticoagulation therapy, especially in patients who have risk factors for stroke. In this sense, it must be considered whether or not there are enough data even to reach an informed consensus. For patients who do not have stroke risk factors (at present, probably most patients who undergo apparently successful ablation of AF), there is consensus that after the blanking period, further anticoagulation with warfarin is not necessary [34–36]. What then for patients who have stroke risk factors? Data from small studies suggest that the stroke incidence is low, but the incidence of AF recurrence, manifest and asymptomatic, is uncertain. Moreover, data indicate there is a late AF recurrence (beyond the first-year post ablation) of at least 5% [37,38]. In addition, the data suggest that not only is recurrence of AF a marker for the need for warfarin therapy, but also, in some patients, as a consequence of radiofrequency ablation to cure AF, there is a reduction of left atrial transport function of up to 30%. The latter may predispose to thromboembolic events despite the presence of sinus rhythm [38].

Because of these considerations and the absence of long-term, randomized, controlled trial data, the Heart Rhythm Society/European Heart Rhythm Association/European Cardiac Arrhythmia Society Expert Consensus Statement on Catheter and Surgical Ablation of Atrial Fibrillation [35] states that discontinuation of warfarin therapy post ablation generally is not recommend in patients who have a CHADS$_2$ score of 2 or more. It also recommends warfarin for all patients for at least 2 months after an AF ablation procedure. Decisions regarding the use of warfarin more than 2 months after the ablation should be based on patients' risk factors for stroke. The Venice Chart International Consensus Document on Atrial Fibrillation [36] makes similar recommendations; the only real difference is that they recommend warfarin be given for at least 3 to 6 months after the ablation procedure.

The following is a considered overview of the author for patients who have risk factors for stroke. (1) For patients who require antiarrhythmic drug therapy after radiofrequency ablation to suppress AF recurrence (ie, despite radiofrequency ablation, cure has not been obtained, but successful therapy seemingly is obtained with the addition of antiarrhythmic drug therapy that was not successful before the ablation), warfarin therapy to maintain an INR in the therapeutic range should be maintained long term. (2) For patients in whom no clinically manifest episodes of AF have been documented 2 months after ostensibly successful radiofrequency ablation to cure AF, warfarin therapy should be maintained for a minimum of 1 year, at which time continued use of warfarin therapy should be reconsidered. (3) For patients who have any documented recurrence of AF after the blanking period, warfarin therapy should be maintained for at least 1 year, at which time, it should be reconsidered. (4) If asymptomatic AF does occur, warfarin therapy should be maintained long term. (5) A recommendation concerning continuation of warfarin therapy beyond 1 year post ablation in patients who have stroke risks must be couched in uncertainties and considered on an individual basis: if there has been no apparent AF recurrence, termination of warfarin therapy may be acceptable, understanding that late recurrence of AF, although likely low, is possible, with its attendant risks; if there is any AF recurrence, continued long-term warfarin therapy is recommended.

References

[1] Wolf PA, Abbott RD, Kannel WB. Atrial fibrillation: a major contributor to stroke in the elderly. The Framingham Study. Arch Intern Med 1987;147:1561–4.
[2] Stroke Prevention in Atrial Fibrillation Investigators. Predictors of thromboembolism in atrial fibrillation: I. Clinical features of patients at risk. Ann Intern Med 1992;116: 1–5.
[3] Atrial Fibrillation Investigators. Risk factors for stroke and efficacy of antithrombotic therapy in atrial fibrillation: analysis of pooled data from five randomized controlled trials. Arch Intern Med 1994;154:1449–57.
[4] Fuster V, Ryden LE, Cannom DS, et al. ACC/AHA/ESC 2006 Guidelines for the management of patients with atrial fibrillation: a report of the American College of Cardiology/ American Heart Association Task Force on Practice Guidelines and the European Society of Cardiology Committee for Practice Guidelines (Writing Committee to revise the 2001 guidelines for the management of patients with atrial fibrillation). J Am Coll Cardiol 2006;48:854–906.
[5] Gage BF, Waterman AD, Shannon W, et al. Validation of clinical classification schemes for predicting stroke: results from a national registry of atrial fibrillation. JAMA 2001;285: 2864–70.
[6] Wang TJ, Massaro JM, Levy D, et al. A risk score for predicting stroke or death in individuals with new-onset atrial fibrillation in the community: the Framingham Heart Study. JAMA 2003;290:1049–56.
[7] Petersen P, Boysen G, Godtfredsen J, et al. Placebo-controlled, randomized trial of warfarin and aspirin for prevention of thromboembolic complications in chronic atrial fibrillation. The Copenhagen AFASAK Study. Lancet 1989;1:175–8.
[8] Stroke Prevention in Atrial Fibrillation Investigators. Stroke Prevention in Atrial Fibrillation Study: Final Results. Circulation 1991;84:527–39.
[9] The Boston Area Anticoagulation Trial for Atrial Fibrillation Investigators. The effect of low dose warfarin on the risk of stroke in patients with nonrheumatic atrial fibrillation. N Engl J Med 1990;323:1505–11.
[10] Connolly S, Laupacis A, Gent M, et al. Canadian Atrial Fibrillation Anticoagulation (CAFA) Study. J Am Coll Cardiol 1991;18:349–55.
[11] Ezekowitz M, Bridgers S, James K, et al. Warfarin in the prevention of stroke associated with nonrheumatic atrial fibrillation. N Engl J Med 1992;327:1406–12.
[12] Albers GW, Sherman DG, Gress DR, et al. Stroke prevention in nonvalvular atrial fibrillation: a review of prospective randomized trials. Ann Neurol 1991;30:511–8.
[13] Anticoagulant coumadin tablets (warfarin sodium tablets, USP crystalline). In: Physicians Desk Reference. 61st edition, 2007; Thomson PDR at Montvale, NJ; pp 898–903.

[14] Hylek E, Skates S, Sheehan M, et al. An analysis of the lowest effective intensity of prophylactic anticoagulation for patients with nonrheumatic atrial fibrillation. N Engl J Med 1996; 335:540–6.

[15] Hylek EM, Go AS, Chang Y, et al. Effect of intensity of oral anticoagulation on stroke severity and mortality in atrial fibrillation. N Engl J Med 2003;349:1019–26.

[16] Fang MC, Chang Y, Hylek EM, et al. Advanced age anticoagulation intensity and risk for intracranial hemorrhage among patients taking warfarin for atrial fibrillation. Ann Intern Med 2004;141:745–52.

[17] Waldo AL, Becker RC, Tapson VF, et al. NABOR Steering Committee. Hospitalized patients with atrial fibrillation and a high risk of stroke are not being provided with adequate anticoagulation. J Am Coll Cardiol 2005;46:1729–36.

[18] Fang MC, Go AS, Hylek EM, et al. Age and the risk of warfarin-associated hemorrhage: the anticoagulation and risk factors in atrial fibrillation study. J Am Geriatr Soc 2006;54: 1231–6.

[19] Garcia D, Hylek E. Stroke prevention in elderly patients with atrial fibrillation. Lancet 2007; 370:460–1.

[20] Hart R, Benavente O, McBridge R, et al. Antithrombotic therapy to prevent stroke in patients with atrial fibrillation: a meta-analysis. Ann Intern Med 1999;131:492–501.

[21] The SPAF Investigators. A differential effect of aspirin on prevention of stroke in atrial fibrillation. J Stroke Cerebrovasc Dis 1993;3:181–8.

[22] Cleland JGF, Kaye GC. Only warfarin has been shown to reduce stroke risk in patients with atrial fibrillation. Br Med J 2001;323:233.

[23] The SPAF Investigators. Adjusted-dose warfarin versus low-intensity, fixed dose warfarin plus aspirin for high-risk patients with atria fibrillation: Stroke Prevention in Atrial Fibrillation III Randomized clinical trial. Lancet 1996;348:633–8.

[24] The SPAF III Writing Committee for the Stroke Prevention in Atrial Fibrillation Investigators. Patients with nonvalvular atrial fibrillation at low risk of stroke during treatment with aspirin. JAMA 1998;279:1273–7.

[25] van Walraven C, Hart RG, Singer DE, et al. All anticoagulants vs aspirin in nonvalvular atrial fibrillation: An individual patient meta-analysis. JAMA 2002;288:2441–8.

[26] Klein AL, Grimm RA, Murray RD, et al. Use of transesophageal echocardiography to guide cardioversion in patients with atrial fibrillation. N Engl J Med 2001;344:1420–41.

[27] Thamilarasan M, Klein AL. Transesophageal echocardiography (TEE) in atrial fibrillation. Cardiol Clin 2000;18:819–31.

[28] Wyse DG, Waldo AL, DiMarco JP, et al. A comparison of rate control and rhythm control in patients with recurrent persistent atrial fibrillation. N Engl J Med 2002;347:1825–33.

[29] Sherman DG, Kim SJ, Boop BS, et al. The occurrence and characteristics of stroke events in the AFFIRM study. Arch Intern Med 2005;105:1185–91.

[30] van Gelder IC, Hagens VE, Bosker HA, et al. A comparison of rate control and rhythm control in patients with recurrent persistent atrial fibrillation. N Engl J Med 2002;347:1834–40.

[31] Rho RW, Page RL. Asymptomatic atrial fibrillation. Prog Cardiovasc Dis 2005;48:79–87.

[32] Israel CW, Gronefeld G, Ehrlich JR, et al. Long-term risk of recurrent atrial fibrillation as documented by an implantable monitoring device: implications for optimal patient care. J Am Coll Cardiol 2004;43:47–52.

[33] Martinek M, Aichinger J, Nesser HJ, et al. New insights into long-term follow-up of atrial fibrillation ablation: full disclosure by an implantable pacemaker device. J Cardiovasc Electrophysiol 2007;18:818–23.

[34] Waldo AL. Guidelines for anticoagulation of atrial fibrillation: is it time for an update? In: Raviele A, editor. Cardiac arrhythmias 2005. Italy: Springer-Verlag Italia; 2006. p. 169–76.

[35] Calkins H, Brugada J, Packer DL, et al. HRS/EHRA/ECAS Expert consensus statement on catheter and surgical ablation of atrial fibrillation: recommendations for personnel, policy, procedures and follow-up. A report of the Heart Rhythm Society (HRS Task Force on Catheter and Surgical Ablation of Atrial Fibrillation). Heart Rhythm 2007;4:816–61.

[36] Natale A, Raviele A, Arentz T, et al. Venice Chart international consensus document on atrial fibrillation ablation. J Cardiovasc Electrophysiol 2007;18:560–80.

[37] Pappone C, Rosario S, Augello G, et al. Mortality, morbidity, and quality of life after circumferential pulmonary vein ablation for atrial fibrillation. Outcomes from a controlled, nonrandomized long term study. J Am Coll Cardiol 2003;42:185–97.

[38] Oral H, Chugh A, Ozaydin M, et al. Risk of thromboembolic events after percutaneous left atrial radiofrequency ablation of atrial fibrillation. Circulation 2006;114:759–65.

ELSEVIER
SAUNDERS

THE MEDICAL
CLINICS
OF NORTH AMERICA

Med Clin N Am 92 (2008) 161–178

The Role of Pacemakers
in the Management of Patients
with Atrial Fibrillation

Gautham Kalahasty, MD*, Kenneth Ellenbogen, MD

Division of Cardiology, Department of Internal Medicine, Virginia Commonwealth University, 1200 East Marshall Street, Richmond, VA 23298, USA

This article reviews the wide range of implantable device–based therapies (mainly pacemakers) that are being used in the management of atrial fibrillation (AF), atrial flutter, and atrial tachycardias (AT). Pacemakers have an important role in the management of some patients with AF. The frequency of their use relative to other non-pharmacologic strategies is likely to increase over time as the incidence and prevalence of AF increases, especially in the elderly. The clinical burden of AF in the elderly population is staggering. In the groups aged 70 to 79 years and 80 to 89 years, the prevalence of AF is at least 4.8% and 8.8%, respectively. By 2050, it is estimated that 50% of the patients with AF will be more than 80 years old [1]. Box 1 summarizes the most common strategies that have been used for device-based management of patients with AF.

The most common indication for pacemaker implantation in the United States is sinus node dysfunction. AF is a common occurrence in patients with sinus node dysfunction. Pacemaker implantation practice patterns in the United States vary from those in Europe. Dual chamber (rather than single chamber) pacemakers are usually implanted in the United States for patients with sick sinus syndrome and paroxysmal AF even if there is no AV conduction abnormality at the time of implantation. The incidence of developing AV block is 8.4% over a period of 34 months [2]. In a European study of patients who received a single chamber (AAI) pacemaker for sick sinus syndrome, there was a 1.7% annual incidence of needing a ventricular lead for AV block [3]. Because the incidence of AV block is not insignificant, in the United States, patients with paroxysmal AF and sick sinus

---

* Corresponding author.
E-mail address: gkalahasty@mcvh-vcu.edu (G. Kalahasty).

0025-7125/08/$ - see front matter © 2008 Elsevier Inc. All rights reserved.
doi:10.1016/j.mcna.2007.09.003   *medical.theclinics.com*

Box 1. Device-related applications for the management of AF

Rate control
    Pacing to facilitate the use of rate-lowering agents
    Pacing in chronic AF
    Pacing for rate regularization
    Pacing in conjunction with atrioventricular (AV) node ablation
      or modification
Rhythm control/maintenance of sinus rhythm
    Pacing to facilitate the use of anti-arrhythmic medication
    Pacing to maintain or promote sinus rhythm
      Algorithms to promote sinus rhythm
      Multi-site pacing (dual site, bi-atrial)
      Novel site pacing
    Pacing/defibrillation to terminate AF

---

syndrome almost universally receive dual chamber pacemakers. Deliberate pacemaker programming and careful pacemaker mode selection with the goal of maintaining "physiologic pacing" becomes critical.

Clinically, AF is described as permanent or chronic if it is long-standing (eg, longer than 1 year) and if cardioversion has failed or has been foregone. AF is called persistent if it lasts more than 7 days regardless of whether cardioversion is needed to restore sinus rhythm; it is considered paroxysmal if episodes of AF terminate spontaneously [4]. Pacemakers have applications in each of these clinical types of AF.

Physiologic pacing

An appreciation of the role of pacemakers in the management of AF (especially in the context of sinus node dysfunction) requires an understanding of the evolution of the meaning of "physiologic pacing." Careful mode selection and proper programming is needed to optimize the beneficial effects and minimize the potentially detrimental effects of pacing. The benefits of dual chamber AV synchronous pacing or atrial-based pacing over single chamber ventricular only pacing in patients with sinus node dysfunction and paroxysmal AF have been well studied and are widely accepted. Hemodynamic parameters, quality of life measures, and clinical endpoints have all been investigated.

Hemodynamic studies have demonstrated that AV synchrony improves stroke volume and cardiac output and reduces right atrial pressure and pulmonary-capillary wedge pressures. A significant number of patients who receive a single chamber ventricular-based pacemaker will develop pacemaker syndrome consisting of symptoms such as fatigue, palpitations, and chest pain. These symptoms resolve after patients are AV synchronously paced [5,6]. When comparisons are made within individual patients rather than between patients, dual chamber AV synchronous pacing is strongly preferred to single chamber ventricular pacing [9].

Table 1 summarizes the key clinical findings in some of the individual studies that have demonstrated the benefits of AV synchronous pacing or atrial-based pacing. These studies have collectively enrolled over 4500 patients. Over a 2.5-year period, AF occurred more frequently with ventricular-based pacing when compared with atrial-based pacing (22.3% versus 3.9%). Interestingly, the two largest trials comparing ventricular-based pacing with AV synchronous pacing failed to demonstrate a benefit of AV synchronous pacing in terms of mortality or stroke risk [10,11]. A recent meta-analysis by Healey and colleagues [12] pooled data from eight randomized trials (including some of those in Table 1) to detect clinically significant outcomes that the individual trials were not powered to detect. The combined data from these trials represents 35,000 patient-years of follow-up and demonstrates that, although the incidence of AF was less with atrial-based pacing when compared with ventricular only pacing, there was no significant benefit in terms of all-cause mortality. Despite the reduced incidence of AF, there was no significant reduction in the risk of stroke.

In a secondary analysis of the MOST data, two additional important findings were reported. Increasing proportions of ventricular pacing was found to be associated with an increased incidence of AF during ventricular backup (VVIR) and dual chamber (DDDR) pacing. Also, greater proportions of ventricular pacing were associated with a greater risk of hospitalization for heart failure [13]. If ventricular pacing occurred more than 40% of the time, there was a twofold increase in the risk for congestive heart failure. This study suggests that the relative benefits of AV synchronous pacing compared with ventricular only pacing are due to the deleterious effects of right ventricular pacing rather than the presumed advantages of AV synchronous pacing. The CTOPP and MOST studies had relatively few patients with true atrial only based pacing (AAI) without the confounding effect of ventricular pacing. In the MADIT II study, patients who received an implantable cardioverter defibrillator (ICD) had higher survival rates but also demonstrated a trend toward increased rates of congestive heart failure; 73 patients (14.9%) in the conventional therapy group and 148 in the defibrillator group (19.9%) were hospitalized with heart failure ($P = .09$) [14]. In the DAVID trial, a composite endpoint of time to death and first hospitalization for congestive heart failure was compared in ICD patients programmed to receive dual chamber pacing (DDDR-70) or ventricular backup pacing (VVI-40) [15]. At 1 year, 83.9% of the patients in the VVI-40 group were free from the composite endpoint compared with 73.3% of patients in the DDDR-70 group. Hospitalization for congestive heart failure occurred in 13.3% of VVI-40 patients compared with 22.6% of DDD-70 patients, trending in favor of the VVI-40 group. Although the DAVID study looked only at an ICD population, it has had

Table 1
Benefits of AV synchronous pacing or atrial-based pacing

Study	Design	Key findings
AAI versus VVI Trial, Andersen et al [7]	AAI versus VVI in 210 patients with sick sinus syndrome	At long-term follow-up (8 years), the incidence of paroxysmal AF and chronic AF was significantly reduced in the AAI group. Overall survival, heart failure, and thromboembolic events were reduced with atrial-based pacing.
Mattioli et al [8]	VVI/VVIR versus AAI/DDD/DDDR/VDD pacing in patients with AV block (100) and sick sinus syndrome (110)	Incidence of AF was 10% at 1 year, 23% at 2 years, and 31% at 5 years. An increase in the incidence of chronic AF was observed in patients with sick sinus syndrome who received ventricular-based pacemakers (VVI/VVIR).
PASE Trial [5]	VVIR or DDDR pacing modes randomly assigned to 407 patients receiving dual chamber pacemakers for sick sinus syndrome, AV block, and other indications	Patients with sick sinus syndrome showed a trend toward a lower incidence of AF and all-cause mortality (AF: 19% versus 28%, $P = .06$; mortality: 12% versus 20%, $P = .09$). Quality of life was not different between the two pacing modes. A significant number of patients (26%) developed pacemaker syndrome when paced in VVIR mode.

CTOPP [10] and sub-study [11]	2568 patients randomized to ventricular pacing (VVI/R) versus physiologic pacing (DDD/R or AAI/R)	The annual rate of AF was less with physiologic pacing. No difference was observed in stroke or cardiovascular death between the two groups. There was a 27% reduction in the annual rate of progression to chronic AF.
MOST [6]	2010 patients randomized to VVIR versus DDDR programming, > 50% had prior AF	AF was reduced in patients randomized to physiologic pacing. No difference in mortality and stroke was observed between physiologic and ventricular-based pacing. Thirty-one percent of patients crossed over from VVIR to DDDR, 49% of which was due to pacemaker syndrome.

a major impact on the programming of dual chamber pacemakers. By high-lighting the deleterious effects of right ventricular pacing, it underscores the importance of mode selection in patients with sinus node dysfunction and paroxysmal AF. The programmed parameters of a pacemaker or ICD should minimize ventricular pacing.

Data from the MADIT II and DAVID studies involved only patients with severe left ventricular dysfunction. This limitation raises the question of whether the detrimental effects of right ventricular pacing (in terms of heart failure and mortality) are seen in patients with lesser degrees of left ventricular dysfunction or normal left ventricular function. There are limited data on which to answer this question.

If physiologic pacing can be thought of as the pacing mode that yields the best outcomes with the least detrimental effects, atrial-based pacing that promotes intrinsic conduction and minimizes right ventricular apical pacing (in patients with no indications for cardiac resynchronization therapy [CRT]) would seem to be the mode of choice. AV synchrony alone is not enough.

Pacemaker diagnostics

Pacemaker diagnostics not only can provide insight into the burden of AF but can also reveal the presence of asymptomatic AF that was not previously suspected [16]. Routine interrogation of a pacemaker implanted for sinus node dysfunction may reveal episodes of AF that are stored in the memory as mode switch episodes or atrial high rate episodes. Mode switch refers to the ability of the pacemaker to change from a dual chamber pacing mode (DDD) to a non-tracking mode (DDI or VVI). This feature is available in current pacemakers and ICDs. Once enabled, it is an automatic event and does not require office-based reprogramming. An atrial arrhythmia that meets a preset duration (a few seconds) and rate (usually > 160 bpm) results in a mode switch. When the atrial arrhythmia terminates, dual chamber pacing is resumed. Mode switching prevents rapid ventricular pacing in response to the tracking of rapid atrial rates. The frequency and duration of atrial arrhythmias including AF and atrial flutter can be recorded. Many pacemakers are capable of storing intracardiac electrograms, sometimes allowing the clinician to distinguish among AF, AT, and atrial flutter. Some devices are only capable of reporting the number and duration of mode switch episodes without storing any associated electrograms. In these cases, an event monitor may be needed to document the atrial arrhythmias. Artifact and oversensing of atrial or far field ventricular events can result in inappropriate mode switch episodes. Appropriate mode switches can have a significant impact on the management of patients in terms of the timely initiation of anticoagulation, reducing the risk of future thromboembolic events.

Fig. 1 shows the interrogation report of a dual chamber pacemaker. It was implanted for symptomatic sinus bradycardia in a 73-year-old patient not previously known to have AF. During the 1 month following implantation, the patient had 186 episodes of atrial high rates, 4 of which were greater than 1 minute in duration. The longest mode switch episode lasted almost 6 hours. These episodes were asymptomatic. Based on these findings, the initiation of warfarin sodium (Coumadin) was discussed with the patient, and the dose of beta-blockers was increased. Fig. 2 shows an example of a stored electrogram of an atrial tachyarrhythmia that resulted in an appropriate mode switch. In addition to mode switch events, it is also important to know the percentage of ventricular pacing in patients with intact AV conduction. The practice of maximizing the AV delay to promote intrinsic AV conduction is supported by data from the DAVID trial, MADIT II trial, and MOST trials.

Chronic or permanent atrial fibrillation

It is not uncommon for patients with chronic AF to require a permanent pacemaker. These patients may develop a slow ventricular response over time resulting in symptomatic bradycardia. Progressively slower conduction is often the result of age-associated degeneration of the conduction system. This process may be gradual, and some elderly patients do not readily

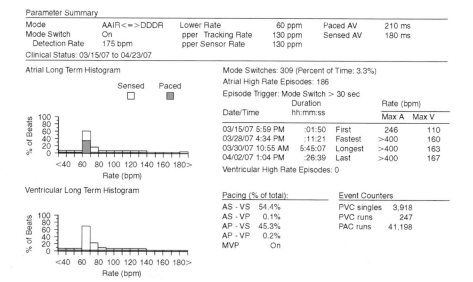

Fig. 1. Interrogation report from a dual chamber pacemaker (Medtronic Adapta ADDR01; Medtronic, Minneapolis, Minnesota). This pacemaker has a feature that allows real-time mode switching from AAI mode to DDD mode (MVP), resulting in minimal ventricular pacing.

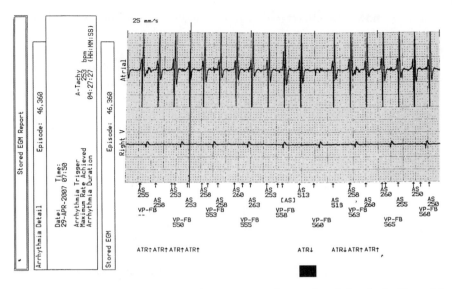

Fig. 2. Example of stored electrograms from an appropriate mode switch episode. The atrial channel shows a rapid irregular atrial rate with a maximum of 253 bpm.

recognize or reveal symptoms of exercise intolerance, dyspnea on exertion, and easy fatigability that can accompany bradycardia and chronotropic incompetence. Physicians and patients frequently dismiss these symptoms as a natural consequence of aging. In addition, comorbid conditions may be present that can result in similar symptoms; therefore, a Holter monitor or event monitor may be needed to truly obtain symptom-rhythm correlation. If this is established, a single chamber rate responsive pacemaker (VVIR) can provide symptom relief and improve functional capacity.

Bradycardia may also be an unavoidable consequence of the medications used to prevent a rapid ventricular response during AF. Beta-blockers, calcium channel blockers, and digoxin are used to blunt rapid ventricular rates during AF but can result in intermittent symptomatic bradycardia or long pauses that can lead to syncope or presyncope. Of note, pauses of up to 2 and 3 seconds during sleep are not unusual and are not solely an indication for pacing; rather, they are a function of the relatively high vagal tone that is present during sleep. Dosage adjustment of medications or the use of beta-blockers with intrinsic sympathomimetic activity can sometimes mitigate bradycardia or pauses but can also result in suboptimal rate control when a patient is active and awake. A pacemaker is indicated to facilitate the use of medications that are considered essential and for which there are no other suitable alternatives.

Regardless of the indication, a rate responsive pacemaker can also provide a chronotropic response appropriate to a patient's physiologic needs. Current pacemakers employ a variety of sensor driven algorithms to increase the heart rate according to the patients needs. The two most common sensors are accelerometers (based on movement) and minute ventilation monitors (based on respiratory rate). Some devices use both. Optimal use of these devices requires routine office-based follow-up and reprogramming.

Regulation of atrioventricular nodal conduction by pacing

During AF, both the rapid ventricular rate and irregular ventricular response contribute to deleterious hemodynamic effects. The irregular ventricular response can result in decreased cardiac output and increased wedge pressure independent of mean rate [17]. It has also been shown that cycle length variability has more influence on ventricular performance at faster heart rates. Ventricular pacing can result in concealed conduction into the AV node and His-Purkinje system, resulting in slowing of AV conduction. Algorithms have been developed that result in pacing slightly faster than the mean ventricular rate but with more regular ventricular response. Despite the expected benefits, clinical trials that have studied these regularization algorithms have yielded mixed and somewhat disappointing results. In the AF Symptoms Study, the effect of ventricular rate regularization on the endpoints of quality of life, AF symptoms, and exercise capacity was evaluated. The investigators reported that ventricular rate regulation had a positive impact on reported symptoms, particularly palpitations, but did not have a significant impact on overall quality of life or functional capacity [18]. Based on these studies, ventricular pacing during chronic rapid AF using regularization algorithms cannot be considered an alternative to AV node ablation or a primary indication for permanent pacemaker implantation.

Atrioventricular node (junction) ablation

It is not possible to achieve typical heart rate targets in many patients with chronic or paroxysmal AF. A resting heart rate of 80 bpm or less, a 24-hour Holter average of 100 bpm or less, and a heart rate less than or equal to 120 bpm with modest activity are reasonable empiric goals for rate control but should be individualized based on symptoms. For patients in whom pharmacologic therapy cannot reach the desired rate targets and for whom there are no other alternatives, ablation of the AV node and pacemaker implantation is the preferred strategy. Although more commonly used in patients with chronic AF, it is also performed in select patients with paroxysmal AF and in whom anti-arrhythmic drugs do not provide adequate rhythm control. These patients should receive a dual chamber pacemaker with a mode switch capability enabled to maintain AV synchrony when the patient is in sinus rhythm. Otherwise, a standard single chamber ventricular rate responsive pacemaker is all that is needed in patients with preserved left ventricular function and chronic AF.

The benefits of AV junction ablation and pacemaker implantation are significant and were summarized in a meta-analysis covering 21 studies that included 1181 patients [19]. Echocardiographic parameters such as the ejection fraction have been shown to improve, as well as the number of office visits, hospital admissions, and the New York Heart Association (NYHA) functional capacity. Quality of life measures such as quality of life scores, activity level, exercise intolerance, symptom frequency, and symptom severity were also improved [19].

Despite the expected advantages, there are some serious disadvantages that should be considered and explained to patients. The most obvious is that AV junction ablation, unlike medications, is generally irreversible and renders the patient pacemaker dependent for life. The procedure itself is generally low risk, nearly 100% successful, and usually not technically difficult. Patients are exposed to a small risk of thromboembolic events while their anticoagulation is stopped for the ablation procedure. There is a small risk of vascular complications such as hematoma and pseudoaneurysm formation. A recurrence rate of 5% has been reported necessitating a redo ablation. Although practice patterns vary widely, there is growing evidence that pacemaker implantation and pacemaker generator replacements can be performed safely while patients are on therapeutic doses of warfarin [20,21]. Most importantly, AV nodal ablation does not obviate the need for long-term anticoagulation. AV synchrony is not preserved, and in patients with significant diastolic dysfunction, the expected symptomatic improvement may be less.

There is a concern that patients are at risk of sudden death following AV node ablation and pacemaker implantation. Based on reported survival data, the risk of sudden death and total mortality is 2% and 6% at 1 year, respectively. Long-term (6 years) mortality is similar in patients undergoing pacing and ablation when compared with continued medical therapy [22]. The increased risk is thought to be due to bradycardia-dependent arrhythmias (torsades de pointes). Programming the lower rate of the pacemaker at 90 bpm for the first month has been shown to minimize this risk [23]. Another concern is the risk associated with lead dislodgement in these patients who are usually pacemaker dependent. Because of these concerns, many physicians will implant the pacemaker several weeks in advance of the ablation procedure. The use of a CRT or standard right ventricular pacing device in patients with significant left ventricular dysfunction is discussed later in this review.

Paroxysmal or persistent atrial fibrillation

The results of the AFFIRM (Atrial Fibrillation Follow-up Investigation of Rhythm Management) trial do not apply to every subset of patients with AF; therefore, rhythm control remains an appropriate strategy in many patients with paroxysmal AF [24]. Factors such as symptoms, quality of life,

and the interplay between AF and comorbidities are important considerations when selecting rhythm control strategies over rate control strategies.
For example, patients with diastolic dysfunction or valvular heart disease
such as aortic or mitral stenosis do not tolerate AF and require aggressive
rhythm control. Some patients are also at risk for congestive heart failure
or tachycardia-induced cardiomyopathy. Despite their limited efficacy and
potential for side effects including proarrhythmia, anti-arrhythmic drugs
have an important role in the treatment of AF. Symptomatic bradycardia
as well as bradycardia-dependent polymorphic ventricular tachycardia has
been reported with amiodarone, sotalol, and propafenone. These medications can also prolong the pauses that are sometimes seen in patients with
sinus node dysfunction. These pauses are often seen immediately following
the termination of AF, before the resumption of sinus node activity. Pacemakers can be used to facilitate the use of these medications.

There has been a great deal of interest in preventing AF in patients with
paroxysmal AF by the use of device-based algorithms designed to address
two aspects of the pathophysiology of AF, triggers and substrate. Clinical
and experimental data suggest that AF may be triggered by atrial premature
complexes. The atria of some patients may be more susceptible to AF due to
inhomogeneous atrial refractoriness. These patients sometimes have atrial
myopathy and often have atrial remodeling and enlargement. Overdrive
pacing, multi-site pacing (dual and bi-atrial), and alternate site pacing are
device-based strategies designed to reduce the AF burden by addressing
these pathophysiologic mechanisms.

Overdrive pacing algorithms seek to reduce atrial premature complexes
and prevent pauses and bradycardia. Fixed rate atrial pacing alone (lower
rate of 70 bpm) has been shown to have no effect on AF burden. All of
the three major device manufacturers have algorithms that attempt to reduce AF recurrence and overall AF burden. The dynamic atrial overdrive
algorithm (DAO; St. Jude Medical, Sylmar, California) is one example
that has been shown to achieve modest reduction in AF burden and has
been given a US Food and Drug Administration labeling for this indication.
Despite extensive studies, the clinical utility of these algorithms is limited.

Multi-site atrial pacing involves placement of one lead in the high right
atrium and another lead near the coronary sinus ostium (dual site) or into
the coronary sinus to pace the left atrium (bi-atrial). Small nonrandomized
studies show conflicting results in terms of reducing AF burden [25,26]. A
prolonged P-wave duration (>120 milliseconds) may be a necessary condition for multi-site pacing to be beneficial when compared single site pacing
[27]. Larger clinical trials have not demonstrated a significant AF burden reduction. In one study, dual site right atrial pacing reduced the recurrence
risk of AF when compared with standard pacing in patients treated with
anti-arrhythmic drugs [28]. Bi-atrial pacing seems to have a limited routine
clinical application when used acutely in postoperative patients. A meta-
analysis involving eight studies enrolling 776 patients reported a significant

reduction in the risk for AF in post heart surgery patients who received temporary bi-atrial pacing using two epicardial wires [29].

The premise of alternate site atrial pacing is that more uniform interatrial conduction can be achieved by pacing at the interatrial septum. The resultant decrease in heterogeneity of atrial refractoriness is expected to reduce AF burden. Pacing can be done from the high atrial septum (Bachmann's bundle) or the low atrial septum (near the coronary sinus os). Studies have yielded conflicting results in a relatively small number of patients.

There are not enough long-term clinical data to support the recommendation of overdrive pacing algorithms, multi-site pacing, or alternate site pacing as primary indications for pacemaker implantation. The results of some of the available studies have likely been confounded by the presence of ventricular pacing.

Cardiac resynchronization therapy and atrial fibrillation

CRT, also known as bi-ventricular pacing, is an important treatment modality in patients with moderate and advanced congestive heart failure. The current American College of Cardiology/American Heart Association/ Heart Rhythm Society (HRS) guidelines indicate that patients with a left ventricular ejection fraction (LVEF) less than or equal to 35%, sinus rhythm, and NYHA class III or ambulatory class IV symptoms despite recommended optimal medical therapy and who have cardiac dysynchrony (currently defined as a QRS duration greater that 120 milliseconds) should receive CRT. Many patients who are candidates for CRT also have a history of paroxysmal or chronic AF. In patients who are candidates for CRT-defibrillators, a history of paroxysmal AF is associated with as much as a 25% incidence of AF within the first 6 months from the time of implant. Patients with a CRT indication are also at high risk of developing AF. The prevalence and incidence of AF increases with increasing severity of heart failure [30]. There are several issues to examine when considering the benefits of CRT in patients with chronic and paroxysmal AF.

First, in patients with existing CRT devices, what is the hemodynamic and clinical impact of the development of AF? The effects parallel those that are seen in patients with heart failure but do not have a CRT device. The most immediate effect on the development of AF in bi-ventricular pacing is the loss of AV synchrony, possibly leading to decompensated heart failure. In one small study of acute hemodynamics, systolic function as measured by dP/dT was worse in heart failure patients with RR irregularity and rapid ventricular rates (120 bpm) but not worse when ventricular rates were in the normal range (80 bpm) [31]. The timing of ventricular pacing is based on sensed or paced atrial events. AV synchrony can be maintained only during sinus rhythm. Most CRT devices have algorithms that promote bi-ventricular pacing even during AF despite the loss of AV synchrony. These algorithms are imperfect, and despite device-reported bi-ventricular pacing of greater than 90%, clinical benefits are less certain owing to variable degrees of fusion between the intrinsic conduction and the paced ventricular complex. Furthermore, these algorithms tend to result in pacing rates that are, on average, faster than during intrinsic conduction (up to the programmed upper pacing rate), raising the concern of tachycardia-induced cardiomyopathies.

A second issue is whether CRT reduces the likelihood of developing AF. As is true in patients with normal left ventricular function, the benefits of bi-ventricular pacing in patients with a CRT device in terms of the reduction of AF burden are mixed and uncertain. In a small cohort study, the annual incidence of AF was 2.8% in the CRT group and 10.2% in the control group ($P = .025$) [32]. In another study, the incidence of AF was not affected by CRT [33].

A third issue is the effect of chronic AF on CRT benefit. Large-scale clinical trial data elucidating the benefits of CRT in patients with AF are limited. The Multisite Stimulation in Cardiomyopathies (MUSTIC) study reported on a limited number of patients with chronic AF who received a CRT device. Both the sinus rhythm group and the AF group in this study showed improvements in heart failure class, 6-minute walk test, and the need for hospitalization [34]. The improvement was greater in the sinus rhythm group. In a study by Molhoek and colleagues [35], patients in normal sinus rhythm and those in chronic AF derived benefit from CRT. Heart failure class, quality of life scores, and exercise capacity were improved in both groups. In the group with AF, patients with previous AV junction ablation derived the most benefit. Patients who had not previously had an AV junction ablation did not show an improvement in quality of life scores at 6 months. There were more non-responders in the AF group than the sinus group (36% versus 20%, $P<.05$). The AVERT-AF trial (Atrioventricular Junction Ablation Followed by Resynchronization Therapy in patients with CHF and AF) is a prospective, randomized, double-blinded, multicenter trial that will be testing the hypothesis that AV junction ablation followed by bi-ventricular pacing significantly improves exercise capacity and functional status when compared with pharmacologic rate control in patients with chronic AF and a depressed ejection fraction, regardless of rate or QRS duration. Enrollment will be completed in 2008 [36].

Another unresolved issue is the timing of implantation of a CRT defibrillator device (CRT-D) versus a standard pacemaker relative to AV junction ablation. Given that there can be an improvement of the LVEF in some patients following AV junction ablation, some practitioners implant a standard dual chamber pacemaker in patients with borderline LVEF (30%–35%) [14,21]. The ejection fraction is then re-evaluated after a period of time (ie, 6 months) and the need for a CRT device is determined [37]. Others elect to implant a CRT-D at initial implantation to avoid the need for another procedure within a relatively short period of time.

A CRT pacemaker without defibrillation capability (CRT-P) is a consideration in patients with a more preserved ejection fraction. The PAVE trial has provided some important insights into the type of pacing that is best in this group of patients. This trial compared chronic bi-ventricular pacing with right ventricular only pacing in patients who underwent AV junction ablation for the management of AF with rapid ventricular rates. The mean LVEF was 46% ± 16% in the two groups. The mean LVEF in the right ventricular pacing group was 45% at the onset of the study and 41% at 6 months ($P<.05$) [38]. There are no guidelines for the use of a CRT-P in patients with moderate left ventricular dysfunction who are undergoing AV junction ablation.

Atrial therapies

Some implantable devices are capable of delivering electrical therapy to manage AF and atrial flutter. These therapies include anti-tachycardia pacing with burst and ramp pacing in the atrium, high-frequency (50 Hz) burst pacing, and atrial defibrillation. All three have been successfully used in terminating AT and atrial flutter.

Pacing therapies are more suitable for relatively slow AT with a regular cycle length. They are not well suited for AF; however, AF has been known to organize into an atrial flutter that is more susceptible to pace termination. There is no evidence that 50-Hz burst pacing has any significant effect in terminating AF or in reducing the overall burden of AF in humans. There are conflicting data with respect to the effect these therapies have on the overall burden of AF. In the ATTEST trial, prevention and termination algorithms were tested prospectively and failed to show a reduction in AF burden [39]. In another prospective trial, atrial therapies resulted in a reduction of atrial tachyarrhythmia burden from a mean of 58.5 to 7.8 h/mo. This study enrolled patients with a standard ICD indication and atrial tachyarrhythmias [40].

Stand-alone implantable atrial defibrillators are not used clinically and are no longer marketed. ICDs with atrial defibrillation capability have been developed, but their use is limited by the painful nature of the shocks. The pain threshold for a defibrillation shock is far less than the threshold for successful atrial defibrillation. The ADSAS 2 study demonstrated that premedication with oral midazolam has been effective in mitigating some of the perceptions of pain [41]. This option can only be used in select, highly motivated patients.

Currently, there are no guidelines that advocate using devices with these features as a primary means to manage atrial tachyarrhythmias. Most physicians use these features as an adjunctive therapy in patients with other standard indications for pacemakers or ICDs. Overall, they have limited utility.

Summary

The role of pacemakers in the management of patients with AF and in the prevention of AF has been extensively studied. Based on well-designed prospective clinical trials, only a few of these strategies can be recommended for routine clinical use in related subpopulations. From the available studies several key considerations are apparent.

1. The definition of physiologic pacing has evolved. It is no longer enough to maintain AV synchrony with a dual chamber atrial-based pacemaker. A single chamber ventricular-based pacemaker should be avoided in patients with paroxysmal AF and sinus node dysfunction. When possible, intrinsic AV conduction should be promoted to minimize the deleterious effects of right ventricular pacing; therefore, mode selection is important (AAI ← →DDD, DDI, or DDD with long AV delays). Unresolved questions include the maximum hemodynamically acceptable AV delay and the best site for right ventricular pacing [42].

2. In appropriate patients, pacemaker implantation and AV junction ablation provide clinical and mortality benefits. This procedure should be considered in any patient with suboptimal rate control and in any patient who is at risk for tachycardia-mediated cardiomyopathy. Although this procedure is most often done in patients with chronic AF, it is also appropriate for some patients with paroxysmal AF.

3. The benefits of pacing in patients with a CRT device may be maximized in those patients with AF who have undergone AV junction ablation. In patients with chronic AF who are receiving a CRT device, AV junction ablation can be recommended. This issue is unresolved in patients with paroxysmal AF who receive a CRT device.

4. Pacing in chronic AF to promote ventricular rate regularization has limited clinical value, and careful attention should be paid to the overall adequacy of rate control. An average ventricular rate above the upper pacing limit may lead to tachycardia-mediated cardiomyopathy and signal the need for more aggressive rate control or AV junction ablation.

5. Pacing algorithms that attempt to prevent AF have limited value. They are not widely accepted as a sole indication nor recommended as a primary indication for pacemaker implantation in patients with paroxysmal or persistent AF [43].

6. Multi-site and novel site pacing strategies do not have broad clinical applications at this time. An exception is the use of short-term multi-site pacing at the time of cardiac surgery.

References

[1] Go AS, Hylek EM, Phillips KA, et al. Prevalence of diagnosed atrial fibrillation in adults. JAMA 2001;285:2370–5.
[2] Sutton R, Kenny RA. The natural history of sick sinus syndrome. Pacing Clin Electrophysiol 1986;9(6 Pt 2):1110–4.
[3] Kristensen L, Nielsen JC, Pedersen AK, et al. AV block and changes in pacing mode during long-term follow-up of 399 consecutive patients with sick sinus syndrome treated with an AAI/AAIR pacemaker. Pacing Clin Electrophysiol 2001;24(3):358–65.

[4] Fuster V, Ryden LE, Asinger RW, et al. ACC/AHA/ESC 2006. A report of the American College of Cardiology/American Heart Association Task Force on Practice Guidelines and the European Society of Cardiology Committee for Practice Guidelines (Writing Committee to revise the 2001 Guidelines for the Management of Patients with Atrial Fibrillation). J Am Coll Cardiol 2006;48:854–906.

[5] Lamas GA, Orav J, Stambler BS, et al, for the Pacemaker Selection in the Elderly Investigators. Quality of life and clinical outcomes in elderly patients treated with ventricular pacing as compared with dual chamber pacing. N Engl J Med 1998;338:1097–104.

[6] Lamas GA, Lee KL, Sweeney MO, et al. Ventricular pacing or dual-chamber pacing for sinus-node dysfunction. N Engl J Med 2002;346:1854–62.

[7] Andersen HR, Nielsen JC, Thomsen PEB, et al. Long-term follow-up of patients from a randomized trial of atrial versus ventricular pacing for sick sinus syndrome. Lancet 1997;350:1210–6.

[8] Mattioli AV, Castellani ET, Vivoli D, et al. Prevalence of atrial fibrillation and stroke in paced patients without prior atrial fibrillation: a prospective study. Clin Cardiol 1998; 21(2):117–22.

[9] Sulke N, Chamber J, Dritsas A, et al. A randomized double blind crossover comparison of four rate-responsive pacing modes. J Am Coll Cardiol 1991;17:696–706.

[10] Connolly SJ, Kerr CR, Gent M, et al. Effects of physiologic pacing versus ventricular pacing on the risk of stroke and death due to cardiovascular causes. N Engl J Med 2000;342: 1385–91.

[11] Skanes AC, Krahn AD, Yee R, et al. Progression to chronic atrial fibrillation after pacing: the Canadian Trial of Physiologic Pacing. J Am Coll Cardiol 2001;38:167–72.

[12] Healey JS, William TD, Gervasio LA, et al. Cardiovascular outcomes with atrial-based pacing compared with ventricular pacing: meta-analysis of randomized trials, using individual patient data. Circulation 2006;114:11–7.

[13] Sweeney MO, Hellkamp AS, Ellenbogen KA, et al. Adverse effect of ventricular pacing on heart failure and atrial fibrillation among patients with normal baseline QRS duration in a clinical trial of pacemaker therapy for sinus node dysfunction. Circulation 2003;107: 2932–7.

[14] Moss AJ, Zareba W, Hall WJ, et al. Prophylactic implantation of a defibrillator in patients with myocardial infarction and reduced ejection fraction. N Engl J Med 2002;346:877–83.

[15] Wilkoff BL, Cook JR, Epstein AE, et al. Dual-chamber pacing or ventricular backup pacing in patients with an implantable defibrillator: the Dual Chamber and VVI Implantable defibrillator (DAVID) Trial. JAMA 2002;288(24):3115–23.

[16] Israel CW, Barold SS. Pacemaker systems as implantable cardiac rhythm monitors. Am J Cardiol 2001;88:442–5.

[17] Popovic ZB, Mowrey KA, Zhang Y, et al. Slow rate during AF improves ventricular performance by reducing sensitivity to cycle length irregularity. Am J Physiol Heart Circ Physiol 2002;283:H2706–13.

[18] Tse HF, Newman D, Ellenbogen KE, et al. Effects of ventricular rate regularization pacing on quality of life and symptoms in patients with atrial fibrillation (Atrial fibrillation symptoms mediated by pacing to mean rates [AF SYMPTOMS study]). Am J Cardiol 2004; 94(7):938–41.

[19] Wood MA, Brown-Mahoney C, Kay GN, et al. Clinical outcomes after ablation and pacing therapy for atrial fibrillation: a meta-analysis. Circulation 2000;101:1138–44.

[20] al-Khadra AS. Implantation of pacemakers and implantable cardioverter defibrillators in orally anticoagulated patients. Pacing Clin Electrophysiol 2003;26(1 Pt 2):511–4.

[21] Giudici MC, Paul DL, Bontu P, et al. Pacemaker and implantable cardioverter defibrillator implantation without reversal of warfarin therapy. Pacing Clin Electrophysiol 2004;27(3): 359–60.

[22] Ozean C, Jahangir A, Friedman PA, et al. Long-term survival after ablation of the atrioventricular node and implantation of a permanent pacemaker in patients with atrial fibrillation. N Engl J Med 2001;334:1043–51.

[23] Geelen P, Brugada J, Andries E, et al. Ventricular fibrillation and sudden death after radio-frequency catheter ablation of the atrioventricular junction. Pacing Clin Electrophysiol 1997;20:343–8.

[24] Wyse DG, Waldo AL, DiMarco JP, et al. Atrial Fibrillation Follow-up Investigation of Rhythm Management (AFFIRM) Investigators. A comparison of rate control and rhythm control in patients with atrial fibrillation. N Engl J Med 2002;347(23):1825–33.

[25] Delfaut P, Saksena S, Prakash K, et al. Long-term outcome of patients with drug-refractory atrial flutter and fibrillation after single- and dual-site right atrial pacing for arrhythmia prevention. J Am Coll Cardiol 1998;32:1900–8.

[26] Levy T, Walker S, Rex S, et al. No incremental benefit of multisite atrial pacing compared with right atrial pacing in patients with drug refractory paroxysmal atrial fibrillation. Heart 2001;85(1):48–52.

[27] Leclercq JF, De Sisti A, Fiorello P, et al. Is dual site better than single site atrial pacing in the prevention of atrial fibrillation? Pacing Clin Electrophysiol 2000;23:2101–7.

[28] Saksena S, Prakash A, Ziegler P, et al. Improved suppression of recurrent atrial fibrillation with dual-site right atrial pacing and antiarrhythmic drug therapy. J Am Coll Cardiol 2002; 40(6):1140–50.

[29] Daoud EG, Snow R, Hummel JD, et al. Temporary atrial epicardial pacing as prophylaxis against atrial fibrillation after heart surgery: a meta-analysis. J Cardiovasc Electrophysiol 2003;14(2):127–32.

[30] Saxon LA, Greenfield RA, Cradnall BG, et al. Results of the multicenter RENEWAL 3 AVT clinic study of cardiac resynchronization defibrillator therapy in patients with paroxysmal atrial fibrillation. J Cardiovasc Electrophysiol 2006;17(5):520–5.

[31] Melenovsky V, Hay I, Fetics BJ, et al. Functional impact of rate irregularity in patients with heart failure and atrial fibrillation receiving cardiac resynchronization therapy. Eur Heart J 2005;26(7):705–11.

[32] Fung J, Yu CM, Chan J, et al. Effects of cardiac resynchronization therapy on the incidence of atrial fibrillation in patients with poor left ventricular systolic function. Am J Cardiol 2005;96:728–31.

[33] Hoppe UC, Casares JM, Eiskjaer H, et al. Effect of cardiac resynchronization on the incidence of atrial fibrillation in patients with severe heart failure. Circulation 2006;114(1): 18–25.

[34] Cazeau S, Leclercq C, Lavergne T, et al. Effects of multisite biventricular pacing in patients with heart failure and intraventricular conduction delay. N Engl J Med 2001;344(12):873–80.

[35] Molhoek SG, Bax JJ, Bleeker GB, et al. Comparison of response to cardiac resynchronization therapy in patients with sinus rhythm versus chronic atrial fibrillation. Am J Cardiol 2004;94(12):1506–9.

[36] Hamdan MH, Freedman RA, Gilbert EM, et al. Atrioventricular junction ablation followed by resynchronization therapy in patients with congestive heart failure and atrial fibrillation (AVERT-AF) study design. Pacing Clin Electrophysiol 2006;29(10):1081–8.

[37] Bruce G, Friedman PA. Device-based therapies for atrial fibrillation. Curr Treat Options Cardiovasc Med 2005;7:359–70.

[38] Doshi RN, Daoud EG, Fellows C, et al. Left ventricular-based cardiac stimulation post AV nodal ablation evaluation (the PAVE Study). J Cardiovasc Electrophysiol 2005;16(11): 1160–5.

[39] Lee MA, Weachter R, Pollak S, et al. The effect of atrial pacing therapies on atrial tachyarrhythmia burden and frequency: results of a randomized trial in patients with bradycardia and atrial tachyarrhythmias. J Am Coll Cardiol 2003;41:1926–32.

[40] Friedman PA, Dijkman B, Warman EN, et al. Atrial therapies reduce atrial arrhythmia burden in defibrillator patients. Circulation 2001;104:1023–8.

[41] Boodhoo L, Mitchell A, Ujhelyi M, et al. Improving the acceptability of the atrial defibrillator: patient-activated cardioversion versus automatic night cardioversion with and without sedation (ADSAS 2). Pacing Clin Electrophysiol 2004;27:910–7.

[42] Barold SS, Herweg B. Right ventricular outflow tract pacing: not ready for prime-time. J Interv Card Electrophysiol 2005;13(1):39–46.

[43] Knight BP, Gersh BJ, Carlson MD, et al. Role of permanent pacing to prevent atrial fibrillation: science advisory from the American Heart Association Council on Clinical Cardiology (Subcommittee on Electrocardiography and Arrhythmias) and the Quality of Care and Outcomes Research Interdisciplinary Working Group, in collaboration with the Heart Rhythm Society. Circulation 2005;111(2):240–3.

ELSEVIER
SAUNDERS

Med Clin N Am 92 (2008) 179–201

THE MEDICAL
CLINICS
OF NORTH AMERICA

Catheter Ablation of Atrial Fibrillation

Thomas D. Callahan IV, MD[a],
Andrea Natale, MD, FACC, FHRS[b],*

[a]*Cardiac Pacing and Electrophysiology, Cleveland Clinic, F15, 9500 Euclid Avenue,*
Cleveland, OH 44195, USA
[b]*Stanford University, Palo Alto, CA*

Atrial fibrillation is a common arrhythmia associated with significant morbidity. It is the most common sustained arrhythmia and affects millions of Americans. The lifetime risk for the development of atrial fibrillation is estimated at 1 in 4 for men and women over the age of 40 [1]. Atrial fibrillation contributes to the development of angina, heart failure, and stroke with an estimated stroke risk of 3% to 5% per year in untreated individuals [2,3]. Furthermore, analysis of Framingham data suggests the mortality rate in patients who have atrial fibrillation is increased 1.5- to twofold compared with the general population [4,5]. Medical therapy for atrial fibrillation remains suboptimal and plagued by significant toxicities and frequent side effects and intolerance. Recurrence rates with medical therapy are estimated at 50% at 6 to 36 months [6].

Whether or not restoration of sinus rhythm should be a goal of therapy is a matter of debate in the literature. Several trials, including the Atrial Fibrillation Follow-Up Investigation of Rhythm Management (AFFIRM) trial, report no benefit of rhythm control over rate control in the treatment of atrial fibrillation [7,8]. These trials, however, examined pharmacologic rhythm control strategies. Further analysis of the AFFIRM data showed that the presence of atrial fibrillation was associated with a 47% increased mortality compared with sinus rhythm. The use of an antiarrhythmic medication was associated with a 49% increased mortality, suggesting that any mortality benefit from the maintenance of sinus rhythm was offset by increased mortality from currently available antiarrhythmics [9]. Catheter

---

* Corresponding author. Section of Pacing and Electrophysiology, Cleveland Clinic, F15, 9500 Euclid Avenue, Cleveland, OH 44195.
E-mail address: natalea@ccf.org (A. Natale).

ablation for atrial fibrillation offers a nonpharmacologic means of restoring sinus rhythm and improves mortality and quality of life compared with patients treated with antiarrhythmic drugs [10,11].

Fundamentals of radiofrequency catheter ablation

In 1979, Vedel and coauthors reported complete heart block after multiple attempts at direct current cardioversion while a recording catheter was positioned at the bundle of His. The investigators hypothesized that current shunting through the recording catheter injured the conduction system leading to heart block [12]. Subsequently, percutaneous catheter ablation for treatment of cardiac arrhythmias was born, and in the infancy of this technique, atrial fibrillation was one of the first arrhythmias to be treated. Patients who had atrial fibrillation and rapid ventricular rates refractory to medical therapy were offered ablation of the atrioventricular (AV) node using high-energy direct current delivered to the region of the AV junction [13,14]. Although effective, this technique was associated with a high rate of life-threatening complications [15].

Use of radiofrequency energy in catheter ablation was found to improve efficacy of ablation and the safety profile and quickly supplanted direct current catheter ablation [16–18]. Radiofrequency catheter ablation uses the delivery of alternating current, typically with frequencies of approximately 500 kHz, which generates myocardial lesions through thermal injury. Current disperses radially from the delivery electrode to a dispersive electrode placed on the skin with impedance, voltage drop, and power dissipation all greatest at the interface of the electrode and tissue. Heating of the tissue in close contact to the delivery electrode is the result of resistance as current passes through it and is referred to as direct heating. Thermal energy from this area is transferred back to the delivery electrode and to the surrounding tissue by conduction. Conductive or indirect heating accounts for a larger volume of thermal injury in the radiofrequency ablation lesion than does resistive or direct heating. Temperature rise is rapid in the zone of resistive heating and immediately adjacent areas; however, temperature rise is slower as the distance the distance from this area increases and can continue to rise at remote sites even after delivery of current has ceased [19].

Lesion size is influenced by several factors. Increasing the length or diameter of the delivery electrode, increasing the contact area, and increasing the source power all result in a larger radius of direct heating and, thus, larger lesion size. Circulating blood results in convective cooling. Although convective cooling within the tissue limits lesion size, cooling of the catheter tip via convection allows improved power delivery, which, in turn, increases lesion size and allows for more rapid lesion formation. Although lesion size is proportional to the peak temperature achieved, at temperatures of 100°C and above, char and coagulum form and can increase impedance dramatically [19]. Within the tissue, temperatures in excess of 100°C cause the sudden production of steam, which can lead to an explosive venting to the endocardial or epicardial surface, called a "pop." Convective cooling of the tissue-catheter interface by circulating blood and, when used, with irrigation of the catheter tip may cause temperatures at this interface to be lower than peak tissue temperatures achieved at within the tissue. As a result, thermal sensors in the catheter tip often underestimate peak, in-lesion temperatures. The authors have found that with nonirrigated catheter tips, measured temperature is not reliable and instead microbubble monitoring with intracardiac echocardiography is a more effective strategy for regulation of energy delivery [20]. Microbubble monitoring is not feasible with open-tip irrigated catheters, and with these, careful limitation of the maximum temperature and power and monitoring of the impedance are used to minimize tissue disruption.

Atrioventricular node ablation

Overview

Like medical therapy for atrial fibrillation, catheter ablation for atrial fibrillation can be divided into two general strategies, rate control and rhythm control. Within the field of catheter ablation, rate control can be achieved by modifying the AV node or ablating the node and implanting a permanent pacemaker. Curative catheter ablation achieves rhythm control by targeting the triggers of atrial fibrillation, restoring sinus rhythm, and preventing future recurrences. The technique of AV node ablation predated the development of curative ablation techniques for atrial fibrillation. AV node modification targets the slow pathway, resulting in increased AV node refractoriness and slower ventricular rates without causing AV block. This technique rarely is used, as complete heart block is common and malignant ventricular arrhythmias can be seen after the procedure. AV node ablation does not cure atrial fibrillation and requires the placement of a permanent pacemaker to ensure adequate ventricular rates. Ideally, the most proximal portion of the AV node is targeted, leaving the distal portion intact. This results in complete heart block, the desired result of the procedure, but maximizes the likelihood of leaving patients with an escape rhythm, which is desirable should a pacemaker malfunction occur. Because of its many limitations, including the requirement of a permanent pacemaker and the failure to address the long-term risk of stroke, and given the possible benefits of restoring sinus rhythm, AV node ablation has a limited role at the authors' institution and is restricted primarily to patients refractory to medical therapy and who have contraindications to curative atrial fibrillation ablation, such as significant comorbidities and poor life expectancy.

Techniques

Before AV node ablation, pacing of the ventricle should be ensured. This can be achieved by implantation of a permanent pacemaker prior to AV node ablation or by the placement of a temporary transvenous pacemaker prior to ablation and subsequent permanent pacemaker implantation immediately after the ablation procedure. The former strategy has the advantage of allowing any possible postimplantation device malfunctions to be addressed prior to AV node ablation. Placement of a dual chamber pacemaker with mode switching capabilities allows for AV synchrony during sinus rhythm or atrial pacing.

Ablation of the AV node usually is performed via the right side of the heart, and radiofrequency ablation is used most often. In approximately 5% to 10% of cases, the AV node can be ablated only through the left side of the heart, necessitating arterial access and a retrograde approach to apply lesions below to the aortic valve [21]. Use of cryoablation is described but does not seem to offer benefit over radiofrequency ablation [22]. Typically, the His bundle is identified. The ablation catheter then is withdrawn toward the right atrium to a site that demonstrates an atrial to ventricular electrogram ratio of 1:1 to 1:2 and a small His signal (Fig. 1). Care should be taken to map adequately and ensure catheter stability as ineffective lesions may result in edema without successful ablation. This may in turn make successful ablation more difficult by obscuring electrograms and increasing the distance to the target tissue. Effective lesions at an appropriate target site often induce an accelerated junctional rhythm early in the radiofrequency application, which subsequently resolves to a slower junctional or ventricular escape as radiofrequency application continues.

Outcomes and limitations

Success rates for AV node ablation are near 100% [23–27]. The procedure improves quality of life and may improve left ventricular ejection fraction

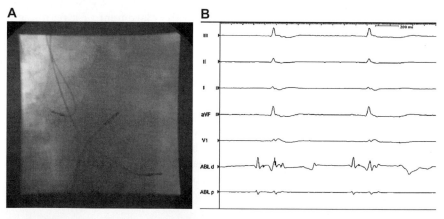

Fig. 1. Fluoroscopy and intracardiac electrograms demonstrating satisfactory catheter position for AV node ablation. The ablation catheter (ABL) is positioned in the region of the slow pathway with approximately equal A and V amplitudes on the distal ablation channel (ABLd) of the intracardiac electrogram. Pacemaker leads are seen in the right atrium (RA) and right ventricle (RV).

modestly, probably from improved rate control [23,24,28–30]. In addition to these benefits, AV node ablation usually can be performed quickly, which may be advantageous for patients unable to endure more protracted ablation procedures. Additionally, the procedure typically can be performed entirely from the right side of the heart and, thus, does not require systemic intraoperative anticoagulation and essentially eliminates the risk for thromboembolic complications. After AV node ablation, there exists a high risk for malignant ventricular arrhythmias. This risk is eliminated by programming a lower rate of at least 80 to 90 beats per minute for the first 4 to 8 weeks post procedure [29,31].

AV node ablation for the treatment of atrial fibrillation suffers from several key limitations. Patients who do not have contraindications must continue on anticoagulation therapy to minimize the risk for the cardioembolic complications of atrial fibrillation. Furthermore, patients may continue to have symptoms from atrial fibrillation, such as shortness of breath, despite regularization of the ventricular rhythm with pacing. In addition, patients are subjected the associated risks for an indwelling cardiac device, including the risk for infection and chronic right ventricular pacing [32]. Patients who have a history of congestive heart failure benefit from biventricular pacing after AV node ablation. No evidence exists, however, to suggest chronic biventricular pacing in the general population is in any way equivalent to native conduction through the His-Purkinje system [33].

Curative catheter ablation for atrial fibrillation

Background and overview

Catheter ablation techniques aimed at curing atrial fibrillation rather than simply controlling the ventricular response target the triggers of atrial fibrillation. Curative catheter ablation techniques initially attempted to mimic the lesions created by the surgical MAZE procedure [34–36]. In 1998, Haissaguerre and colleagues described focal firing as an important source of ectopic beats, which could lead to atrial fibrillation, and reported that these foci respond to ablation. It is believed that as many as 94% of such triggers originate from the pulmonary veins [37,38]. This finding led to focal ablation within the pulmonary veins to eliminate these triggers. Further studies propelled the evolution of the technique to the circumferential isolation of the pulmonary veins, which has since become the cornerstone of curative atrial fibrillation ablation. Patients who have paroxysmal atrial fibrillation and a structurally normal heart may expect a high rate of cure from isolation of the pulmonary veins alone. This represents, however, a small minority of patients who have atrial fibrillation presenting for ablation. Most patients, especially those who have dilated or scarred atria and chronic atrial fibrillation, do not have the same rate of cure with simple isolation of the pulmonary veins [39]. Areas of focal firing outside the pulmonary veins in the left and right atria also initiate atrial fibrillation [40].

Ablation of additional triggers outside the pulmonary veins and addition of lesions to interrupt the maintenance of atrial fibrillation may be required to improve long-term success in these substrate modification populations. These adjunctive lesion sets have become an integral component of curative atrial fibrillation ablation for most patients.

Current techniques for curative atrial fibrillation ablation can be categorized broadly as anatomic ablation or electrogram-guided isolation. Anatomic ablation currently relies on electroanatomic mapping systems to create a 3-dimensional representation of the left atrium and pulmonary veins. The position of the ablation catheter can be visualized within this representation and the location of ablation points marked with respect to the anatomy. Ablation lesions are placed circumferentially around the pulmonary veins, individually or often encircling two ipsilateral pulmonary veins simultaneously. Local electrograms can be measured from the ablation catheter and can help determine the duration of each lesion. Careful inspection for gaps allowing persistent conduction between the left atrium and the pulmonary veins is not performed, however. Persistent conduction between the pulmonary veins and left atrium can be demonstrated in up to 60% of the pulmonary veins after anatomic ablation [41,42].

In contrast to this technique, electrogram-guided isolation relies on a second, mapping catheter with a ring-shaped array of electrodes. This array is placed at the ostium of each pulmonary vein during isolation. At the authors' institution, lesions are delivered circumferentially around the antrum of each individual pulmonary vein. The ring catheter then is used to interrogate the circumference of the pulmonary vein antra, looking for gaps that can be closed (Fig. 2). Electrogram guidance of pulmonary vein antrum isolation (PVAI) improves long-term success compared with a purely anatomic approach [41,43].

Patient selection

As with any invasive procedure, patient selection is critical to optimizing the safety and success of PVAI. Although some data suggest increased mortality associated with atrial fibrillation and antiarrhythmic medications, much more remains to be done to elucidate the magnitude of these risks and the impact PVAI might have on them. Therefore, the diagnosis of atrial fibrillation alone is not sufficient to warrant PVAI. Furthermore, PVAI, like all invasive procedures, carries inherent risks that may be increased by patients' age and comorbidities. Finally, patient features are demonstrated to have an impact on the likelihood of success. All of this plays an important role in determining the appropriateness of PVAI.

Although some data suggest PVAI may be superior to medical therapy for first-line therapy of atrial fibrillation, current guidelines recommend most patients fail at least one antiarrhythmic drug prior to consideration of atrial fibrillation ablation [44]. Current indications include symptomatic

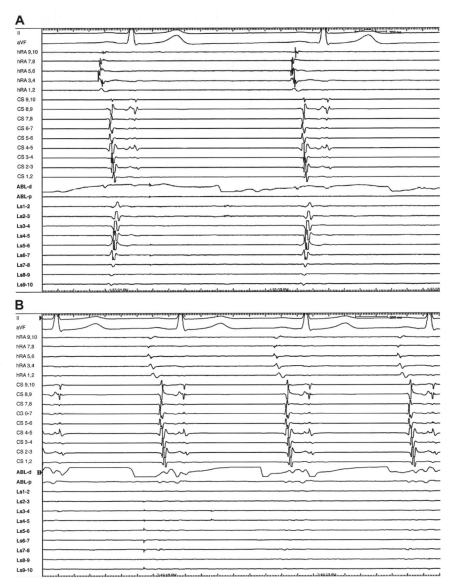

Fig. 2. Intracardiac electrograms demonstrating potentials within the right inferior pulmonary vein pre-isolation (A) and absence of potentials on the mapping ring catheter (LS 1–10) post isolation (B).

atrial fibrillation refractory to or intolerant of medical therapy. Additionally, patients in whom anticoagulation is indicated secondary to atrial fibrillation, but who cannot tolerate or whose occupations or activities preclude long-term anticoagulation, may be considered candidates for PVAI regardless of the presence of symptoms. Finally, patients who desire not to take antiarrhythmics or long-term anticoagulation sometimes are considered for PVAI.

No patient should be considered for PVAI if she cannot reasonably be expected to tolerate the procedure. For instance, patients who have severe dementia or decompensated heart failure are unlikely to be able to endure a potentially long procedure that requires patient cooperation and that they remain supine. As the procedure requires aggressive intraoperative anticoagulation, active bleeding or a history of a severe bleeding diathesis serves as a contraindication. Patients in persistent or permanent atrial fibrillation should not undergo PVAI if they would not be considered candidates for cardioversion. Adequate anticoagulation of sufficient duration should be ensured just as it would be prior to cardioversion. If patients have a history of prior ablations or open heart surgery, structural abnormalities, such as pulmonary vein stenosis, should be ruled out. Congenital heart defects, including repaired atrial septal defects, can add to the technical difficulty but are not absolute contraindications in the hands of experienced centers.

Certain patient features are found to be associated with increased or decreased likelihood of success and may help in patient selection and counseling. Patients who have atrial fibrillation that is shorter in duration and paroxysmal and patients who have normal-sized atria are more likely to be cured of their atrial fibrillation by PVAI. Conversely, patients who have long-standing, permanent atrial fibrillation and patients who have dilated atria or known atrial scarring are less likely to achieve complete cure after PVAI [45,46].

The preoperative assessment should include a careful history and physical examination. Patients who have allergies to intravenous contrast dye should be prepared according to standard procedures. Many operators obtain preoperative CT scan or MRI optimized for imaging of the pulmonary veins prior to PVAI; however, this is not absolutely necessary unless patients have a history of a prior ablation in the left heart. Antiarrhythmic medications can suppress spontaneous firing and fractionation of the electrograms that are used to guide ablation. Therefore, antiarrhythmic medications should be discontinued with approximately a 5 half-lives washout period prior to the procedure. Continued full anticoagulation with warfarin therapy decreases the risk for periprocedure thromboembolic events and is not interrupted for PVAI at the authors' institution. Patients not previously on chronic anticoagulation are started on warfarin with a goal international normalized ratio of 2 to 3 at least 3 weeks prior to PVAI, and this is continued for at least 3 to 6 months after the procedure. Patients must remain in a fasting state prior to the procedure and should be instructed to expect an overnight hospital admission for observation after the procedure.

Technical aspects

Pulmonary veins are approached via a transseptal approach, necessitating multiple venous sheaths for the delivery of catheters. Transseptal catheters are delivered through sheaths typically placed in the right femoral vein. Additionally, an intracardiac echocardiogram (ICE) probe may be introduced through the left or right femoral vein. Placement of a coronary sinus catheter provides an additional fluoroscopic landmark to guide catheter positioning and is used as a reference point for certain electroanatomic mapping systems. Additionally, a coronary sinus catheter may help differentiate left- versus right-sided arrhythmogenic triggers [47]. This typically is placed via the right internal jugular vein. Electrogram-guided ablation requires an ablation and a mapping catheter be placed into the left atrium; thus, two transseptal sheaths are needed. Fluoroscopic and ICE visualization of the transseptal needle and the anatomic landmarks should guide transseptal puncture. Care must be taken to ensure that punctures are performed through the inferior interatrial septum, where it is thinner and easier to cross, than the more muscular superior septum. Additionally, placing transseptal puncture posteriorly places the catheters close to the posterior left atrium and the pulmonary veins facilitating reach of the catheters to these targets (Fig. 3). Before the transseptal puncture, unfractionated heparin should be bolused and a drip initiated. A target activated clotting time (ACT) of 350 to 400 seconds is used at the authors' institution and decreases perioperative thromboembolic events compared with lower targets [48].

The muscular sleeves of the pulmonary veins are the most common site of triggers of atrial fibrillation [37,38]. Although early approaches used focal lesions within individual pulmonary veins to ablate these foci, they were associated with an increased rate of pulmonary vein stenosis and higher rates of recurrence compared with circumferential isolation [49]. Discrete

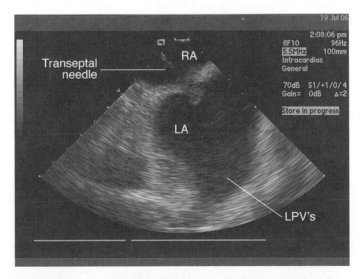

Fig. 3. ICE showing tenting of the intra-atrial septum with the transseptal needle at a satisfactory location on the septum across from the left pulmonary veins (LPVs). The right atrial (RA) and left atrial (LA) are shown.

electrical connections between the left atrium and the pulmonary veins often can be identified; however, a segmental approach that targets only these connections has a higher rate of recurrence than circumferential techniques [38,50–53]. Occasionally, individual pulmonary veins may be identified as the triggers of atrial fibrillation in a given patient. It may be tempting to isolate only the veins identified as harboring triggers in these cases. Failure to isolate all the pulmonary veins, however, yields a lower long-term success rate and, if done at all, probably should be reserved for younger patients [54–56]. As discussed previously, purely anatomic ablation is associated with a high incidence of persistent conduction between the pulmonary veins and left atrium and is associated with rates of success inferior to electrogram-guided isolation [41–43]. Thus, the authors believe that electrogram-guided isolation is preferred over anatomic techniques.

Although it is known that most triggers of atrial fibrillation arise from the muscular sleeves of the pulmonary veins, the junction of the pulmonary veins with the left atrium is not a discrete ostium. Instead, these junctions are conically shaped and the triggers found within the pulmonary veins often exist proximally in this junction. This understanding has shaped the development of catheter ablation for atrial fibrillation at the authors' institution from a distal ablation procedure isolating the pulmonary veins at the ostium, what is commonly known as pulmonary vein isolation (PVI), to a more proximal isolation of the entire pulmonary vein antrum, referred to as PVAI (Figs. 4 and 5). The pulmonary vein antra isolated by this technique encompass the pulmonary veins, the left atrial roof, the left atrial posterior wall, and a portion of the interatrial septum in anterior to the right pulmonary veins (Fig. 6) [57,58].

Adjunctive curative ablation techniques

In addition to isolation of the pulmonary veins, adjunctive targets often are ablated in an attempt to prevent short-term and long-term recurrences of atrial fibrillation and prevent the development of other atrial arrhythmias. The left atrial posterior wall, the interatrial septum, and the ligament of Marshall all are identified as sites of ectopic beats initiating atrial fibrillation [59]. Ablation in these areas may improve overall success especially in patients who have permanent atrial fibrillation. Initiation of atrial flutter, left-sided atrial flutter, atrial tachycardia, and microreentrant atrial flutter may complicate atrial fibrillation ablation. Ablation lines placed on the posterior wall and roof of the left atrium, typically connecting the left superior pulmonary vein to the right superior pulmonary vein, decrease the risk for developing left atrial arrhythmias, decrease inducibility of atrial fibrillation, and improve long-term success after atrial fibrillation ablation [60,61]. In addition, mitral valve isthmus lines decrease likelihood of recurrent atrial fibrillation in patients who have permanent atrial fibrillation. This may be secondary to compartmentalization of the left atrium or substrate

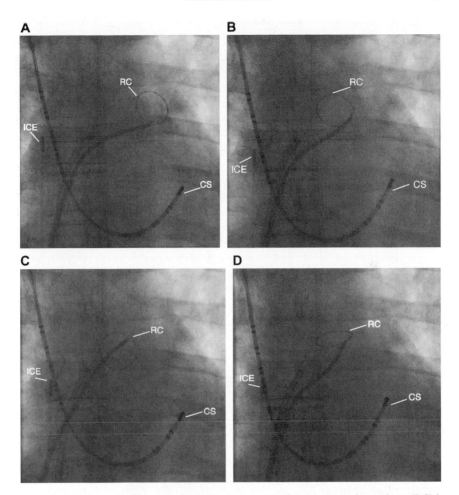

Fig. 4. (*A–D*) Fluoroscopic images illustrating movement of the ring mapping catheter (RC) in the antrum of the left superior pulmonary vein, including the os (*A*), superoposterior antrum (*B*), inferoposterior antrum (*C*), and roof (*D*). The coronary sinus catheter (CS) and ICE probe are seen.

modification in the region of the ligament of Marshal and around the coronary sinus [62]. In addition to these sites, areas of complex fractionated electrograms are implicated in the development of atrial fibrillation. These are found most commonly in the pulmonary veins, on the interatrial septum and the left atrial roof, and at the coronary sinus ostium. Limited data suggest ablation at the sites of complex fractionated electrograms as a stand-alone strategy may be associated with a relatively high rate of success in the elimination of atrial fibrillation [63,64]. Finally, some investigators advocate ablation to target the autonomic innervation of the left atrium and pulmonary veins. In patients who demonstrate autonomic effect while ablating

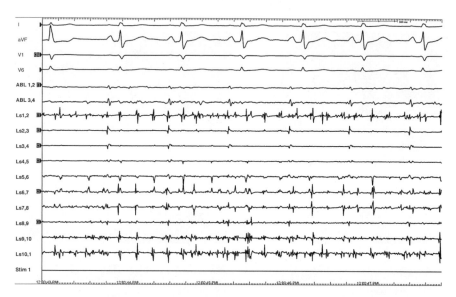

Fig. 5. Intracardiac electrogram obtained after isolation of the right superior pulmonary vein demonstrating fibrillation within the vein recorded by the ring catheter (LS 1–10) whereas the atria remain in sinus rhythm as recorded on the surface leads (I, aVF, V1, and V6).

around one or more of the pulmonary veins, denervation of the pulmonary veins, as demonstrated by abolition of the evoked vagal reflex, may improve freedom from atrial fibrillation recurrence [65,66].

Additional ablation sites within the right atrium may improve the efficacy of PVAI in certain populations. The superior vena cava (SVC) is a common site of atrial fibrillation triggers. Isolation of the SVC by creation of a circumferential ablation line at the junction of the right atrium and SVC may improve the success of atrial fibrillation ablation, especially in patients who have permanent atrial fibrillation (Fig. 7) [59,67–69]. The crista terminalis and the coronary sinus ostium are identified as sites of ectopic beats triggering atrial fibrillation [59]. Empiric ablation of the coronary sinus, however, does not seem to improve the overall success of PVAI [70].

At the authors' institution, inclusion of adjunctive lesions has been an important component of the PVAI technique for some time. Early experience led to incorporating the isolation of the SVC, and as discussed previously the antrum approach includes isolation of the posterior wall, the left atrial roof, and the interatrial septum and extends anterior to the right pulmonary veins. Additionally, in patients who have permanent atrial fibrillation, the left atrium routinely is interrogated for areas of complex fractionated electrograms, and the septal ablation is extended to include the mitral valve annulus. Challenge with high doses of isoproterenol is considered to uncover additional triggers, especially in nonparoxysmal atrial fibrillation.

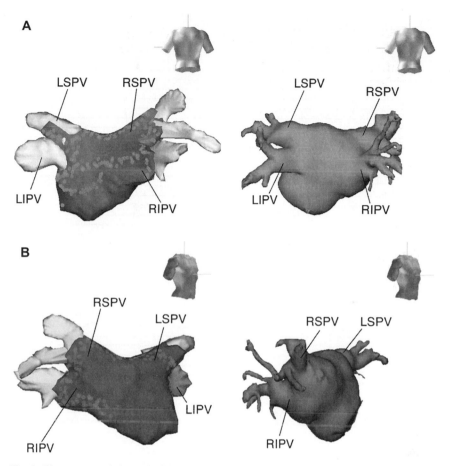

Fig. 6. Electroanatomic images of the left atrium with (*A*) and without (*B*) PVAI lesions as seen from PA and RAO perspectives.

Endpoints

The procedural endpoint depends on the strategy used for ablation. This includes entry block around the ostium or the antrum of the pulmonary veins for electrogram-guided atrial fibrillation ablation. A ring or circular mapping catheter with tightly spaced electrodes is used to detect any electrical gaps within the encircling lesions and confirms block of atrial signal into the pulmonary veins. Confirmation of exit block from the pulmonary veins is documented by pacing within the pulmonary veins or when independent firing in the pulmonary veins is found [23]. During circumferential anatomic ablation, the endpoint is abolition of local electrograms as detected by the ablation catheter. Electrical isolation of the pulmonary veins is not required and not achieved in the majority of the pulmonary veins. Limited and contradictory data exist associating termination of atrial fibrillation during

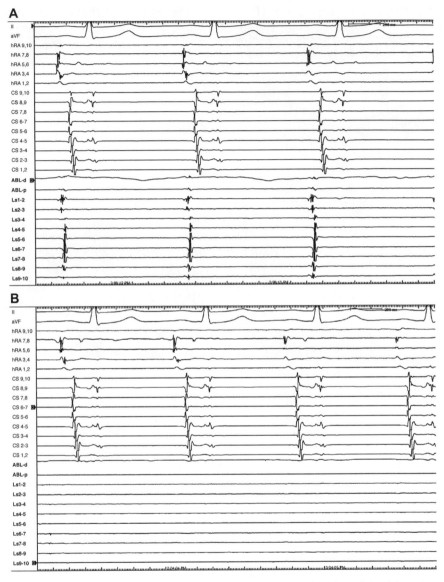

Fig. 7. Intracardiac electrograms demonstrating potentials at the junction of the right atrium and SVC pre-isolation (*A*) and absence of potentials on the mapping catheter channels (LS 1–10) post isolation (*B*).

ablation and the inability to induce atrial fibrillation further with improved long-term success [71–73].

Outcomes and limitations

Curative catheter ablation for atrial fibrillation has evolved to enjoy a high overall success rate and low rate of complications. Studies examining the cost-effectiveness of atrial fibrillation ablation suggest that cost-equivalency of curative atrial fibrillation ablation to medical management is reached after approximately 5 years [74]. Success rates are highest when treating patients who have paroxysmal atrial fibrillation. In this population, it is reasonable to expect a success rate of 80% to 85% [43,60,75]. When recurrences occur, they often are related to focal areas of recovery, leading to conduction gaps across previous ablation lines [76–79]. A second procedure to reisolate the pulmonary veins often provides cure in these patients. Success rates in patients who have permanent atrial fibrillation generally are reported closer to 50% to 60% with a single procedure [67,71,80,81]. Repeat ablation for those who have recurrences improves the overall success in these patients to rates approaching 75% to 90% [67,81]. As with most technical procedures, experience is an important factor in attaining optimal outcomes, and centers with higher volumes achieve higher rates of cure [82]. Assessment of recurrences varies in the literature, with some investigators relying solely on symptoms, whereas others routinely performing ambulatory rhythm monitoring to capture asymptomatic recurrences. Some data suggest that asymptomatic recurrences after atrial fibrillation ablation are uncommon, occurring only in approximately 2% of the population [83]. Others report higher rates of asymptomatic recurrences. In general, studies with higher reported rates included patients who were continued long term on antiarrhythmic drugs, which may mask symptoms of recurrences. The authors' practice is to discontinue all antiarrhythmic drugs 4 weeks after ablation and not to use amiodarone after the procedure. Although success, defined as freedom from atrial fibrillation, may not be achieved in all patients, those who have recurrence of atrial fibrillation still may benefit from an improvement in symptoms through a reduction in the frequency of episodes or by an improved response to previously ineffective antiarrhythmic medications.

Perhaps the greatest challenge associated with PVAI is the technical difficulty of creating circumferential isolation using multiple discrete ablation points. Electroanatomic mapping systems may help overcome this to some extent; however, operator skill and experience are essential for success. Other challenges associated with PVAI could arise from the transseptal puncture or problems with patient cooperation. Placement of transseptal punctures posteriorly on the interatrial septum is critical to optimizing the reach of the catheters to the veins on the posterior wall of the left atrium. At times, the septum may be thickened or fibrous making it extremely resistant to puncture. ICE is invaluable in the visualization of the septum and left atrial structures, thus improving optimal placement of the transseptal punctures. Ability of patients to cooperate also may pose important challenges during atrial fibrillation ablation. Deep respirations can diminish catheter stability severely, often drawing catheters from an ostial location into the pulmonary veins. Careful titration of sedation to optimize patient comfort while permitting cooperation especially during critical stages of the procedure can minimize this difficulty.

In addition to these challenges, radiation exposure is an important consideration for patients and operators during atrial fibrillation ablation. Duration of fluoroscopy can vary widely depending on patient characteristics, technique used, and operator experience. Fluoroscopy times of 60 to 70 minutes are not uncommon. Electroanatomic mapping systems reduce fluoroscopic times [84–88]. Common practices to reduce radiation dose by decreasing frame rates, reducing magnification, and reducing the field with shutters should be used. The development of atrial arrhythmias, such as atrial flutter, also may add to the challenge of successful PVI. Depending on the ablation approach, from 3% to as many as 30% of patients are reported to develop small-loop atrial reentry, which can be difficult to map [89,90].

The overall rate of major complications associated with ostial PVI is reported at 4% to 6% [81,82,91]. Perforation leading to tamponade may occur in approximately 1% of cases [82]. This most often is amenable to treatment with a percutaneous pericardial drain but rarely requires thoracotomy and pericardial window. Posterior perforation and formation of a left atrial-esophageal fistula are reported. Power titration using the detection of microbubbles on ICE is reported to prevent this complication. In addition, use of a radio-opaque esophageal temperature probe allows visualization of the esophageal course and monitoring of esophageal temperatures during ablation. Radiofrequency current delivery should be terminated when the esophageal temperature increases and not resumed in that location until temperatures return to baseline. No cases of left atrial-esophageal fistula formation have been reported when this technique is used. Others use ingested barium paste to localize the esophagus and help avoid this complication. Phrenic nerve injury leading to diaphragmatic paralysis or gastric emptying syndrome is reported at a rate of 0.1% to 0.48%. This is associated most commonly with ablation in the regions of the right superior pulmonary vein, left atrial appendage, and the SVC. Recovery is seen in approximately 66% of cases [82,92]. Fluoroscopic visualization of the diaphragm while ablating in these areas may reveal diaphragmatic stimulation during radiofrequency ablation and allow termination of energy delivery before permanent injury to the phrenic nerve occurs. Before delivery of radiofrequency current over the lateral aspects of the SVC–right atrial junction, pacing at high output may reveal phrenic nerve stimulation evidenced by diaphragmatic stimulation, indicating that ablation in that region is unsafe. Cerebrovascular accidents and transient ischemic attacks are feared complications of any left-sided ablation procedure, including PVAI. Rates generally are reported at approximately 0.5% to 2.5% [82,93,94]. Targeting an ACT of 350 to 400 seconds significantly reduces the risk for thromboembolic events during PVAI compared with lower ACT targets, with a reported event rate of less than 0.5% [48].

Severe, symptomatic pulmonary vein stenosis may complicate PVI but has become rare, as the technique has moved from ablating distally within the pulmonary veins to a much more proximal approach of isolation of the pulmonary vein antra. Mild to moderate pulmonary stenosis does not limit flow significantly and is not associated with symptoms. Severe stenosis is reported in 15% to 20% of patients undergoing ablation within the pulmonary veins [95]. Isolation at the pulmonary vein ostium rather than focal ablation within the pulmonary veins is associated with rates of pulmonary vein stenosis of 1% to 2% [82,95–97]. Use of ICE to visualize the pulmonary veins and isolation even more proximally in the pulmonary vein antra reduces the risk for PV stenosis further (Fig. 8) [20,95]. Even when severe, pulmonary vein stenosis often is asymptomatic. When symptoms do occur, angioplasty and stenting are effective treatment options and only a fraction of patients are left with chronic symptoms [82,98].

Follow-up

Postablation follow-up should assess the efficacy of the procedure, screen for complications, and address postablation medical therapy for atrial fibrillation. At the authors' institution, patients are discharged with a transtelephonic monitor, with instructions to transmit rhythm strips whenever they feel symptoms consistent with a recurrence. Additionally, routine transmissions scheduled several times weekly screen for recurrence. Recurrences of atrial fibrillation and episodes of atrial tachycardia or atypical atrial flutter are common within the first few weeks after PVAI. These early recurrences often are related to inflammation from the ablation and resolve completely

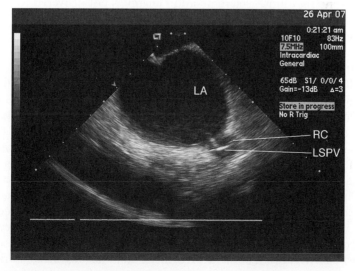

Fig. 8. ICE demonstrating left atrium (LA) and the ring catheter (RC) at the ostium of the left superior pulmonary vein (LSPV).

as inflammation subsides. As a result, recurrences within the first 6 to 8 weeks are not considered an indication of failure of the procedure. For this same reason, antiarrhythmic medications typically are restarted immediately after PVAI and discontinued after 8 weeks. Twenty-four–hour holter monitoring is performed at 3 months' follow-up and every 3 months thereafter to screen further for asymptomatic recurrences. Patients routinely are scheduled for outpatient follow-up 3 months after PVAI. At this time, they are evaluated for symptomatic recurrence and a CT scan is obtained to assess for pulmonary vein stenosis. If even mild stenosis is detected, the CT scan is repeated at the next follow-up visit. Warfarin is continued perioperatively and at least until the 3- to 6-month follow-up visit. Discontinuation of warfarin after PVAI currently is being studied. The decision to terminate anticoagulation after PVAI must be made on an individual basis after careful assessment of patient risk for recurrence and discussion with patients regarding the potential risks.

Future advances

Much of the effort in the advancement of curative atrial fibrillation ablation is directed toward meeting the challenges of the technical demands of isolating the pulmonary veins. Balloon catheters, alternative ablative energy sources, and remote catheter manipulation all strive to diminish these technical demands. Balloon catheters, theoretically, could assist operators in stabilizing a catheter in a pulmonary vein and allow circumferential delivery of ablative energy. These catheters, however, must be able to accommodate the widely variable anatomy found in the pulmonary veins. Additionally, they must ensure ablation energy is not delivered too distally in to the pulmonary veins. High-intensity ultrasound, cryotherapy, and diode laser are potential alternatives to radiofrequency ablation and potentially could be married to balloon catheter technology to create circumferential lesions with a few applications, further reducing the technical challenge of circumferential isolation and potentially reducing the time required for ablation. These sources must be able to produce lesions at a consistent depth reliably and must at least equal the safety profile of radiofrequency energy to serve as viable alternatives. Large magnets may be used to steer a soft-tipped catheter allowing remote guidance of lesion delivery. Robotic catheter navigation systems also allow remote manipulation of catheters. Both promise to reduce radiation exposure to operators dramatically and potentially improve catheter stability and fine manipulation. When combined with electroanatomic mapping, these systems conceivably could automate much of the ablation procedure. To gain widespread use, however, these systems must meet demands of time saving, ease of use, and cost-effectiveness. The field of catheter ablation for atrial fibrillation has grown and evolved rapidly over recent years and this trend is expected to continue in the near future.

References

[1] Lloyd-Jones DM, Wang TJ, Leip EP, et al. Lifetime risk for development of atrial fibrillation: the Framingham Heart Study. Circulation 2004;110(9):1042–6.

[2] Risk factors for stroke and efficacy of antithrombotic therapy in atrial fibrillation. Analysis of pooled data from five randomized controlled trials. Arch Intern Med 1994;154(13): 1449–57.

[3] Wolf PA, Abbott RD, Kannel WB. Atrial fibrillation as an independent risk factor for stroke: the Framingham Study. Stroke 1991;22(8):983–8.

[4] Benjamin EJ, Wolf PA, D'Agostino RB, et al. Impact of atrial fibrillation on the risk of death: the Framingham Heart Study. Circulation 1998;98(10):946–52.

[5] Kannel WB, Wolf PA, Benjamin EJ, et al. Prevalence, incidence, prognosis, and predisposing conditions for atrial fibrillation: population-based estimates. Am J Cardiol 1998;82(8A): 2N–9N.

[6] Chung MK. Atrial fibrillation: rate control is as good as rhythm control for some, but not all. Cleve Clin J Med 2003;70(6):567–73.

[7] Van Gelder IC, Hagens VE, Bosker HA, et al. A comparison of rate control and rhythm control in patients with recurrent persistent atrial fibrillation. N Engl J Med 2002;347(23): 1834–40.

[8] Wyse DG, Waldo AL, DiMarco JP, et al. A comparison of rate control and rhythm control in patients with atrial fibrillation. N Engl J Med 2002;347(23):1825–33.

[9] Corley SD, Epstein AE, DiMarco JP, et al. Relationships between sinus rhythm, treatment, and survival in the Atrial Fibrillation Follow-Up Investigation of Rhythm Management (AFFIRM) Study. Circulation 2004;109(12):1509–13.

[10] Wazni OM, Marrouche NF, Martin DO, et al. Radiofrequency ablation vs antiarrhythmic drugs as first-line treatment of symptomatic atrial fibrillation: a randomized trial. JAMA 2005;293(21):2634–40.

[11] Pappone C, Rosanio S, Augello G, et al. Mortality, morbidity, and quality of life after circumferential pulmonary vein ablation for atrial fibrillation: outcomes from a controlled nonrandomized long-term study. J Am Coll Cardiol 2003;42(2):185–97.

[12] Vedel J, Frank R, Fontaine G, et al. [Permanent intra-hisian atrioventricular block induced during right intraventricular exploration]. Arch Mal Coeur Vaiss 1979;72(1):107–12 [in French].

[13] Gallagher JJ, Svenson RH, Kasell JH, et al. Catheter technique for closed-chest ablation of the atrioventricular conduction system. N Engl J Med 1982;306(4):194–200.

[14] Scheinman MM, Morady F, Hess DS, et al. Catheter-induced ablation of the atrioventricular junction to control refractory supraventricular arrhythmias. JAMA 1982;248(7):851–5.

[15] Evans GT Jr, Scheinman MM, Scheinman MM, et al. The Percutaneous Cardiac Mapping and Ablation Registry: final summary of results. Pacing Clin Electrophysiol 1988;11(11 Pt 1): 1621–6.

[16] Chen SA, Tsang WP, Hsia CP, et al. Catheter ablation of free wall accessory atrioventricular pathways in 89 patients with Wolff-Parkinson-White syndrome—comparison of direct current and radiofrequency ablation. Eur Heart J 1992;13(10):1329–38.

[17] Morady F, Calkins H, Langberg JJ, et al. A prospective randomized comparison of direct current and radiofrequency ablation of the atrioventricular junction. J Am Coll Cardiol 1993;21(1):102–9.

[18] Olgin JE, Scheinman MM. Comparison of high energy direct current and radiofrequency catheter ablation of the atrioventricular junction. J Am Coll Cardiol 1993;21(3):557–64.

[19] Haines DE. The biophysics of radiofrequency catheter ablation in the heart: the importance of temperature monitoring. Pacing Clin Electrophysiol 1993;16(3 Pt 2):586–91.

[20] Marrouche NF, Martin DO, Wazni O, et al. Phased-array intracardiac echocardiography monitoring during pulmonary vein isolation in patients with atrial fibrillation: impact on outcome and complications. Circulation 2003;107(21):2710–6.

[21] Kalbfleisch SJ, Williamson B, Man KC, et al. A randomized comparison of the right- and left-sided approaches to ablation of the atrioventricular junction. Am J Cardiol 1993; 72(18):1406–10.

[22] Dubuc M, Khairy P, Rodriguez-Santiago A, et al. Catheter cryoablation of the atrioventricular node in patients with atrial fibrillation: a novel technology for ablation of cardiac arrhythmias. J Cardiovasc Electrophysiol 2001;12(4):439–44.

[23] Weerasooriya R, Davis M, Powell A, et al. The Australian Intervention Randomized Control of Rate in Atrial Fibrillation Trial (AIRCRAFT). J Am Coll Cardiol 2003;41(10): 1697–702.

[24] Verma A, Newman D, Geist M, et al. Effects of rhythm regularization and rate control in improving left ventricular function in atrial fibrillation patients undergoing atrioventricular nodal ablation. Can J Cardiol 2001;17(4):437–45.

[25] Wood MA, Kay GN, Ellenbogen KA. The North American experience with the Ablate and Pace Trial (APT) for medically refractory atrial fibrillation. Europace 1999;1(1):22–5.

[26] Brignole M, Menozzi C, Gianfranchi L, et al. Assessment of atrioventricular junction ablation and VVIR pacemaker versus pharmacological treatment in patients with heart failure and chronic atrial fibrillation: a randomized, controlled study. Circulation 1998;98(10):953–60.

[27] Fitzpatrick AP, Kourouyan HD, Siu A, et al. Quality of life and outcomes after radiofrequency His-bundle catheter ablation and permanent pacemaker implantation: impact of treatment in paroxysmal and established atrial fibrillation. Am Heart J 1996;131(3):499–507.

[28] Natale A, Zimerman L, Tomassoni G, et al. Impact on ventricular function and quality of life of transcatheter ablation of the atrioventricular junction in chronic atrial fibrillation with a normal ventricular response. Am J Cardiol 1996;78(12):1431–3.

[29] Wood MA, Brown-Mahoney C, Kay GN, et al. Clinical outcomes after ablation and pacing therapy for atrial fibrillation: a meta-analysis. Circulation 2000;101(10):1138–44.

[30] Natale A, Zimerman L, Tomassoni G, et al. AV node ablation and pacemaker implantation after withdrawal of effective rate-control medications for chronic atrial fibrillation: effect on quality of life and exercise performance. Pacing Clin Electrophysiol 1999;22(11):1634–9.

[31] Geelen P, Brugada J, Andries E, et al. Ventricular fibrillation and sudden death after radiofrequency catheter ablation of the atrioventricular junction. Pacing Clin Electrophysiol 1997;20(2 Pt 1):343–8.

[32] Wilkoff BL, Cook JR, Epstein AE, et al. Dual-chamber pacing or ventricular backup pacing in patients with an implantable defibrillator: the Dual Chamber and VVI Implantable Defibrillator (DAVID) Trial. JAMA 2002;288(24):3115–23.

[33] Doshi RN, Daoud EG, Fellows C, et al. Left ventricular-based cardiac stimulation post AV nodal ablation evaluation (the PAVE study). J Cardiovasc Electrophysiol 2005;16(11): 1160–5.

[34] Cox JL, Canavan TE, Schuessler RB, et al. The surgical treatment of atrial fibrillation. II. Intraoperative electrophysiologic mapping and description of the electrophysiologic basis of atrial flutter and atrial fibrillation. J Thorac Cardiovasc Surg 1991;101(3):406–26.

[35] Padanilam BJ, Prystowsky EN. Should atrial fibrillation ablation be considered first-line therapy for some patients? Should ablation be first-line therapy and for whom? The antagonist position. Circulation 2005;112(8):1223–9 [discussion: 1230].

[36] Packer DL, Asirvatham S, Munger TM. Progress in nonpharmacologic therapy of atrial fibrillation. J Cardiovasc Electrophysiol 2003;14(Suppl 12):S296–309.

[37] Haissaguerre M, Jais P, Shah DC, et al. Spontaneous initiation of atrial fibrillation by ectopic beats originating in the pulmonary veins. N Engl J Med 1998;339(10):659–66.

[38] Chen SA, Hsieh MH, Tai CT, et al. Initiation of atrial fibrillation by ectopic beats originating from the pulmonary veins: electrophysiological characteristics, pharmacological responses, and effects of radiofrequency ablation. Circulation 1999;100(18):1879–86.

[39] Verma A, Wazni OM, Marrouche NF, et al. Pre-existent left atrial scarring in patients undergoing pulmonary vein antrum isolation: an independent predictor of procedural failure. J Am Coll Cardiol 2005;45(2):285–92.

[40] Natale A, Pisano E, Beheiry S, et al. Ablation of right and left atrial premature beats following cardioversion in patients with chronic atrial fibrillation refractory to antiarrhythmic drugs. Am J Cardiol 2000;85(11):1372–5.

[41] Kanagaratnam L, Tomassoni G, Schweikert R, et al. Empirical pulmonary vein isolation in patients with chronic atrial fibrillation using a three-dimensional nonfluoroscopic mapping system: long-term follow-up. Pacing Clin Electrophysiol 2001;24(12):1774–9.

[42] Hocini M, Sanders P, Jais P, et al. Prevalence of pulmonary vein disconnection after anatomical ablation for atrial fibrillation: consequences of wide atrial encircling of the pulmonary veins. Eur Heart J 2005;26(7):696–704.

[43] Mantovan R, Verlato R, Calzolari V, et al. Comparison between anatomical and integrated approaches to atrial fibrillation ablation: adjunctive role of electrical pulmonary vein disconnection. J Cardiovasc Electrophysiol 2005;16(12):1293–7.

[44] Fuster V, Reyen LE, Cannom DS, et al. ACC/AHA/ESC 2006 Practice Guidelines for the Management of Patients with Atrial Fibrillation. J Am Coll Cardiol 2006;48(4):e149–246.

[45] Kannel WB, Abbott RD, Savage DD, et al. Epidemiologic features of chronic atrial fibrillation: the Framingham study. N Engl J Med 1982;306(17):1018–22.

[46] Oral H, Knight BP, Tada H, et al. Pulmonary vein isolation for paroxysmal and persistent atrial fibrillation. Circulation 2002;105(9):1077–81.

[47] Ashar MS, Pennington J, Callans DJ, et al. Localization of arrhythmogenic triggers of atrial fibrillation. J Cardiovasc Electrophysiol 2000;11(12):1300–5.

[48] Wazni OM, Rossillo A, Marrouche NF, et al. Embolic events and char formation during pulmonary vein isolation in patients with atrial fibrillation: impact of different anticoagulation regimens and importance of intracardiac echo imaging. J Cardiovasc Electrophysiol 2005; 16(6):576–81.

[49] Robbins IM, Colvin EV, Doyle TP, et al. Pulmonary vein stenosis after catheter ablation of atrial fibrillation. Circulation 1998;98(17):1769–75.

[50] Nilsson B, Chen X, Pehrson S, et al. Recurrence of pulmonary vein conduction and atrial fibrillation after pulmonary vein isolation for atrial fibrillation: a randomized trial of the ostial versus the extraostial ablation strategy. Am Heart J 2006;152(3):537, e531–8.

[51] Oral H, Scharf C, Chugh A, et al. Catheter ablation for paroxysmal atrial fibrillation: segmental pulmonary vein ostial ablation versus left atrial ablation. Circulation 2003;108(19):2355–60.

[52] Hocini M, Haissaguerre M, Shah D, et al. Multiple sources initiating atrial fibrillation from a single pulmonary vein identified by a circumferential catheter. Pacing Clin Electrophysiol 2000;23(11 Pt 2):1828–31.

[53] Haissaguerre M, Shah DC, Jais P, et al. Electrophysiological breakthroughs from the left atrium to the pulmonary veins. Circulation 2000;102(20):2463–5.

[54] Oral H, Chugh A, Good E, et al. A tailored approach to catheter ablation of paroxysmal atrial fibrillation. Circulation 2006;113(15):1824–31.

[55] Katritsis DG, Ellenbogen KA, Panagiotakos DB, et al. Ablation of superior pulmonary veins compared to ablation of all four pulmonary veins. J Cardiovasc Electrophysiol 2004;15(6):641–5.

[56] Gerstenfeld EP, Callans DJ, Dixit S, et al. Incidence and location of focal atrial fibrillation triggers in patients undergoing repeat pulmonary vein isolation: implications for ablation strategies. J Cardiovasc Electrophysiol 2003;14(7):685–90.

[57] Kanj M, Wazni O, Natale A. Pulmonary vein antrum isolation. Heart Rhythm 2007; 4(Suppl 3):S73–9.

[58] Kanj MH, Wazni OM, Natale A. How to do circular mapping catheter-guided pulmonary vein antrum isolation: the Cleveland Clinic approach. Heart Rhythm 2006;3(7):866–9.

[59] Lin WS, Tai CT, Hsieh MH, et al. Catheter ablation of paroxysmal atrial fibrillation initiated by non-pulmonary vein ectopy. Circulation 2003;107(25):3176–83.

[60] Hocini M, Jais P, Sanders P, et al. Techniques, evaluation, and consequences of linear block at the left atrial roof in paroxysmal atrial fibrillation: a prospective randomized study. Circulation 2005;112(24):3688–96.

[61] Pappone C, Manguso F, Vicedomini G, et al. Prevention of iatrogenic atrial tachycardia after ablation of atrial fibrillation: a prospective randomized study comparing circumferential
pulmonary vein ablation with a modified approach. Circulation 2004;110(19):3036–42.

[62] Fassini G, Riva S, Chiodelli R, et al. Left mitral isthmus ablation associated with PV Isolation: long-term results of a prospective randomized study. J Cardiovasc Electrophysiol 2005;
16(11):1150–6.

[63] Rostock T, Rotter M, Sanders P, et al. High-density activation mapping of fractionated electrograms in the atria of patients with paroxysmal atrial fibrillation. Heart Rhythm 2006;3(1):27–34.

[64] Nademanee K, McKenzie J, Kosar E, et al. A new approach for catheter ablation of atrial
fibrillation: mapping of the electrophysiologic substrate. J Am Coll Cardiol 2004;43(11):
2044–53.

[65] Bauer A, Deisenhofer I, Schneider R, et al. Effects of circumferential or segmental pulmonary vein ablation for paroxysmal atrial fibrillation on cardiac autonomic function. Heart
Rhythm 2006;3(12):1428–35.

[66] Pappone C, Santinelli V, Manguso F, et al. Pulmonary vein denervation enhances long-term
benefit after circumferential ablation for paroxysmal atrial fibrillation. Circulation 2004;
109(3):327–34.

[67] Calo L, Lamberti F, Loricchio ML, et al. Left atrial ablation versus biatrial ablation for persistent and permanent atrial fibrillation: a prospective and randomized study. J Am Coll Cardiol 2006;47(12):2504–12.

[68] Goya M, Ouyang F, Ernst S, et al. Electroanatomic mapping and catheter ablation of breakthroughs from the right atrium to the superior vena cava in patients with atrial fibrillation.
Circulation 2002;106(11):1317–20.

[69] Tsai CF, Tai CT, Hsieh MH, et al. Initiation of atrial fibrillation by ectopic beats originating
from the superior vena cava: electrophysiological characteristics and results of radiofrequency ablation. Circulation 2000;102(1):67–74.

[70] Muelet J, Phillips K, Barrett C, et al. Empiric coronary sinus ablation during pulmonary venous isolation does not improve the success of AF ablation. Heart Rhythm, in press.

[71] Richter B, Gwechenberger M, Filzmoser P, et al. Is inducibility of atrial fibrillation after ra-
dio frequency ablation really a relevant prognostic factor? Eur Heart J 2006;27(21):2553–9.

[72] Oral H, Chugh A, Lemola K, et al. Noninducibility of atrial fibrillation as an end point of left
atrial circumferential ablation for paroxysmal atrial fibrillation: a randomized study. Circulation 2004;110(18):2797–801.

[73] Haissaguerre M, Sanders P, Hocini M, et al. Changes in atrial fibrillation cycle length and
inducibility during catheter ablation and their relation to outcome. Circulation 2004;
109(24):3007–13.

[74] Khaykin Y. Cost-effectiveness of catheter ablation for atrial fibrillation. Curr Opin Cardiol
2007;22(1):11–7.

[75] Liu X, Long D, Dong J, et al. Is circumferential pulmonary vein isolation preferable to stepwise segmental pulmonary vein isolation for patients with paroxysmal atrial fibrillation? Circ
J 2006;70(11):1392–7.

[76] Mesas CE, Augello G, Lang CC, et al. Electroanatomic remodeling of the left atrium in patients undergoing repeat pulmonary vein ablation: mechanistic insights and implications for
ablation. J Cardiovasc Electrophysiol 2006;17(12):1279–85.

[77] Rostock T, O'Neill MD, Sanders P, et al. Characterization of conduction recovery across left
atrial linear lesions in patients with paroxysmal and persistent atrial fibrillation. J Cardiovasc
Electrophysiol 2006;17(10):1106–11.

[78] Ouyang F, Antz M, Ernst S, et al. Recovered pulmonary vein conduction as a dominant factor for recurrent atrial tachyarrhythmias after complete circular isolation of the pulmonary
veins: lessons from double Lasso technique. Circulation 2005;111(2):127–35.

[79] Cappato R, Negroni S, Pecora D, et al. Prospective assessment of late conduction recurrence
across radiofrequency lesions producing electrical disconnection at the pulmonary vein
ostium in patients with atrial fibrillation. Circulation 2003;108(13):1599–604.

[80] Oral H, Pappone C, Chugh A, et al. Circumferential pulmonary-vein ablation for chronic atrial fibrillation. N Engl J Med 2006;354(9):934–41.

[81] Cheema A, Dong J, Dalal D, et al. Long-term safety and efficacy of circumferential ablation with pulmonary vein isolation. J Cardiovasc Electrophysiol 2006;17(10):1080–5.

[82] Cappato R, Calkins H, Chen SA, et al. Worldwide survey on the methods, efficacy, and safety of catheter ablation for human atrial fibrillation. Circulation 2005;111(9):1100–5.

[83] Oral H, Veerareddy S, Good E, et al. Prevalence of asymptomatic recurrences of atrial fibrillation after successful radiofrequency catheter ablation. J Cardiovasc Electrophysiol 2004; 15(8):920–4.

[84] Estner HL, Deisenhofer I, Luik A, et al. Electrical isolation of pulmonary veins in patients with atrial fibrillation: reduction of fluoroscopy exposure and procedure duration by the use of a non-fluoroscopic navigation system (NavX). Europace 2006;8(8):583–7.

[85] Tondo C, Mantica M, Russo G, et al. A new nonfluoroscopic navigation system to guide pulmonary vein isolation. Pacing Clin Electrophysiol 2005;28(Supp 1):S102–5.

[86] Karch MR, Zrenner B, Deisenhofer I, et al. Freedom from atrial tachyarrhythmias after catheter ablation of atrial fibrillation: a randomized comparison between 2 current ablation strategies. Circulation 2005;111(22):2875–80.

[87] Wood MA, Christman PJ, Shepard RK, et al. Use of a non-fluoroscopic catheter navigation system for pulmonary vein isolation. J Interv Card Electrophysiol 2004;10(2): 165–70.

[88] Macle L, Jais P, Scavee C, et al. Pulmonary vein disconnection using the LocaLisa three-dimensional nonfluoroscopic catheter imaging system. J Cardiovasc Electrophysiol 2003; 14(7):693–7.

[89] Cummings JE, Schweikert R, Saliba W, et al. Left atrial flutter following pulmonary vein antrum isolation with radiofrequency energy: linear lesions or repeat isolation. J Cardiovasc Electrophysiol 2005;16(3):293–7.

[90] Deisenhofer I, Estner H, Zrenner B, et al. Left atrial tachycardia after circumferential pulmonary vein ablation for atrial fibrillation: incidence, electrophysiological characteristics, and results of radiofrequency ablation. Europace 2006;8(8):573–82.

[91] Stabile G, Bertaglia E, Senatore G, et al. Feasibility of pulmonary vein ostia radiofrequency ablation in patients with atrial fibrillation: a multicenter study (CACAF pilot study). Pacing Clin Electrophysiol 2003;26(1 Pt 2):284–7.

[92] Sacher F, Monahan KH, Thomas SP, et al. Phrenic nerve injury after atrial fibrillation catheter ablation: characterization and outcome in a multicenter study. J Am Coll Cardiol 2006; 47(12):2498–503.

[93] Mansour M, Ruskin J, Keane D. Efficacy and safety of segmental ostial versus circumferential extra-ostial pulmonary vein isolation for atrial fibrillation. J Cardiovasc Electrophysiol 2004;15(5):532–7.

[94] Zhou L, Keane D, Reed G, et al. Thromboembolic complications of cardiac radiofrequency catheter ablation: a review of the reported incidence, pathogenesis and current research directions. J Cardiovasc Electrophysiol 1999;10(4):611–20.

[95] Saad EB, Rossillo A, Saad CP, et al. Pulmonary vein stenosis after radiofrequency ablation of atrial fibrillation: functional characterization, evolution, and influence of the ablation strategy. Circulation 2003;108(25):3102–7.

[96] Purerfellner H, Cihal R, Aichinger J, et al. Pulmonary vein stenosis by ostial irrigated-tip ablation: incidence, time course, and prediction. J Cardiovasc Electrophysiol 2003;14(2): 158–64.

[97] Kato R, Lickfett L, Meininger G, et al. Pulmonary vein anatomy in patients undergoing catheter ablation of atrial fibrillation: lessons learned by use of magnetic resonance imaging. Circulation 2003;107(15):2004–10.

[98] Saad EB, Marrouche NF, Saad CP, et al. Pulmonary vein stenosis after catheter ablation of atrial fibrillation: emergence of a new clinical syndrome. Ann Intern Med 2003;138(8):634–8.

THE MEDICAL
CLINICS
OF NORTH AMERICA

ELSEVIER
SAUNDERS

Med Clin N Am 92 (2008) 203–215

Surgical Approaches for Atrial Fibrillation

A. Marc Gillinov, MD[a],*,
Adam E. Saltman, MD, PhD[b]

[a]Department of Thoracic and Cardiovascular Surgery, The Cleveland Clinic Foundation,
9500 Euclid Avenue, Desk F24, Cleveland, OH 44195, USA
[b]Division of Cardiothoracic Surgery, Maimonides Medical Center, 4802 Tenth Avenue,
Brooklyn, NY 11219, USA

Although it long has been recognized that atrial fibrillation (AF) is common in patients presenting for mitral valve and other forms of cardiac surgery, routine ablation of AF in such patients is a recent phenomenon. This change in surgical practice is attributable to new data clarifying the pathogenesis and dangers of untreated AF and development of new ablation technologies that facilitate ablation. For cardiac surgery patients presenting with AF, surgeons now offer a more complete operation that corrects the structural heart disease and the AF. With this comprehensive approach, it is estimated that surgeons will perform more than 10,000 ablation procedures in 2007. In addition, surgeons rapidly are developing minimally invasive epicardial approaches for stand-alone AF ablation. The purposes of this review are to (1) review the rationale for surgical ablation of AF in cardiac surgery patients, (2) describe the classic maze procedure and its results, (3) detail new approaches to surgical ablation of AF, (4) emphasize the importance of management of the left atrial appendage (LAA), and (5) consider

This work was supported by the Atrial Fibrillation Innovation Center, a Third Frontier Project Funded by the State of Ohio.

Dr. Gillinov has received honoraria for speaking from Medtronic, St. Jude Medical, Edwards Lifesciences, and Guidant Corporation. He is a former consultant to AtriCure. He receives research support from the Atrial Fibrillation Innovation Center, a Third Frontier project funded by the State of Ohio. He has received research support from Medtronic.

Dr. Saltman is a consultant to and has received honoraria for speaking from Boston Scientific/Guidant Cardiac Surgery. He has received research support from Guidant, Medical CV, and ESTECH LICS.

* Corresponding author.
E-mail address: gillinom@ccf.org (A.M. Gillinov).

doi:10.1016/j.mcna.2007.08.004

medical.theclinics.com

challenges and future directions in the ablation of AF in cardiac surgery patients.

Rationale for surgical ablation

Atrial fibrillation prevalence

AF is present in up to 50% of patients undergoing mitral valve surgery and in 1% to 6% of patients presenting for coronary artery bypass grafting (CABG) or aortic valve surgery [1–4]. Because AF is common particularly in patients who have mitral valve dysfunction, most studies examining concomitant ablation focus on this group. As in the general population, the prevalence of AF in patients who have mitral valve disease increases with increasing patient age. In patients who have mitral valve dysfunction, AF is a marker of advanced cardiovascular disease. Compared with mitral valve patients who do not have AF, those who have AF have higher New York Heart Association functional class, more severe left ventricular dysfunction, and greater left atrial size [4–8].

Atrial fibrillation dangers

AF is associated with increased mortality and morbidity in mitral valve and CABG patients. In patients who have degenerative mitral valve disease, AF is an independent risk factor for cardiac mortality and morbidity [1–4]. In patients undergoing mitral valve surgery, persistence of postoperative AF is a marker and a risk factor for increased mortality; in addition, AF is associated with morbidity that includes stroke, other thromboembolism, and anticoagulant-related hemorrhage. In some patients, AF causes symptomatic tachycardia, reduced cardiac output, and tachycardia-induced cardiomyopathy. This is deleterious particularly in patients who have structural heart disease and reduced cardiac output. For these reasons, the presence of AF should be addressed by the operative strategy in cardiac surgery patients.

The onset of AF is a relative indication for mitral valve surgery in those who have mitral valve dysfunction [2]. In most instances, however, mitral valve surgery alone does not ablate AF [5–7,9]. When duration of preoperative AF exceeds 6 months, 70% to 80% of patients have AF if they undergo mitral valve surgery alone [5,6,9]. In contrast, when AF is present for 3 months or less, particularly if it is paroxysmal, mitral valve surgery results in 80% conversion to sinus rhythm [5,6]. Therefore, ablation should be added to the mitral valve procedure in any patients who have AF of greater than 6 months' duration or in any patients who have AF that is not paroxysmal.

Atrial fibrillation mechanisms and implications for surgical ablation

The pathogenesis of AF in cardiac surgery patients is understood incompletely, and there is no consensus concerning ablation strategy in these patients. Clinical presentation of AF varies between individuals, and current guidelines account for this by classifying AF as paroxysmal, persistent, or permanent [10]. Alternatively, AF may be classified as intermittent or continuous [11]. It is certain that like clinical presentation, the pathogenesis of AF varies between patients; however, the extent to which mechanisms of focal activity and re-entry contribute to the initiation and maintenance of AF is unclear [12]. Although the electrophysiologic causes of AF require further investigation, the anatomic basis of AF is increasingly clear.

Endocardial electrophysiologic mapping demonstrates that the pulmonary veins and posterior left atrium are critical anatomic sites in humans who have isolated AF [13,14]. Available mapping studies also support the importance of the left atrium as the driving chamber in mitral valve patients [15–20]. In many mitral valve patients who have permanent AF, regular and repetitive activation can be identified in the posterior left atrium in the regions of the pulmonary vein orifices and LAA [15–19]. The spectrum of AF is more complex than this, however, as such foci are not identified in all mapped patients, and some patients also manifest right atrial focal or re-entrant activation [15].

Although routine real-time intraoperative mapping currently is not available to guide AF ablation in cardiac surgery patients [20], an anatomic approach to ablation based on the understanding of pathophysiology and empiric results is reasonable. Such an anatomic (rather than map-guided) approach rapidly is becoming the foundation for catheter-based ablation of AF [21–23]. A left atrial procedure that includes a box-like lesion around all four pulmonary veins and a lesion to the mitral annulus seems to eliminate AF in 70% to 90% of mitral valve patients [19,24–27]. The addition of right atrial lesions in these patients is controversial [28,29]. Omission of a right atrial isthmus lesion, however, leaves some patients at risk for typical atrial flutter and others at risk for continued AF [30]. Therefore, because creation of right atrial lesions is simple and does not increase appreciably operative time, AF ablation in cardiac surgery patients should include a biatrial lesion set.

The maze procedure

The Cox maze III operation, or maze procedure, is the gold standard for surgical treatment of AF. The maze procedure is the most effective curative therapy for AF yet devised [31–33]. In the maze procedure, multiple left and right atrial incisions and cryolesions are placed to interrupt the multiple re-entrant circuits of AF (Fig. 1). The maze procedure includes isolation of the pulmonary veins and posterior left atrium and excision of the LAA; these maneuvers are critical to the efficacy of the maze procedure in restoration of sinus rhythm and reduction of the risk for thromboembolism.

Although the maze procedure is a complex operation that requires 45 to 60 minutes of cardiopulmonary bypass and cardiac arrest, experienced surgeons have performed the classic operation in large numbers of patients

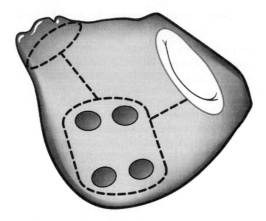

Fig. 1. Left atrial lesion set of the maze procedure. Small circles represent pulmonary vein orifices and white oval represents the mitral valve. Dashed lines represent surgical incisions. (Reprinted with permission of The Cleveland Clinic Center for Medical Art & Photography © Copyright 2007. All rights reserved.)

having concomitant cardiac surgery [1–3,5,33]. The addition of a maze procedure does not increase operative mortality or morbidity [34–36]. It is associated, however, with a 5% to 10% need for implantation of a permanent pacemaker, most commonly in those who have pre-existing sinus node dysfunction or in patients having multivalve surgery. Recent data demonstrate that the maze procedure has equivalent long-term efficacy in patients undergoing lone operations and concomitant procedures. Results of a concomitant maze procedure vary somewhat between different groups; successful restoration of sinus rhythm has been achieved in 70% to 96% of patients [34–36].

Early postoperative AF is common after a maze procedure, usually abating by 3 months [34–36]. Over time, however, some patients develop recurrent AF. The pathogenesis of this is unclear, but risk factors have been identified. Increasing left atrial diameter, longer duration of preoperative AF, and advanced patient age all increase the late prevalence of AF. Thus, 5 years after a concomitant maze procedure, the predicted prevalence of AF is only 5% in mitral valve patients who have a 4-cm left atrium; in contrast, the predicted prevalence is 15% in similar patients who have a 6-cm left atrium. Others have identified similar risk factors for AF after the maze procedure, suggesting the possibility that earlier operation and left atrial size reduction in those who have left atrial enlargement (>6 cm) might improve results [37–40].

The temporal pattern of AF (paroxysmal, persistent, or permanent) does not have an impact on the results of the maze procedure [36]. Similarly, in mitral valve patients, etiology of mitral valve dysfunction does not influence results, and there is general agreement that the maze procedure is effective in patients who have rheumatic valve disease and in those who have degenerative mitral valve disease [41,42]. Even in patients who have rheumatic disease, biatrial contraction usually is restored [41].

The maze procedure is associated with important clinical benefits in patients who have mitral valve disease. Recent data suggest that restoration of sinus rhythm improves survival in patients who have AF and mitral valve disease [43]. Other advantages of the maze procedure in mitral valve patients who have AF are well documented, including reduced risks for stroke, other thromboembolism, and anticoagulant-related hemorrhage [43–46].

The reduced risk for late stroke after a maze procedure deserves particular emphasis. In the largest series focusing on this outcome, Cox and colleagues [46] noted a single late stroke at a mean follow-up of 5 years in 300 patients who had a classic maze procedure. This remarkable late freedom from late stroke likely is attributable to restoration of sinus rhythm in the majority of patients and to excision of the LAA, an integral component of the maze procedure.

These results confirm the safety of the maze procedure, its efficacy at restoring sinus rhythm, and the resulting clinical benefits, most notably the virtual elimination of late strokes. Despite these excellent results, the maze procedure has been underused, and today, it is almost obsolete. Most surgeons are reluctant to add a maze procedure to the operative course of patients who are having mitral valve or other cardiac surgery. With recent advances in the understanding of the pathogenesis of AF and development of new ablation technologies, however, surgeons increasingly are likely to ablate AF using simple techniques that require only a few minutes of operative time.

New approaches to surgical ablation of atrial fibrillation

Lesion sets

Like recent approaches to catheter-based ablation, new surgical techniques for AF ablation are focused anatomically, concentrating on the creation of lines of conduction block in the left atrium [47–49]. Because the left atrium is opened for mitral valve procedures, precise creation of lesions is possible. A variety of lesion sets has been used to ablate AF in patients who have mitral valve disease. Most include pulmonary vein isolation, excision or exclusion of the LAA, and linear left atrial connecting lesions [47–51]. The pulmonary veins may be isolated with a box-like lesion, as in the maze procedure or, alternatively, with separate right- and left-sided ovals around the pulmonary veins. With the advantage of direct vision, surgeons easily can create a lesion from the left pulmonary veins to the mitral annulus; this lesion improves results, particularly in patients who have permanent AF and mitral valve disease [52]. In patients who have left atrial enlargement (> 6 cm), the authors recommend left atrial reduction, as this may increase restoration of sinus rhythm.

The issue concerning the creation of biatrial lesions (more closely mimicking the Cox maze III set) versus creating left atrial lesions alone remains contentious. It clearly is easier and faster to create a more limited lesion set; yet recent data indicate that patients undergoing right and left atrial treatment have a better long-term result at maintaining sinus rhythm [29]. Through the judicious selection of a technology or multiple technologies (discussed later), it is becoming possible to create right-sided lesions without opening the right atrium or prolonging cardiopulmonary bypass time or aortic cross-clamp time. In this manner, the largest number of patients can be treated in the most efficacious and safest fashion.

Surgical ablation for lone atrial fibrillation

When considering the number of patients presenting to operating rooms with AF in combination with coronary or valvular disease, even if all undergo concomitant ablation, it is unlikely that more than 40,000 patients would be treated annually. This is a small fraction of the total number of people suffering from this disease. A much larger patient population, therefore, could benefit from stand-alone AF ablation. It is difficult, however, to justify using cardiopulmonary bypass and cardioplegic arrest, especially through a sternotomy, to open the heart for exposure and access for the surgical treatment of lone AF: witness the relatively poor adoption of the Cox maze procedure over the last 20 years.

To bring an effective therapy to the largest number of patients, therefore, there has been much recent activity directed toward developing an epicardial approach to ablation that can be performed on a beating heart, preferably through small (minimally invasive) access incisions or ports. Such an approach should be able to overcome the disadvantages associated with the traditional Cox maze operation and the endocardial, catheter-based techniques (indirect visualization, ablation within a flowing blood pool, and an inability to manage the LAA).

The first report of such a minimally invasive, epicardial ablation performed on a beating heart appeared in 2003 [53]. Since then, three main technologies have been developed and used that provide less invasive approaches: robotics [54], thoracoscopy (endoscopy) [55–57], and minithoracotomy [58,59]. Each has its own advantages and disadvantages but all provide physicians with access to the entire atrial epicardium of a beating heart, whereupon lesions can be placed with precision and immediate visual feedback. Pulmonary vein isolation, for example, easily is accomplished in this manner. In addition, LAA management is straightforward in the majority of cases.

At this point, it is not possible to state conclusively which approach or which ablative technology used in a minimally invasive setting provides superior results. The numbers of patients treated are still small and there are technologic hurdles to be overcome (mitral annular and tricuspid isthmus lesion creation, for example). Refinements in approach and technology are progressing rapidly and new tools and methods are becoming available.

A review of the available energy sources

The classic lesion creation method is cutting and sewing tissue. Once the healing process is complete, there remains a scar composed mostly of collagen and little cellular material. It is not electrically conductive and the lesion is, by definition, "transmural." The goal of any energy source, therefore, is to create a similar scar by exposing tissue to extremes of temperature, inducing thermal injury, coagulation necrosis, and healing.

To produce such an injury, the tissue must be either heated to 50°C or frozen to –60°C [60,61]. The quantity of tissue injured usually is directly proportional to the duration of time for which the tissue is held at either temperature. The various energy sources differ mainly in the method by which they transfer energy to the tissue and how deeply that energy is conducted into the tissue. Heat-based energy sources include radiofrequency (RF), laser, microwave, and high-intensity focused ultrasound. As of 2007, these devices are Food and Drug Administration–labeled for the ablation of soft tissues or cardiac tissue but not for the treatment of AF. The specific treatment of AF is considered, therefore, off-label usage.

Despite clearly different energy forms and application methods when applied with the left atrium open, from the endocardial aspect with full cold cardioplegic arrest, there seems little difference in the safety or efficacy of any one device over the others [62]. The most extensive experience has been with the dry unipolar RF devices, mainly ESTECH's Cobra probe. Surveying its use in 16 studies including 1187 patients, Khargi and colleagues [62] found that dry unipolar RF was effective at freeing patients from AF 78% of the time (reported success ranged from 42% to 92%). There have been several complications attributed to the use of the probe; the most worrisome were esophageal injuries, resulting in death 60% of the time [63,64].

Adverse events can occur with any technology when applied incorrectly [65], but as more experience is gained and safer methods of ablation developed, such as placing a cold, wet sponge between the posterior wall of the left atrium and the esophagus or shielding the probe in nonconducting sheaths, these injuries have become an extreme rarity.

The left atrial appendage

Because 60% to 90% of stroke-causing emboli in patients who have AF originate from the LAA, this structure has been termed, "our most lethal human attachment" [66,67]. Therefore, excision or exclusion of the LAA is a critical component of operations to treat AF; this may explain in part the exceedingly low risk for stroke after the maze procedure. Ligation of the LAA in mitral valve patients who have AF reduces the late risk for thromboembolic events even if patients do not have intraoperative ablation [62].

Surgical technique has an impact on results of LAA ligation, with incomplete ligation increasing the risk for thromboembolism [68,69]. Currently used techniques include exclusion by suture ligation or noncutting stapler and excision with suture closure or stapling [69]. The authors currently favor surgical excision of the appendage with standard cut-and-sew techniques. Development of devices designed specifically for management of the LAA will facilitate this procedure. Published preclinical experience with a LAA clip is promising, and clinical trials are anticipated in the fourth quarter of 2007 (Fig. 2) [70].

Challenges and future directions

Advances necessary to improve AF ablation in cardiac surgery patients include uniform definitions and methodology for reporting results, improved technology to facilitate ablation and its intraoperative assessment, and refinement of minimally invasive procedures.

Reporting results

Standard terminology and methodology for reporting results is absent from the cardiac surgery and electrophysiology literature, and current reporting is haphazard and subject to criticism [71–73]. Although there are guidelines for categorizing the clinical pattern of AF, these are applied inconsistently. Techniques for postablation rhythm assessment vary, with no generally accepted standard. Ideally, simple and convenient technology for long-term and continuous rhythm monitoring will be developed. Data obtained with such systems could be analyzed in uniform fashions to

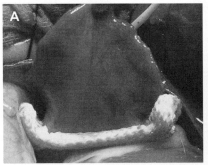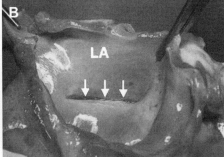

Fig. 2. Exclusion of the LAA with a specially designed, cloth-covered clip. (*A*) Clip placed on canine LAA. (*B*) View of orifice of the excluded LAA from inside the left atrium 90 days after clip application.

determine (1) absolute freedom from AF, (2) AF burden in individual patients, and (3) prevalence of AF in treated populations [71–73].

Ablation technology and intraoperative assessment

Current surgical ablation technology has several limitations. No single ablation device enables creation of all lesions from the epicardial aspect with ease of use, absence of collateral damage, and guaranteed lesion transmurality [74,75]. In addition, because there is not yet the capability to perform real-time, epicardial mapping in the operating room, ablation cannot be tailored to patients' particular electrophysiologic characteristics. Although anatomically based approaches usually are successful, it is likely that a strategy based on anatomic and electrophysiologic findings will improve results.

Minimally invasive approaches

Although most operations that include mitral valve surgery and ablation are performed through a sternotomy, it now is possible to perform minimally invasive procedures. This may be achieved via a small right thoracotomy or through a partial upper sternotomy. These procedures have been performed with bipolar RF, unipolar heat-based systems, and cryothermy [76,77]. They are technically challenging, however, as minimally invasive or keyhole approaches using current technology are hampered by difficult access to the posterior left atrium and LAA. Refinement in ablation technology is necessary to facilitate widespread application of minimally invasive cardiac surgery with ablation.

Summary

AF is common in patients presenting for cardiac surgery. Left untreated, AF increases morbidity and jeopardizes survival. Recent data demonstrate that AF ablation improves outcomes in these patients. Therefore, virtually all cardiac surgery patients who have AF should have AF ablation. The cut-and-sew maze procedure is obsolete, replaced by operations that use alternate energy sources to create lines of conduction block rapidly with little risk for bleeding. Minimally invasive cardiac surgery with AF ablation now is possible. Continued progress will facilitate tailored ablation approaches for individual patients and improve results. Development of new devices to facilitate minimally invasive exclusion of the LAA may offer a new alternative to patients who have AF and are at risk for stroke.

References

[1] Cox JL. Intraoperative options for treating atrial fibrillation associated with mitral valve disease. J Thorac Cardiovasc Surg 2001;122:212–5.
[2] Ad N, Cox JL. Combined mitral valve surgery and the Maze III procedure. Semin Thorac Cardiovasc Surg 2002;14:206–9.

[3] Grigioni F, Avierinos JF, Ling LH, et al. Atrial fibrillation complicating the course of degenerative mitral regurgitation: determinants and long-term outcome. J Am Coll Cardiol 2002; 40:84–92.

[4] Quader MA, McCarthy PM, Gillinov AM, et al. Does preoperative atrial fibrillation reduce survival after coronary artery bypass grafting? Ann Thorac Surg 2004;77:1514–22.

[5] Obadia JF, el Farra M, Bastien OH, et al. Outcome of atrial fibrillation after mitral valve repair. J Thorac Cardiovasc Surg 1997;114:179–85.

[6] Chua YL, Schaff HV, Orszulak TA, et al. Outcome of mitral valve repair in patients with preoperative atrial fibrillation. Should the maze procedure be combined with mitral valvuloplasty? J Thorac Cardiovasc Surg 1994;107:408–15.

[7] Lim E, Barlow CW, Hosseinpour AR, et al. Influence of atrial fibrillation on outcome following mitral valve repair. Circulation 2001;104:I59–63.

[8] Jessurun ER, van Hemel NM, Kelder JC, et al. Mitral valve surgery and atrial fibrillation: is atrial fibrillation surgery also needed? Eur J Cardiothorac Surg 2000;17:530–7.

[9] Kalil RA, Maratia CB, D'Avila A, et al. Predictive factors for persistence of atrial fibrillation after mitral valve operation. Ann Thorac Surg 1999;67:614–7.

[10] Fuster V, Ryden LE, Asinger RW, et al. ACC/AHA/ESC guidelines for the management of patients with atrial fibrillation. A report of the American College of Cardiology/American Heart Association Task Force on Practice Guidelines and the European Society of Cardiology Committee for Practice Guidelines and Policy Conferences (Committee to develop guidelines for the management of patients with atrial fibrillation) developed in collaboration with the North American Society of Pacing and Electrophysiology. Eur Heart J 2001;22: 1852–923.

[11] Cox JL. Atrial fibrillation I: a new classification system. J Thorac Cardiovasc Surg 2003;126: 1686–92.

[12] Wu TJ, Kerwin WF, Hwang C, et al. Atrial fibrillation: focal activity, re-entry, or both? Heart Rhythm 2004;1:117–20.

[13] Haissaguerre M, Jais P, Shah DC, et al. Spontaneous initiation of atrial fibrillation by ectopic beats originating in the pulmonary veins. N Engl J Med 1998;339:659–66.

[14] Todd DM, Skanes AC, Guiraudon G, et al. Role of the posterior left atrium and pulmonary veins in human lone atrial fibrillation: electrophysiological and pathological data from patients undergoing atrial fibrillation surgery. Circulation 2003;108:3108–14.

[15] Nitta T, Ishii Y, Miyagi Y, et al. Concurrent multiple left atrial focal activations with fibrillatory conduction and right atrial focal or reentrant activation as the mechanism in atrial fibrillation. J Thorac Cardiovasc Surg 2004;127:770–8.

[16] Yamauchi S, Ogasawara H, Saji Y, et al. Efficacy of intraoperative mapping to optimize the surgical ablation of atrial fibrillation in cardiac surgery. Ann Thorac Surg 2002;74: 450–7.

[17] Harada A, Konishi T, Fukata M, et al. Intraoperative map guided operation for atrial fibrillation due to mitral valve disease. Ann Thorac Surg 2000;69:446–50 [discussion: 450–1].

[18] Harada A, Sasaki K, Fukushima T, et al. Atrial activation during chronic atrial fibrillation in patients with isolated mitral valve disease. Ann Thorac Surg 1996;61:104–11 [discussion: 111–2].

[19] Sueda T, Imai K, Ishii O, et al. Efficacy of pulmonary vein isolation for the elimination of chronic atrial fibrillation in cardiac valvular surgery. Ann Thorac Surg 2001;71:1189–93.

[20] Schuessler RB. Do we need a map to get through the maze? J Thorac Cardiovasc Surg 2004; 127:627–8.

[21] Pappone C, Santinelli V, Manguso F, et al. Pulmonary vein denervation enhances long-term benefit after circumferential ablation for paroxysmal atrial fibrillation. Circulation 2004;109: 327–34.

[22] Oral H, Scharf C, Chugh A, et al. Catheter ablation for paroxysmal atrial fibrillation: segmental pulmonary vein ostial ablation versus left atrial ablation. Circulation 2003;108: 2355–60.

[23] Marrouche NΓ, Dresing T, Cole C, et al. Circular mapping and ablation of the pulmonary vein for treatment of atrial fibrillation: impact of different catheter technologies. J Am Coll Cardiol 2002;40:464–74.

[24] Kondo N, Takahashi K, Minakawa M, et al. Left atrial maze procedure: a useful addition to other corrective operations. Ann Thorac Surg 2003;75:1490–4.

[25] Gaita F, Gallotti R, Calo L, et al. Limited posterior left atrial cryoablation in patients with chronic atrial fibrillation undergoing valvular heart sugery. J Am Coll Cardiol 2000;36: 159–66.

[26] Tuinenburg AE, Van Gelder IC, Tieleman RG, et al. Mini-maze suffices as adjunct to mitral valve surgery in patients with preoperative atrial fibrillation. J Cardiovasc Electrophysiol 2000;11:960–7.

[27] Kalil RA, Lima GG, Leiria TL, et al. Simple surgical isolation of pulmonary veins for treating secondary atrial fibrillation in mitral valve disease. Ann Thorac Surg 2002;73:1169–73.

[28] Deneke T, Khargi K, Grcwe PH, et al. Left atrial versus bi-atrial Maze operation using intraoperatively cooled-tip radiofrequency ablation in patients undergoing open-heart surgery: safety and efficacy. J Am Coll Cardiol 2002;39:1644–50.

[29] Barnett SD, Ad N. Surgical ablation as treatment of the elimination of atrial fibrillation: a meta-analysis. J Thorac Cardiovasc Surg 2006;131:1029–35.

[30] Usui A, Inden Y, Mizutani S, et al. Repetitive atrial flutter as a complication of the left-sided simple maze procedure. Ann Thorac Surg 2002;73:1457–9.

[31] Cox JL, Schuessler RB, Boineau JP. The development of the Maze procedure for the treatment of atrial fibrillation. Semin Thorac Cardiovasc Surg 2000;12:2–14.

[32] McCarthy PM, Gillinov AM, Castle L, et al. The Cox-Maze procedure: the Cleveland Clinic experience. Semin Thorac Cardiovasc Surg 2000;12:25–9.

[33] Schaff HV, Dearani JA, Daly RC, et al. Cox-Maze procedure for atrial fibrillation: Mayo Clinic experience. Semin Thorac Cardiovasc Surg 2000;12:30–7.

[34] Prasad SM, Maniar HS, Camillo CJ, et al. The Cox maze III procedure for atrial fibrillation: long-term efficacy in patients undergoing lone versus concomitant procedures. J Thorac Cardiovasc Surg 2003;126:1822–88.

[35] Gillinov AM. Ablation of atrial fibrillation in mitral valve surgery. Curr Opin Cardiol 2005; 20:107–14.

[36] Gillinov AM, Sirak J, Blackstone EH, et al. The Cox maze procedure in mitral valve disease: predictors of recurrent atrial fibrillation. J Thorac Cardiovasc Surg 2005;130:1653–60.

[37] Scherer M, Dzemali O, Aybek T, et al. Impact of left atrial size reduction on chronic atrial fibrillation in mitral valve surgery. J Heart Valve Dis 2003;12:469–74.

[38] Gaynor SL, Schuessler RB, Bailey MS, et al. Surgical treatment of atrial fibrillation: predictors of late recurrence. J Thorac Cardiovasc Surg 2005;129:104–11.

[39] Isobe F, Kawashima Y. The outcome and indications of the Cox maze III procedure for chronic atrial fibrillation with mitral valve disease. J Thorac Cardiovasc Surg 1998;116:220–7.

[40] Kosakai Y, Kawaguchi AT, Fumitaka I, et al. Modified maze procedure for pateints with atrial fibrillation undergoing simultaneous open heart surgery. Circulation 1995;92:359–64.

[41] Lee JW, Park NH, Choo SJ, et al. Surgical outcome of the maze procedure for atrial fibrillation in mitral valve disease: rheumatic versus degenerative. Ann Thorac Surg 2003;75: 57–61 [discussion: 61].

[42] Jatene MB, Marcial MB, Tarasoutchi F, et al. Influence of the maze procedure on the treatment of rheumatic atrial fibrillation—evaluation of rhythm control and clinical outcome in a comparative study. Eur J Cardiothorac Surg 2000;17:117–24.

[43] Bando K, Kasegawa H, Okada Y, et al. The impact of pre- and postoperative atrial fibrillation on outcome after mitral valvuloplasty for nonischemic mitral regurgitation. J Thorac Cardiovasc Surg 2005;129:1032–40.

[44] Bando K, Kobayashi J, Kosakai Y, et al. Impact of Cox maze procedure on outcome in patients with atrial fibrillation and mitral valve disease. J Thorac Cardiovasc Surg 2002;124: 575–83.

[45] Handa N, Schaff HV, Morris JJ, et al. Outcome of valve repair and the Cox maze procedure for mitral regurgitation and associated atrial fibrillation. J Thorac Cardiovasc Surg 1999; 118:628–35.

[46] Cox JL, Ad N, Palazzo T. Impact of the maze procedure on the stroke rate in patients with atrial fibrillation. J Thorac Cardiovasc Surg 1999;118:833–40.

[47] Gillinov AM, Blackstone EH, McCarthy PM. Atrial fibrillation: current surgical options and their assessment. Ann Thorac Surg 2002;74:2210–7.

[48] Gillinov AM, McCarthy PM. Advances in the surgical treatment of atrial fibrillation. Cardiol Clin 2004;22:147–57.

[49] Gillinov AM, McCarthy PM, Marrouche N, et al. Contemporary surgical treatment for atrial fibrillation. Pacing Clin Electrophysiol 2003;26:1–4.

[50] Raman J, Ishikawa S, Storer MM, et al. Surgical radiofrequency ablation of both atria for atrial fibrillation: results of a multicenter trial. J Thorac Cardiovasc Surg 2003;126:1357–66.

[51] Sie HT, Beukema WP, Elvan A, et al. Long-term results of irrigated radiofrequency modified maze procedure in 200 patients with concomitant cardiac surgery: six years experience. Ann Thorac Surg 2004;77:512–6 [discussion: 516–7].

[52] Luria DM, Nemec J, Etheridge SP, et al. Intra-atrial conduction block along the mitral valve annulus during accessory pathway ablation: evidence for a left atrial "isthmus". J Cardiovasc Electrophysiol 2001;12:744–9.

[53] Saltman AE, Rosenthal LS, Francalancia NA, et al. A completely endoscopic approach to microwave ablation for atrial fibrillation. Heart Surg Forum 2003;6:E38–41.

[54] Reade CC, Johnson JO, Bolotin G, et al. Combining robotic mitral valve repair and microwave atrial fibrillation ablation: techniques and initial results. Ann Thorac Surg 2005;79: 480–4.

[55] Salenger R, Lahey SJ, Saltman AE. The completely endoscopic treatment of atrial fibrillation: report on the first 14 patients with early results. Heart Surg Forum 2004;7:E555–8.

[56] Pruitt JC, Lazzara RR, Dworkin GH, et al. Totally endoscopic ablation of lone atrial fibrillation: initial clinical experience. Ann Thorac Surg 2006;81:1325–30.

[57] Bisleri G, Manzato A, Argenziano M, et al. Thoracoscopic epicardial pulmonary vein ablation for lone paroxysmal atrial fibrillation. Europace 2005;7:145–8.

[58] Wolf RK, Schneeberger EW, Osterday R, et al. Video-assisted bilateral pulmonary vein isolation and left atrial appendage exclusion for atrial fibrillation. J Thorac Cardiovasc Surg 2005;130:797–802.

[59] Cox JL, Ad N. The importance of cryoablation of the coronary sinus during the Maze procedure. Semin Thorac Cardiovasc Surg 2000;12:20–4.

[60] Nath S, Lynch C, Whayne JG, et al. Cellular electrophysiological effects of hyperthermia on isolated guinea pig papillary muscle. Implications for catheter ablation. Circulation 1993;88: 1826–31.

[61] Lustgarten DL, Keane D, Ruskin J. Cryothermal ablation: mechanism of tissue injury and current experience in the treatment of tachyarrhythmias. Prog Cardiovasc Dis 1999;41:481–98.

[62] Khargi K, Hutten BA, Lemke B, et al. Surgical treatment of atrial fibrillation; a systematic review. Eur J Cardiothorac Surg 2005;27:258–65.

[63] Gillinov AM, Pettersson G, Rice TW. Esophageal injury during radiofrequency ablation for atrial fibrillation. J Thorac Cardiovasc Surg 2001;122:1239–40.

[64] Doll N, Borger MA, Fabricius A, et al. Esophageal perforation during left atrial radiofrequency ablation: Is the risk too high? J Thorac Cardiovasc Surg 2003;125:836–42.

[65] Manasse E, Medici D, Ghiselli S, et al. Left main coronary arterial lesion after microwave epicardial ablation. Ann Thorac Surg 2003;76:276–7.

[66] Johnson WD, Ganjoo AK, Stone CD, et al. The left atrial appendage: our most lethal human attachment! Surgical implications. Eur J Cardiothorac Surg 2000;17:718–22.

[67] Garcia-Fernandez MA, Perez-David E, Quiles J, et al. Role of left atrial appendage obliteration in stroke reduction in patients with mitral valve prosthesis: a transesophageal echocardiographic study. J Am Coll Cardiol 2003;42:1253–8.

[68] Rosenzweig BP, Katz E, Kort S, et al. Thromboembolus from a ligated left atrial appendage. J Am Soc Echocardiogr 2001;14:396–8.

[69] Gillinov AM, Pettersson G, Cosgrove DM 3rd. Stapled excision of the left atrial appendage. J Thorac Cardiovasc Surg 2004;129:679–80.

[70] Kamohara K, Fukamachi K, Ootaki Y, et al. A novel device for left atrial appendage exclusion. J Thorac Cardiovasc Surg 2005;130:1639–44.

[71] Pacifico A, Henry PD. Ablation for atrial fibrillation: are cures really achieved? J Am Coll Cardiol 2004;43:1940–2.

[72] Gillinov AM, McCarthy PM, Blackstone EH, et al. Surgical ablation of atrial fibrillation with bipolar radiofrequency. J Thorac Cardiovasc Surg 2004;129:1322–9.

[73] Shemin RJ, Cox JL, Gillinov AM, et al. Guidelines for reporting data and outcomes for the surgical treatment of atrial fibrillation. Ann Thorac Surg 2007;83:1225–30.

[74] Gillinov AM, Saltman AE. Ablation of atrial fibrillation with concomitant cardiac surgery [review]. Semin Thorac Cardiovasc Surg 2007;19:25–32.

[75] Gillinov AM. Advances in the surgical treatment of atrial fibrillation [review]. Stroke 2007; 38(Suppl 2):618–23.

[76] Doll N, Kiaii BB, Fabricius AM, et al. Intraoperative left atrial ablation (for atrial fibrillation) using a new argon cryocatheter: early clinical experience. Ann Thorac Surg 2003;76: 1711–5 [discussion: 1715].

[77] Mohr FW, Fabricius AM, Falk V, et al. Curative treatment of atrial fibrillation with intraoperative radiofrequency ablation: short-term and midterm results. J Thorac Cardiovasc Surg 2002;123:919–27.

ELSEVIER
SAUNDERS

THE MEDICAL
CLINICS
OF NORTH AMERICA

Med Clin N Am 92 (2008) 217–235

Atrial Fibrillation: Goals of Therapy and Management Strategies to Achieve the Goals

Benzy J. Padanilam, MD, Eric N. Prystowsky, MD*

The Care Group, LLC, 8333 Naab Road Suite 400, Indianapolis, IN 46260-1919, USA

Atrial fibrillation (AF) may be associated with disabling symptoms and complications, such as stroke and tachycardia-induced cardiomyopathy. Although AF per se rarely is a life-threatening arrhythmia, it was associated with a decreased overall survival in the Framingham Heart Study [1]. The three major therapeutic strategies in managing AF include prevention of stroke, rate control, and rhythm control. Anticoagulation with warfarin reduces the risk for stroke. Therapies used to achieve control of symptoms or to prevent tachycardia-mediated cardiomyopathy often are similar. For example, ventricular rate control during AF or maintenance of sinus rhythm may improve symptoms or prevent cardiomyopathy. When clinical goals are not met using one strategy, an alternate strategy can be pursued in the same patient. Current therapies do not show survival benefits, and future research needs to focus on the goals of improving survival and on the primary prevention of AF. Currently, prevention of complications and control of symptoms may be considered the primary goals of AF management (Box 1).

Goals of therapy

Prevention of thromboembolism

AF, with its accompanying loss of organized atrial contraction, can lead to stagnation of blood, especially in the left atrial appendage, with resultant thrombus formation and embolism. There is some evidence that AF is associated with a hypercoagulable state, further promoting thromboembolism [2,3]. Stroke, the most common thromboembolic event in AF, occurs at

---

* Corresponding author.
E-mail address: eprystow@thecaregroup.com (E.N. Prystowsky).

0025-7125/08/$ - see front matter © 2008 Elsevier Inc. All rights reserved.
doi:10.1016/j.mcna.2007.08.006

Box 1. Goals of atrial fibrillation therapy

Prevention of stroke (thromboembolism)
Prevention of tachycardia-induced cardiomyopathy
Symptom relief
Improved survival
Primary prevention

---

a higher frequency in individuals who have AF, and approximately 36% of all strokes in individuals ages 80 to 89 years are attributed to AF [4]. Furthermore, strokes occurring in patients who have AF have a higher degree of severity [5]. Individuals who have AF are not at equal risk for thromboembolic events and several predisposing clinical factors can identify those patients at high risk (discussed later). Anticoagulation with warfarin is the current standard of therapy for preventing thromboembolism in patients at high risk for stroke. The goal of anticoagulation is to prevent AF-related thromboembolic complications without increasing the risks for bleeding significantly. There is evidence that suggests warfarin therapy is underused [6,7]; more widespread use of warfarin therapy in appropriate patients is another goal to be achieved. An important lesson learned from recent clinical trials of AF management is that patients at high risk for stroke who seem to be maintaining sinus rhythm while receiving antiarrhythmic medications still require warfarin therapy [8,9]. These patients have a continued risk for stroke, possibly from clinically unrecognized episodes of AF.

Prevention of tachycardia-induced cardiomyopathy

Untreated AF often is associated with rapid ventricular rates of more than 120 beats per minute. In experimental models, ventricular dysfunction can occur as soon as 24 hours and continue to deteriorate for 3 to 5 weeks with rapid pacing rates. Recovery of ventricular function with cessation of pacing starts within 48 hours and normalization can occur within 1 to 2 weeks [10]. Patients who have AF and prolonged periods of rapid ventricular rates may develop left ventricular (LV) dysfunction, although the severity and temporal course of its onset varies significantly between individuals. In a study of AV node ablation and permanent pacemaker placement for AF refractory to medical therapy, 37% (105 of 282) of patients had LV ejection fraction of 40% or less [11], indicating a high prevalence of cardiomyopathy in such patients. Control of ventricular rates, by rate or rhythm control strategies, when undertaken early after AF onset, can prevent subsequent development of cardiomyopathy. If patients already have developed tachycardia-induced ventricular dysfunction at presentation, the immediate goal is to reverse this process with aggressive rate control or cardioversion to sinus rhythm. In such patients, particular attention should be paid to avoid recurrent AF with prolonged periods of rapid ventricular rates, because quick development of LV failure and incidents of sudden death are reported in the literature [12].

Control of symptoms

Patients who have AF exhibit a panoply of clinical presentations, ranging from none to disabling symptoms. Common symptoms include anxiety, palpitations, dyspnea, dizziness, chest pain, and fatigue. Several hemodynamic derangements, including rapid ventricular rates, loss of organized atrial contraction, irregularity of cardiac rhythm, and bradycardia (resulting particularly from sinus pauses when AF episodes terminate) may be the underlying cause of the symptoms related to AF. Although the Atrial Fibrillation Follow-up Investigation of Rhythm Management (AFFIRM) trial [8] demonstrated that symptoms can be controlled equally well with a rate control or rhythm control strategy in selected older patients, clinicians managing patients who have AF encounter many patients who need sinus rhythm to feel better. This may be relevant particularly in younger patients and those who have paroxysmal AF. The loss of regularity and fine autonomic control of cardiac rhythm and the loss of atrial contribution to ventricular filling are postulated as playing a bigger role in these patients, accounting for the lack of success of rate control. When a rate control strategy is selected, it is important to allow adequate time for symptoms to improve, because in many patients it can take several months for good symptom relief after achieving rate control. Control of symptoms rather than elimination of all symptoms may be an acceptable goal in many patients based on a risks/benefits analysis of the available therapeutic options.

Future goals

Improvement in survival should be a goal of AF therapy. Elucidation of basic mechanisms of the disease and targeted therapy that does not have significant adverse effects (eg, atrial specific antiarrhythmic drugs) [13], continued anticoagulation in patients taking antiarrhythmic drugs for rhythm control [14], and catheter ablation strategies to cure AF could improve patient survival. Preliminary data comparing ablation with antiarrhythmic medications show favorable outcomes for the ablation strategy [15,16].

Primary prevention of AF is an important public health goal as it affects an estimated 2.2 million people in the United States [17] and its prevalence is rising [18]. Preliminary data suggest that the use of medications, such as angiotensin-converting enzyme inhibitors, angiotensin receptor blockers, and 3-hydroxy-3-methylglutaryl coenzyme A (HMG-CoA) reductase inhibitors, and dietary intake of fish and n-3 polyunsaturated fatty acids may reduce AF incidence [13]. Whether or not treatment of disease states, such as hypertension and heart failure, that have a known association with AF could lead to a decreased incidence of AF also needs evaluation.

Therapeutic options

Anticoagulation

Risk stratification

Because anticoagulation therapy inherently is associated with an increased risk for bleeding complications, such therapy is limited to patients who have AF and who are deemed at high risk for thromboembolism. Collective information from various clinical trials of anticoagulation therapy has identified several risk factors that predispose persons who have AF to thromboembolism [19]. Gage and colleagues [20] developed a scoring system for stroke risk prediction, called $CHADS_2$, using these risk factors. Each of the letters in this acronym represents a risk factor—congestive heart failure, hypertension, age, diabetes, and stroke. Previous stroke or transient ischemic attack (TIA) is the strongest predictor of stroke and, therefore, carries 2 points, whereas the other risk factors carry 1 point each. The American College of Cardiology/American Heart Associaion/European Society of Cardiology (ACC/AHA/ESC) guidelines on AF management use the $CHADS_2$ scoring for risk factor classification [21]. Box 2 summarizes the ACC/AHA/ESC system of dividing predisposing factors into less validated

---

Box 2. Risk factors for thromboembolism

Less validated risk
Female gender
Age 65–74 y
Coronary artery disease
Thyrotoxicosis

Moderate risk
Age ≥75 y
Hypertension
LV ejection fraction ≤35%
Heart failure
Diabetes mellitus

High risk
Previous stroke, TIA, embolism
Mitral stenosis
Prosthetic heart valve

or weaker risk factors, moderate risk factors, and high risk factors. Patients who have any high risk factor or more than one moderate risk factor are considered at high risk ($>4\%$ annual risk) for stroke and warfarin is recommended for them, whereas those who have no risk factors are considered low risk ($<2\%$ annual risk) for stroke and are prescribed aspirin (Box 3). Patients who have one moderate risk factor have an intermediate risk (2.8% annual risk) for stroke [20,21]. Treatment decisions are individualized in these latter patients and warfarin or aspirin may be used [21].

Warfarin

Warfarin therapy is highly effective, compared with placebo, in reducing (by 61%) the stroke risk in patients who have AF [22]. Strokes occurring in AF patients while they are taking warfarin therapy also are less severe [23]. In clinical studies, an international normalized ratio (INR) between 2.0 and 3.0 correlates to maximum protection against strokes with minimum bleeding risks [24]. Warfarin has several drawbacks, including a 1% to 1.5% risk for major bleeding complications [19]. The risk for bleeding may be higher in women and in the elderly, who also are at the highest risk for embolic stroke from AF [25,26]. The risk for bleeding seems higher at initiation of warfarin, and a recent study has noted a threefold increase in bleeding risk during the first 3 months of therapy [27].

Alternatives to warfarin

Aspirin is significantly less effective than warfarin, with a stroke reduction of 19% [22]. Aspirin, however, is recommended in lower-risk patients because of its favorable side-effect profile and ease of use. In a clinical study of high-risk patients, a combination of aspirin and clopidogrel was inferior to warfarin for stroke prevention [28]. Ximelagatran (an oral direct thrombin inhibitor) did not meet United States Food and Drug Administration approval because of concerns regarding its hepatotoxicity and clinical trial design [29]. Nonpharmacologic stroke prevention, a consideration only in high-risk patients who are not candidates for warfarin, has not been well studied. Approaches include surgical left atrial appendage removal and catheter-based left atrial appendage occlusion [30,31].

Anticoagulation management before cardioversion

The use of anticoagulation before and after cardioversion (electrical or pharmacologic) requires special consideration because of increased risk

---

Box 3. Risk category and recommended therapy

No risk factors: aspirin (81 mg or 325 mg daily)
One moderate risk factor: aspirin or warfarin
Any high risk factor or >1 moderate risk factors: warfarin

for stroke noted in retrospective studies after cardioversion [32]. According to the current guidelines [21], patients may be cardioverted without anticoagulation if the duration of AF is less than 48 hours. When the duration of AF is unknown or greater than 48 hours, anticoagulation with warfarin should be instituted with a therapeutic INR for at least 3 weeks before and 4 weeks after the cardioversion [21]. An alternative approach is a transesophageal echocardiogram-based cardioversion followed by at least 4 weeks of warfarin anticoagulation [33]. In this approach, patients who do not have a therapeutic INR may be given intravenous unfractionated heparin or subcutaneous low molecular weight heparin to achieve immediate anticoagulation at the time of cardioversion [33,34].

Rate control and rhythm control

The two basic therapeutic options to control symptoms in AF are rhythm control, where sinus rhythm is re-established, and rate control, where patients remain in AF with control of ventricular rates. Pharmacologic and nonpharmacologic options are available for both of these strategies.

Although the rhythm control strategy intuitively seems superior, because it is aimed at re-establishing the normal rhythm, clinical studies show no significant difference in major clinical outcomes between this strategy and that of rate control. Five randomized clinical trials looked at total mortality, thromboembolic events, hemorrhage, and symptomatic improvement and found no statistically significant differences in outcomes between the pharmacologic rate control and rhythm control strategies [8,9,35–37]. The mean age of participants in the largest of these trials (AFFIRM) was 69.7 years, leading many clinicians to choose rate control as a preferred strategy in older less symptomatic patients.

The reasons for the lack of advantage of sinus rhythm maintenance are not clear, but could relate to the toxicity associated with antiarrhythmic medications, negating the advantages of sinus rhythm, and to discontinuation of anticoagulation in patients, seemingly maintaining sinus rhythm. One of the important messages from rate control versus rhythm control trials is the need for continued anticoagulation therapy in high-risk patients while they are taking antiarrhythmic medications. A retrospective subanalysis of the on-treatment outcomes in AFFIRM study suggests that a strategy to maintain sinus rhythm without the adverse effects of antiarrhythmic medications may confer a survival advantage [14]. Radiofrequency ablation trials also shed some light on this debate. In a nonrandomized study, Pappone and colleagues [15] compared the outcomes in a selected group of 589 patients who underwent circumferential pulmonary vein ablation with 582 age- and gender-matched cohort patients who received antiarrhythmic medications to maintain sinus rhythm. After a median follow-up of 900 days, the observed survival was longer and the quality-of-life better for patients who underwent ablation. Radiofrequency pulmonary vein isolation was a superior first-line therapy compared with antiarrhythmic drug therapy in a small, randomized trial of 70 patients [16]. Finally, in heart failure patients, ablation resulted in improved heart function even when heart rates were well controlled before ablation [38,39]. Thus, future use of antiarrhythmic medications with a better side-effect profile and advancements in ablation techniques could lead to demonstration of better outcomes with rhythm control strategy.

Choice of strategy

The choice of a particular strategy should be dictated by the clinical scenario, with a preference toward rate control in less symptomatic elderly patients. Rate control also may be preferred in patients who are noncompliant or decline hospitalizations and cardioversions, because the rhythm control strategy may require a higher number of hospitalizations [8]. Patients in whom the only antiarrhythmic choice is amiodarone also are potential candidates for an initial rate control strategy. Initial rhythm control strategy may be appropriate in younger symptomatic patients, newly diagnosed patients who have lone AF, and those who have AF believed secondary to a precipitating event. Although there is a suggestion of improved survival by maintaining sinus rhythm in heart failure patients [8,40,41], results of further studies [42] are awaited before recommending rhythm control as a primary strategy in this group of patients. In the end, clinical judgment needs to be exercised and care individualized for each patient.

Definition of rate control

The best parameters for rate control in AF are not well defined, but the AFFIRM study criteria generally are recommended [8,21] (≤ 80 beats/minute ventricular rate at rest and maximum of <110 beats/minute during a 6-minute walk or an average heart rate of <100 beats/minute during 24-hour ambulatory monitoring with no heart rate $>110\%$ of maximal age-predicted exercise heart rate). It is unclear whether or not very strict heart rate control is essential for good outcomes, especially in patients who do not have LV dysfunction and significant symptoms. Cooper and colleagues [43] analyzed the outcomes in different quartiles of heart rate control in the AFFIRM study (heart rate quartiles at rest: 44–69, 70–78, 79–87, and 88–148 beats/minute and heart rate quartiles with 60-minute walk: 53–82, 83–92, 93–106 and 107–220 beats/minute) and found no differences in overall survival or quality of life. These data may indicate that very strict heart rate control may not be essential for good outcomes. At the authors' institution, we prefer to regulate heart rate for AF in each patient's normal daily activity profile. To accomplish this, the daily heart rate trend graphs from 24-hour ECG recordings are used and medications adjusted to maintain average rates for each hour of less than 100 beats per minute and for the 24-hour period approximately 70 to 80 beats per minute [44].

Therapeutic options for rate control

β-Blockers, nondihydropyridine calcium channel blockers, and digoxin are the usual pharmacologic agents used for rate control. Digoxin is less effective than β-blockers and calcium channel blockers, particularly during exercise, but has a synergistic effect when added to them [45]. β-Blockers are preferred as an initial AV blocking agent when there is LV dysfunction associated with AF [46,47]. Verapamil and diltiazem in a sustained released form often are well tolerated and useful for rate control. At times, it is useful to give smaller doses of two classes of drugs to minimize adverse effects. Amiodarone and clonidine also has been used for rate control purposes in limited situations [21,48]. AV junction ablation with permanent pacemaker implantation (ablate and pace strategy) is a highly effective method for rate control but usually reserved for situations where pharmacologic options are ineffective. Clinical studies have demonstrated improvement in quality of life and LV function with such an approach [49,50]. Concerns with this approach include patients becoming pacemaker dependent, provocation of fatal ventricular arrhythmias, and the more recently described deleterious effects of permanent right ventricular pacing [51]. Consideration may be given to biventricular pacing for patients who have significant LV dysfunction undergoing AV junction ablation for AF rate control to address the potential deleterious effects of right ventricular pacing in that situation [52–54].

Rhythm control with antiarrhythmic medications

Antiarrhythmic medications, by changing the electrophysiologic properties of atrial tissue, can terminate AF or prevent its recurrence. The Vaughan-Williams classification divides these agents into class IA, IB, and IC (sodium channel blockers); class II (β-blockers); class III (potassium channel blockers); and class IV (calcium channel blockers). Only class I and class III agents are referred to as antiarrhythmic medications in this article, because β-blockers and calcium channel blockers do not have the ability to cardiovert AF or maintain sinus rhythm after cardioversion of AF.

Choice of antiarrhythmic medication

Selection of antiarrhythmic agents should be directed by a safety-based approach (Fig. 1). The class IC agent, flecainide, increased mortality in the setting of previous myocardial infarction and ventricular ectopy in the Cardiac Arrhythmia Suppression Trial [55]. Based on this information, flecainide and propafenone are considered contraindicated in AF patients who have ischemic heart disease [21]. Class IC agents do not increase mortality in patients who have structurally normal hearts [56], however, making them one of the initial agents of choice for treatment of AF. Class III (sotalol and dofetelide) and class IA (quinidine, procainamide, and disopyramide) agents prolong cardiac repolarization and, therefore, can be associated with torsades de pointes form of ventricular tachycardia. Although many patients at risk can be identified by monitoring for early proarrhythmia and QT prolongation on ECG, late

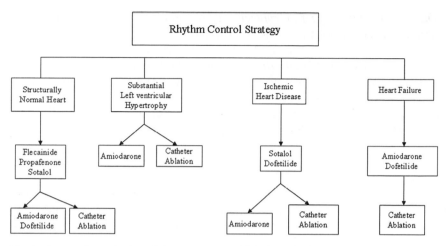

Fig. 1. Approach to selection of therapy to re-establish sinus rhythm in patients who have AF.

episodes of torsades de pointes can occur, particularly in the setting of hypoka-
lemia, bradycardia, or renal dysfunction [57]. Amiodarone is a multi-ion
channel blocking agent (included in class III) and prolongs QT interval but
has a very low risk for causing torsades de pointes. Amiodarone is the most effective antiarrhythmic drug available and, in the Canadian Trial of Atrial Fibrillation, only 35% of patients taking amiodarone had recurrent AF
compared with 63% of those taking propafenone or sotalol during a mean
follow-up of 468 ($\pm$ 150) days [58]. Amiodarone, however, has many organ toxicities—thyroid, pulmonary, neurologic, hepatic, optic neuropathy (rare), and
dermatologic effects [59]—that limit its usefulness. In a metanalysis of 44 antiarrhythmic medication trials (11,322 patients), sotalol, dofetelide, or amiodarone did not show any significant change in mortality compared with placebo
and the same review showed an increased mortality associated with the use of
class IA drugs compared with placebo [56].

When selecting an antiarrhythmic medication for AF treatment, first determine if the heart structurally is normal. The initial choice of an antiarrhythmic medication in patients who have normal hearts is flecainide,
propafenone, or sotalol. In the presence of LV hypertrophy (>1.4 cm),
amiodarone is the preferred initial therapy because of the perceived potential for proarrhythmia with other agents [21]. Only amiodarone and dofetelide are demonstrated to not decrease survival in the setting of heart failure,
making them the preferred agents for these patients. Patients who have ischemic heart disease usually are given sotalol or dofetilide as initial agents.
Sotalol and dofetelide are excreted through kidneys and should be avoided
in patients who have significant renal dysfunction. Bradycardia accentuates
QT prolonging effects of sotalol and dofetelide, and patients may require
permanent pacing to facilitate the use of these agents in this scenario. Finally, consider avoiding these latter medications in patients who have

complex medical regimens, particularly if significant variations in serum electrolytes could occur.

Outpatient initiation of antiarrhythmic medications

Dofetilide therapy always is initiated in a hospital with daily 12-lead ECGs and telemetry monitoring for at least 3 days. All other antiarrhythmic medications can be initiated in an outpatient setting in patients who have no or minimal heart disease per current guidelines [21]. In the presence of heart disease, the authors recommend starting sotalol during constant heart rhythm monitoring in a hospital. Patients who are in AF at the time of therapy initiation also are candidates for inpatient treatment, because they may have unidentified sinus node dysfunction, leading to significant bradycardia with conversion of AF to sinus rhythm. One exception is amiodarone initiation at low doses of 200 to 600 mg per day. Here, drug loading takes several weeks and it is impractical to monitor patients in hospital. When drugs are initiated on an outpatient basis, the authors recommend 12-lead ECGs 2 to 3 days after each dose change. Electrocardiograms are analyzed for excessive prolongation of QT interval (QTc > 500 ms) with sotalol and for prolongation of PR interval and QRS duration with flecainide or propafenone.

Cardioversion

Conversion of AF to sinus rhythm can be done using synchronized external shocks or antiarrhythmic medications at loading doses. Anticoagulation issues must be addressed prior to pharmacologic or electrical cardioversions. AF, unlike atrial flutter, is not a rhythm that can be terminated with overdrive pacing. A "pill-in-the-pocket" strategy of outpatient cardioversion may be attempted using loading doses of propafenone or flecainide in some patients [60]. The first such attempt, however, should be done in a hospital setting [21] to establish safety. Administration of β-blockers or calcium channel blockers is recommended at least 30 minutes before high-dose propafenone or flecainide to prevent development of atrial flutter with 1:1 AV conduction leading to potentially life-threatening ventricular rates [21].

Nonpharmacologic rhythm control

When rhythm maintenance is needed and antiarrhythmic medications are ineffective, radiofrequency catheter ablation approaches may be considered. Recent observations from Haissaguerre and colleagues [61,62] have demonstrated that the initiators of AF typically originate in the pulmonary veins, and electrical isolation of these veins often prevents AF. Many different ablation techniques subsequently have been described, and the best AF ablation technique to eliminate AF in individual patients has yet to be defined [63]. The surgical maze procedure to cure AF is highly effective, but this typically is reserved for patients who have failed the catheter ablation approach or for patients undergoing another open-heart procedure, where it is added onto the primary procedure [64].

Management strategies based on clinical presentations

Initial approach to any patients who have atrial fibrillation

History, physical examination, laboratory tests

Initial evaluation of AF should include clinical history regarding the time of onset and the nature of patients' symptoms (Fig. 2). Attention should be directed to identifying a possible precipitating event that led to AF. Symptoms suggestive of complications, such as heart failure and stroke, also should be part of the history. Physical examination is directed to vital signs and cardiovascular and other system examinations, especially to further the information obtained from the history. Initial laboratory testing should include a complete blood count, a metabolic panel, and renal and thyroid function evaluations. A 2-D echocardiogram is indicated in most patients to identify causative factors for AF and to evaluate for LV dysfunction.

Hemodynamics

Initial attention is directed to the hemodynamic stability of patients. AF, particularly with rapid ventricular rates, can result in severe hemodynamic

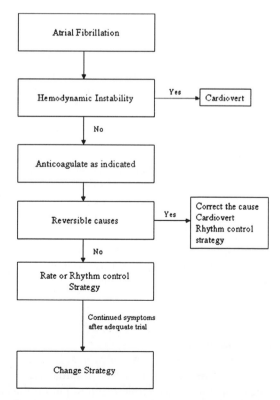

Fig. 2. General approach to patients presenting with AF.

compromise, especially in patients who have heart disease where cardiac output is heavily dependent on the atrial contribution and diastolic filling time of the ventricle. Examples include hypertrophic cardiomyopathy with its associated noncompliant ventricles, diastolic dysfunction, and severe mitral stenosis. Significant hemodynamic instability also can occur in scenarios where there is pre-existing hemodynamic compromise, such as sepsis, myocardial infarction, or pulmonary embolism. Patients who have life-threatening hemodynamic compromise need emergent cardioversion without consideration to anticoagulation status. These patients also are at risk for recurrent AF after the cardioversion and may need treatment with intravenous antiarrhythmic drugs, such as amiodarone, to maintain sinus rhythm or to control ventricular rates during AF. Digoxin is another agent that can give rate control without causing hypotension; however, its effectiveness is minimized in these states of high sympathetic tone.

Precipitating factors

Once the hemodynamic status is addressed, potential precipitating events that caused AF are evaluated. Examples of cardiac disorders that may underlie AF include pericarditis, heart failure, thoracic surgery, Wolff-Parkinson-White syndrome, and mitral stenosis. Several noncardiac conditions also can precipitate AF, for example, pneumonia, pulmonary embolism, acute hypoxia, thyrotoxicosis, and alcohol binge drinking. Although AF may not recur when precipitating factors are eliminated, there is a distinct possibility that AF episodes may continue to occur and the correlation was coincidental or the precipitating event simply brought out the underlying causative AF pathophysiology. Therefore, AF in patients who have possible precipitating events initially is managed the same way as is AF in other patients with regards to anticoagulation. Anticoagulation should be considered in all high-risk patients with the understanding that it can be discontinued if there are no clinical AF recurrences during follow-up. For moderate-risk patients in whom warfarin anticoagulation is optional, waiting to see if AF recurs in the absence of the initial precipitating event before initiating anticoagulation treatment is reasonable. A rhythm control rather than a rate control approach is preferred because of the distinct possibility of long-term sinus rhythm maintenance without antiarrhythmic medications. Short-term antiarrhythmic therapy may be considered if the initial AF episode is persistent.

Newly diagnosed atrial fibrillation

Persistent atrial fibrillation

In patients presenting with new-onset symptoms, it may be worth waiting at least 24 hours to determine if the AF self-terminates. At least one attempt at establishing sinus rhythm is reasonable in most patients who have a new diagnosis of AF, because patients may maintain sinus rhythm for prolonged periods after an initial cardioversion. Older asymptomatic patients who have no precipitating events for AF may be managed with rate control from the beginning. When AF is diagnosed for the first time in a patient, the time of onset of the arrhythmia may or may not be clear based on clinical history. Because it has an impact on anticoagulation decisions for cardioversion, meticulous attention should be paid to establish the time at which AF started. History of palpitations and dyspnea are unreliable particularly in elderly patients and these may signify AF-related heart failure symptoms rather than the onset of the arrhythmia itself. It may be wise to err on the side of indeterminate time of onset in elderly patients and patients who have multiple stroke risk factors and have the patients undergo 3 weeks of anticoagulation or transesophageal echocardiogram before cardioversion. If the time of onset is clear and less than 48 hours from history, particularly in young patients, cardioversion (electrical or pharmacologic) may be considered without anticoagulation.

Paroxysmal atrial fibrillation

Because AF episodes are self-terminating, cardioversion is unnecessary. Antiarrhythmic medications should be avoided until a pattern of recurrent symptomatic episodes is established. Rate control may be needed and should be guided by symptoms. Patients who have minimally symptomatic and infrequent episodes may not need any treatment other than anticoagulation considerations.

Recurrent atrial fibrillation

In the overwhelming majority of patients, persistent or paroxysmal AF recurs after the initial event. Anticoagulation decisions are made based on the risk profile for stroke and are not affected by the persistent or paroxysmal nature of AF. The decision of pursuing a rhythm or rate control strategy depends on individual patient factors. In general, based on general principles (discussed previously), rate control is favored in older, less symptomatic patients. For patients who have infrequent but highly symptomatic persistent AF episodes, a pill-in-the-pocket strategy may be appropriate and help reduce the risk for side effects related to long-term antiarrhythmic therapy. Catheter ablation is an option for persistent and paroxysmal AF, when antiarrhythmic therapy is ineffective in controlling symptoms.

Permanent atrial fibrillation

Permanent AF is a term applied to cases where patients are allowed to remain in AF without further attempts at rhythm control, because rhythm control is deemed unnecessary or not attainable with reasonable risk/benefit ratio. Anticoagulation should be administered when indicated based on risk factors. Ventricular rate control must be addressed in all cases.

Tachycardia-bradycardia syndrome

Patients who have paroxysmal AF may have high ventricular rates during AF episodes and bradycardia during sinus rhythm. Similarly, patients who have persistent or permanent AF may present with uncontrolled high ventricular rates at times and symptomatic slow ventricular rates at other times. These two situations, where tachycardia and bradycardia are present in the same patient, present a scenario where rate control and antiarrhythmic medications are difficult to use. Permanent pacemaker implantation usually is necessary to facilitate appropriate therapy. Sinus node dysfunction may resolve after a successful catheter ablation of AF and may be a consideration, particularly in young patients, to avoid the need for permanent pacing [65].

Atrial fibrillation with heart failure

Patients presenting with heart failure (systolic or diastolic dysfunction) resulting from AF generally have high ventricular rates. Cardioversion to sinus rhythm and initiation of an antiarrhythmic medication (dofetelide or amiodarone) usually are needed, because such patients often do not tolerate β-blockers or calcium channel blockers for rate control. The need for cardioversion is less clear when ventricular rates are controlled at presentation (issues regarding rate control versus rhythm control in this situation are discussed previously).

Postoperative atrial fibrillation

AF occurs in approximately one third of patients after open-heart surgery [66]. It is an important risk factor for postoperative stroke and anticoagulation should be instituted despite the increased bleeding risk inherent in this setting [66–68]. A metanalysis of 42 clinical trials showed benefits of β-blockers, sotalol, and amiodarone in reducing the incidence of postoperative AF [69]. β-Blockers are recommended routinely for patients undergoing cardiac surgery and amiodarone may be considered for patients at high risk for postoperative AF [21].

Atrial fibrillation and Wolff-Parkinson-White syndrome

Wolff-Parkinson-White syndrome presents two specific clinical problems with AF. First, an accessory pathway–mediated atrioventricular reentry tachycardia can degenerate into AF. Second, in some patients who have accessory pathways capable of rapid conduction to the ventricle, the AF may degenerate into ventricular fibrillation and cause sudden death [70]. Electrical cardioversion is necessary if patients are hemodynamically unstable. In stable patients, intravenous procainamide or amiodarone can be used to slow conduction over the accessory pathway. Intravenous β-blockers and calcium channel blockers could result in hypotension and accelerated conduction over the accessory pathway and are contraindicated in this setting. Digoxin also is contraindicated in this setting because of concerns of accelerated conduction over the accessory pathway and paradoxic effect of increased ventricular rates from AV node blockade [21]. Definitive therapy is radiofrequency ablation of the accessory pathway.

Summary

The primary goals in the management of patients who have AF are the prevention of stroke and cardiomyopathy and the amelioration of symptoms. Each patient presents to a physician with a specific constellation of symptoms and signs, but, fortunately, most patients can be assigned to broad categories of therapy. For some, anticoagulation and rate control suffice, whereas others require more aggressive attempts to restore and maintain sinus rhythm. Physicians and patients need to be willing to alter therapeutic plans if an initial strategy of rate or rhythm control is unsuccessful.

References

[1] Benjamin EJ, Wolf PA, D'Agostino RB, et al. Impact of atrial fibrillation on the risk of death: the Framingham Heart Study. Circulation 1998;98(10):946–52.

[2] Heppell RM, Berkin KE, McLenachan JM, et al. Haemostatic and haemodynamic abnormalities associated with left atrial thrombosis in non-rheumatic atrial fibrillation. Heart 1997;77(5):407–11.

[3] Conway DS, Pearce LA, Chin BS, et al. Prognostic value of plasma von Willebrand factor and soluble P-selectin as indices of endothelial damage and platelet activation in 994 patients with nonvalvular atrial fibrillation. Circulation 2003;107(25):3141–5.

[4] Wolf PA, Abbott RD, Kannel WB. Atrial fibrillation as an independent risk factor for stroke: the Framingham Study. Stroke 1991;22(8):983–8.

[5] Lin HJ, Wolf PA, Kelly-Hayes M, et al. Stroke severity in atrial fibrillation. The Framingham Study. Stroke 1996;27(10):1760–4.

[6] Stafford RS, Singer DE. National patterns of warfarin use in atrial fibrillation. Arch Intern Med 1996;156(22):2537–41.

[7] Waldo AL, Becker RC, Tapson VF, et al. NABOR Steering Committee. Hospitalized patients with atrial fibrillation and a high risk of stroke are not being provided with adequate anticoagulation. J Am Coll Cardiol 2005;46(9):1729–36.

[8] Wyse DG, Waldo AL, DiMarco JP, et al, Atrial Fibrillation Follow-up Investigation of Rhythm Management (AFFIRM) Investigators. A comparison of rate control and rhythm control in patients with atrial fibrillation. N Engl J Med 2002;347(23):1825–33.

[9] Van Gelder IC, Hagens VE, Bosker HA, et al, Rate Control versus Electrical Cardioversion for Persistent Atrial Fibrillation Study Group. A comparison of rate control and rhythm control in patients with recurrent persistent atrial fibrillation. N Engl J Med 2002;347(23): 1834–40.

[10] Shinbane JS, Wood MA, Jensen DN, et al. Tachycardia-induced cardiomyopathy: a review of animal models and clinical studies. J Am Coll Cardiol 1997;29(4):709–15.

[11] Ozcan C, Jahangir A, Friedman PA, et al. Significant effects of atrioventricular node ablation and pacemaker implantation on left ventricular function and long-term survival in patients with atrial fibrillation and left ventricular dysfunction. Am J Cardiol 2003;92(1): 33–7.

[12] Nerheim P, Birger-Botkin S, Piracha L, et al. Heart failure and sudden death in patients with tachycardia-induced cardiomyopathy and recurrent tachycardia. Circulation 2004;110(3): 247–52.

[13] Padanilam BJ, Prystowsky EN. New antiarrhythmic agents for the prevention and treatment of atrial fibrillation. J Cardiovasc Electrophysiol 2006;17:S62–6.

[14] Corley SD, Epstein AE, DiMarco JP, et al, AFFIRM Investigators. Relationships between sinus rhythm, treatment, and survival in the Atrial Fibrillation Follow-Up Investigation of Rhythm Management (AFFIRM) Study. Circulation 2004;109(12):1509–13.

[15] Pappone C, Rosanio S, Augello G, et al. Mortality, morbidity, and quality of life after circumferential pulmonary vein ablation for atrial fibrillation: outcomes from a controlled non-randomized long-term study. J Am Coll Cardiol 2003;42(2):185–97.

[16] Wazni OM, Marrouche NF, Martin DO, et al. Radiofrequency ablation vs antiarrhythmic drugs as first-line treatment of symptomatic atrial fibrillation: a randomized trial. JAMA 2005;293(21):2634–40.

[17] Feinberg WM, Blackshear JL, Laupacis A, et al. Prevalence, age distribution, and gender of patients with atrial fibrillation. Analysis and implications. Arch Intern Med 1995;155(5): 469–73.

[18] Wolf PA, Benjamin EJ, Belanger AJ, et al. Secular trends in the prevalence of atrial fibrillation: the Framingham Study. Am Heart J 1996;131(4):790–5.

[19] Anonymous. Risk factors for stroke and efficacy of antithrombotic therapy in atrial fibrillation. Analysis of pooled data from five randomized controlled trials. Arch Intern Med 1994; 154(13):1449–57.

[20] Gage BF, Waterman AD, Shannon W, et al. Validation of clinical classification schemes for predicting stroke: results from the National Registry of Atrial Fibrillation. JAMA 2001; 285(22):2864–70.

[21] Fuster V, Ryden LE, Cannom DS, et al, American College of Cardiology/American Heart Association Task Force on Practice Guidelines. European Society of Cardiology Committee for Practice Guidelines. European Heart Rhythm Association. Heart Rhythm Society. ACC/AHA/ESC 2006 Guidelines for the Management of Patients with Atrial Fibrillation: a report of the American College of Cardiology/American Heart Association Task Force on Practice Guidelines and the European Society of Cardiology Committee for Practice Guidelines (Writing Committee to Revise the 2001 Guidelines for the Management of Patients With Atrial Fibrillation): developed in collaboration with the European Heart Rhythm Association and the Heart Rhythm Society. Circulation 2006;114(7): e257–354.

[22] Hart RG, Halperin JL. Atrial fibrillation and thromboembolism: a decade of progress in stroke prevention. Ann Intern Med 1999;131(9):688–95.

[23] Singer DE, Albers GW, Dalen JE, et al. Antithrombotic therapy in atrial fibrillation: the Seventh ACCP Conference on Antithrombotic and Thrombolytic Therapy. Chest 2004;126(3 Suppl):429S–56S.

[24] Hylek EM, Go AS, Chang Y, et al. Effect of intensity of oral anticoagulation on stroke severity and mortality in atrial fibrillation. N Engl J Med 2003;349(11):1019–26.

[25] Hart RG, Halperin JL, Pearce LA, et al, Stroke Prevention in Atrial Fibrillation Investigators. Lessons from the stroke prevention in atrial fibrillation trials. Ann Intern Med 2003; 138(10):831–8.

[26] Friberg J, Scharling H, Gadsboll N, et al, Copenhagen City Heart Study. Comparison of the impact of atrial fibrillation on the risk of stroke and cardiovascular death in women versus men (The Copenhagen City Heart Study). Am J Cardiol 2004;94(7):889–94.

[27] Hylek EM, Evans-Molina C, Shea C, et al. Major hemorrhage and tolerability of warfarin in the first year of therapy among elderly patients with atrial fibrillation. Circulation 2007; 115(21):2689–96.

[28] Connolly S, Pogue J, Hart R, et al, ACTIVE Writing Group on behalf of the ACTIVE Investigators. Clopidogrel plus aspirin versus oral anticoagulation for atrial fibrillation in the

Atrial fibrillation Clopidogrel Trial with Irbesartan for prevention of Vascular Events (ACTIVE W): a randomised controlled trial. Lancet 2006;367(9526):1903–12.

[29] Kaul S, Diamond GA, Weintraub WS. Trials and tribulations of non-inferiority: the ximelagatran experience. J Am Coll Cardiol 2005;46(11):1986–95.

[30] Blackshear JL, Johnson WD, Odell JA, et al. Thoracoscopic extracardiac obliteration of the left atrial appendage for stroke risk reduction in atrial fibrillation. J Am Coll Cardiol 2003; 42(7):1249–52.

[31] Ostermayer SH, Reisman M, Kramer PH, et al. Percutaneous left atrial appendage transcatheter occlusion (PLAATO system) to prevent stroke in high-risk patients with non-rheumatic atrial fibrillation: results from the international multi-center feasibility trials. J Am Coll Cardiol 2005;46(1):9–14.

[32] Arnold AZ, Mick MJ, Mazurek RP, et al. Role of prophylactic anticoagulation for direct current cardioversion in patients with atrial fibrillation or atrial flutter. J Am Coll Cardiol 1992;19(4):851–5.

[33] Klein AL, Grimm RA, Murray RD, et al, Assessment of Cardioversion Using Transesophageal Echocardiography Investigators. Use of transesophageal echocardiography to guide cardioversion in patients with atrial fibrillation. N Engl J Med 2001;344(19):1411–20.

[34] Stellbrink C, Nixdorff U, Hofmann T, et al, ACE (Anticoagulation in Cardioversion using Enoxaparin) Study Group. Safety and efficacy of enoxaparin compared with unfractionated heparin and oral anticoagulants for prevention of thromboembolic complications in cardioversion of nonvalvular atrial fibrillation: the Anticoagulation in Cardioversion using Enoxaparin (ACE) trial. Circulation 2004;109(8):997–1003.

[35] Carlsson J, Miketic S, Windeler J, et al, STAF Investigators. Randomized trial of rate-control versus rhythm-control in persistent atrial fibrillation: the Strategies of Treatment of Atrial Fibrillation (STAF) study. J Am Coll Cardiol 2003;41(10):1690–6.

[36] Hohnloser SH, Kuck KH, Lilienthal J. Rhythm or rate control in atrial fibrillation—pharmacological intervention in atrial fibrillation (PIAF): a randomised trial. Lancet 2000; 356(9244):1789–94.

[37] Opolski G, Torbicki A, Kosior DA, et al, Investigators of the Polish How to Treat Chronic Atrial Fibrillation Study. Rate control vs rhythm control in patients with nonvalvular persistent atrial fibrillation: the results of the Polish How to Treat Chronic Atrial Fibrillation (HOT CAFE) Study. Chest 2004;126(2):476–86.

[38] Hsu LF, Jais P, Sanders P, et al. Catheter ablation for atrial fibrillation in congestive heart failure. N Engl J Med 2004;351(23):2373–83.

[39] Gentlesk PJ, Sauer WH, Gerstenfeld EP, et al. Reversal of left ventricular dysfunction following ablation of atrial fibrillation. J Cardiovasc Electrophysiol 2007;18(1):9–14.

[40] Deedwania PC, Singh BN, Ellenbogen K, et al. Spontaneous conversion and maintenance of sinus rhythm by amiodarone in patients with heart failure and atrial fibrillation: observations from the veterans affairs congestive heart failure survival trial of antiarrhythmic therapy (CHF-STAT). The Department of Veterans Affairs CHF-STAT Investigators. Circulation 1998;98(23):2574–9.

[41] Pedersen OD, Bagger H, Keller N, et al. Efficacy of dofetilide in the treatment of atrial fibrillation-flutter in patients with reduced left ventricular function: a Danish investigations of arrhythmia and mortality on dofetilide (diamond) substudy. Circulation 2001;104(3):292–6.

[42] Rationale and design of a study assessing treatment strategies of atrial fibrillation in patients with heart failure: the Atrial Fibrillation and Congestive Heart Failure (AF-CHF) trial. Am Heart J 2002;14:597–607.

[43] Cooper HA, Bloomfield DA, Bush DE, et al, for the AFFIRM Study Investigators. Relation between achieved heart rate and outcomes in patients with atrial fibrillation (from the Atrial Fibrillation Follow-up Investigation of Rhythm Management (AFFIRM) Study). Am J Cardiol 2004;93:1247–53.

[44] Prystowsky EN. Assessment of rhythm and rate control in patients with atrial fibrillation. J Cardiovasc Electrophysiol 2006;17(2):S7–10.

[45] Bjerregaard P, Bailey WB, Robinson SE. Rate control in patients with chronic atrial fibrillation. Am J Cardiol 2004;93(3):329–32.
[46] Meng F, Yoshikawa T, Baba A, et al. Beta-blockers are effective in congestive heart failure patients with atrial fibrillation. J Card Fail 2003;9(5):398–403.
[47] Khand AU, Rankin AC, Martin W, et al. Carvedilol alone or in combination with digoxin for the management of atrial fibrillation in patients with heart failure? J Am Coll Cardiol 2003;42(11):1944–51.
[48] Scardi S, Humar F, Pandullo C, et al. Oral clonidine for heart rate control in chronic atrial fibrillation. Lancet 1993;341(8854):1211–2.
[49] Wood MA, Brown-Mahoney C, Kay GN, et al. Clinical outcomes after ablation and pacing therapy for atrial fibrillation: a meta-analysis. Circulation 2000;101(10):1138–44.
[50] Weerasooriya R, Davis M, Powell A, et al. The Australian intervention randomized control of rate in atrial fibrillation trial (AIRCRAFT). J Am Coll Cardiol 2003;41(10):1697–702.
[51] Wilkoff BL, Cook JR, Epstein AE, et al, Dual Chamber and VVI Implantable Defibrillator Trial Investigators. Dual-chamber pacing or ventricular backup pacing in patients with an implantable defibrillator: the dual chamber and VVI implantable defibrillator (DAVID) trial. JAMA 2002;288(24):3115–23.
[52] Simantirakis EN, Vardakis KE, Kochiadakis GE, et al. Left ventricular mechanics during right ventricular apical or left ventricular-based pacing in patients with chronic atrial fibrillation after atrioventricular junction ablation. J Am Coll Cardiol 2004;43(6):1013–8.
[53] Garrigue S, Bordachar P, Reuter S, et al. Comparison of permanent left ventricular and biventricular pacing in patients with heart failure and chronic atrial fibrillation: prospective haemodynamic study. Heart 2002;87(6):529–34.
[54] Doshi RN, Daoud EG, Fellows C, et al, PAVE Study Group. Left ventricular-based cardiac stimulation post AV nodal ablation evaluation (the PAVE study). J Cardiovasc Electrophysiol 2005;16(11):1160–5.
[55] Preliminary report: effect of encainide and flecainide on mortality in a randomized trial of arrhythmia suppression after myocardial infarction. N Engl J Med 1989;321:406–12.
[56] Lafuente-Lafuente C, Mouly S, Longas-Tejero MA, et al. Antiarrhythmic drugs for maintaining sinus rhythm after cardioversion of atrial fibrillation: a systematic review of randomized controlled trials [review] [63 refs]. Arch Intern Med 2006;166(7):719–28.
[57] Roden DM, Woosley RL, Primm RK. Incidence and clinical features of the quinidine-associated long QT syndrome: implications for patient care. Am Heart J 1986;111(6):1088–93.
[58] Roy D, Talajic M, Dorian P, et al. Amiodarone to prevent recurrence of atrial fibrillation. Canadian Trial of Atrial Fibrillation Investigators. N Engl J Med 2000;342(13):913–20.
[59] Zimetbaum P. Amiodarone for atrial fibrillation. N Engl J Med 2007;356(9):935–41.
[60] Alboni P, Botto GL, Baldi N, et al. Outpatient treatment of recent-onset atrial fibrillation with the "pill-in-the-pocket" approach. N Engl J Med 2004;351(23):2384–91.
[61] Haissaguerre M, Jais P, Shah DC, et al. Spontaneous initiation of atrial fibrillation by ectopic beats originating in the pulmonary veins. N Engl J Med 1998;339(10):659–66.
[62] Haissaguerre M, Jais P, Shah DC, et al. Electrophysiological end point for catheter ablation of atrial fibrillation initiated from multiple pulmonary venous foci. Circulation 2000;101(12):1409–17.
[63] Padanilam BJ, Prystowsky EN. Should ablation be first-line therapy and for whom: The antagonist position. Circulation 2005;112(8):1223–9.
[64] Cox J, Schuessler R, Lappas D. An 8 ½-year clinical experience with surgery for atrial fibrillation. Ann Surg 1996;224(3):267–75.
[65] Hocini M, Sanders P, Deisenhofer I, et al. Reverse remodeling of sinus node function after catheter ablation of atrial fibrillation in patients with prolonged sinus pauses. Circulation 2003;108(10):1172–5.
[66] McKeown PP, Gutterman D. Executive summary: American College of Chest Physicians guidelines for the prevention and management of postoperative atrial fibrillation after cardiac surgery. Chest 2005;128(2 Suppl):1S–5S.

[67] Stamou SC, Hill PC, Dangas G, et al. Stroke after coronary artery bypass: incidence, predictors, and clinical outcome. Stroke 2001;32(7):1508–13.

[68] Taylor GJ, Malik SA, Colliver JA, et al. Usefulness of atrial fibrillation as a predictor of stroke after isolated coronary artery bypass grafting. Am J Cardiol 1987;60(10):905–7.

[69] Crystal E, Connolly SJ, Sleik K, et al. Interventions on prevention of postoperative atrial fibrillation in patients undergoing heart surgery: a meta-analysis. Circulation 2002;106(1): 75–80.

[70] Klein GJ, Bashore TM, Sellers TD, et al. Ventricular fibrillation in the Wolff-Parkinson-White syndrome. N Engl J Med 1979;301(20):1080–5.

ELSEVIER
SAUNDERS

Med Clin N Am 92 (2008) 237–258

THE MEDICAL
CLINICS
OF NORTH AMERICA

Atrial Fibrillation: Unanswered Questions and Future Directions

Vivek Y. Reddy, MD[a,b,*]

[a]Cardiac Arrhythmia Service and Heart Center, Massachusetts General Hospital,
55 Fruit Street, GRB-109, Boston, MA 02114, USA
[b]Harvard Medical School, Boston, MA, USA

Just over a decade ago, Haissaguerre and colleagues [1] provided the seminal demonstration of the role of pulmonary vein (PV) triggers in the pathogenesis of atrial fibrillation (AF) and the potential therapeutic role of catheter ablation to treat patients who have paroxysmal AF. This initial observation ushered in the modern era of catheter ablation to treat patients who have AF, and tremendous progress has been made in understanding its pathogenesis and the catheter approaches to treating this rhythm. Although the current state of AF catheter ablation is well described earlier in this issue, this article reflects on some of the major unanswered questions about AF management, and the future technological and investigational directions being explored in the nonpharmacologic management of AF.

Catheter ablation of paroxysmal atrial fibrillation

After the initial demonstration that the PVs harbor most of the triggers for paroxysmal AF, the approach to catheter ablation in this patient population evolved considerably. The initial approaches centered on inducing and identifying the specific AF triggering sites within the PVs and targeting these for catheter ablation [1,2]. From a safety and efficacy perspective, empiric isolation of all PVs was clearly a much more suitable strategy [3–6].

This work was supported in part by the Deane Institute for Integrative Research in Atrial Fibrillation and Stroke. Dr. Reddy has received grant support or served as a consultant to Biosense-Webster, Inc., CardioFocus, Inc., Cryocath Technologies Inc., GE Medical Systems, Inc., Hansen Medical, Inc., Philips Medical Systems, Inc., ProRhythm, Inc., St. Jude Medical, Inc., and Stereotaxis, Inc.

* Cardiac Arrhythmia Service, Massachusetts General Hospital, 55 Fruit Street, GRB-109, Boston, MA 02114.

E-mail address: vreddy@partners.org

The poor efficacy of ablating AF triggers stems from the difficulty in inducing these initiating foci during any given electrophysiology ablation procedure. Thus, during these early procedures, electrophysiologists would often spend many hours with multiple catheters positioned in various PVs waiting for AF-initiating premature ectopic depolarizations to occur. Beyond this prolonged case duration, these procedures were often followed by clinical recurrences related to additional initiating foci at sites completely unelicited during the index ablation procedure. However, by empirically ablating around the PV ostia to electrically isolate all veins, one could ensure that no PV triggers would affect the left atrium, proper.

Empiric PV isolation also has one very important safety advantage compared with focal ablation of AF triggers. Briefly, ablation deep within the PVs could result in pulmonary vein stenosis, a dreaded complication that has a strong tendency to recur as restenosis after balloon venoplasty. However, if the circumferential isolating ablation lesion set is placed outside the PVs, the risk for stenosis can be minimized.

Based on the improved efficacy and safety of empiric PV isolation, several approaches have been forwarded to achieve this electrophysiologic end point. These approaches include using contrast angiography to identify and target the PV ostia, targeting the ostia using electroanatomic mapping systems to localize the catheter tip (with or without the incorporation of preacquired three-dimensional CT or MR images), and using intracardiac echocardiography to position a circular mapping catheter at the PV ostia and target the electrograms for ablation. Regardless of the approach used during the index procedure, the mechanism of arrhythmia recurrence is virtually always caused by electrical PV reconnection [7]. That is, point-to-point ablation lesions are placed to completely encircle the PVs during the initial ablation procedure. However, because the ablation lesions cannot be directly visualized, a surrogate marker for lesion integrity is used: the lack of electrical conduction across the ablation lesions at the end of the procedure. However, if the tissue at one of these sites is damaged but not fully necrotic from the ablation, PV to left atrial conduction can recur several weeks later after tissue healing is complete, leading to clinical AF recurrences. The difference in clinical outcome after ablation of paroxysmal AF is very likely related directly to the ability of the operator to manipulate and stably position the ablation catheter with the requisite force to generate effective ablation lesions.

Thus, the most important goal during catheter ablation of paroxysmal AF is to achieve *permanent* PV isolation. To improve the technical feasibility of the procedure and thereby improve the continuity of the isolating ablation lesion sets, extensive effort has been made to improve the ablation technology. These various technologic advances can be broadly separated into two groups: (1) remote navigation technology to provide for precise navigation with the hope that this translates to improved lesion contiguity, and (2) balloon ablation catheter technology using various ablation energy sources designed to isolate the PVs in a facile manner.

Remote navigation technology

Currently two remote navigation systems are available for clinical use: (1) a magnetic navigation system (the Niobe II system, manufactured by Stereotaxis, Inc.) and (2) a robotic navigation system (the Sensei system, manufactured by Hansen Medical, Inc.).

Remote magnetic navigation

The magnetic navigation system (Fig. 1) uses two large external magnets positioned on either side of the fluoroscopy table to generate a uniform magnetic field (0.08 Tesla) of approximately 15 cm diameter within the patient's chest [8]. Specialized ablation catheters are used with this system; briefly, these catheters are extremely floppy along their distal end, and have magnets embedded at the tip of the catheter. Thus, when placed within the patient's heart, the catheter tip will align with the orientation of the generated magnetic field. The operator uses a software interface to manipulate the magnetic field, and by extension, the tip of the ablation catheter. This ability to manipulate the magnetic field provides the first level of freedom of movement with this system. The other level of freedom of movement is the ability to remotely advance or retract the catheter tip. This function is possible using a computer-controlled catheter advancer system consisting of a disposable plastic unit positioned at the femoral catheter insertion site. The catheter shaft is affixed to this unit where it enters the sheath, and can transduce the remote operator instructions to advance or retract the catheter appropriately. This combination of remote catheter advancement/retraction and

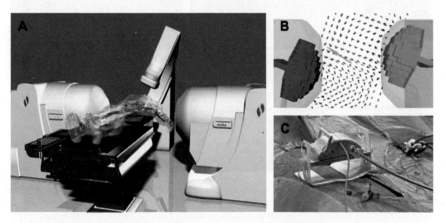

Fig. 1. The magnetic navigation system uses two large magnets positioned on either side of the fluoroscopy table (*A*). These magnets can generate a uniform magnetic field in virtually any direction (*B*) so that magnetically enabled catheters will orient in the same direction as the field. A disposable catheter advancement system (*C*) is positioned at the femoral puncture site to remotely advance or retract the catheter. (*Courtesy of* Stereotaxis, St. Louis, Missouri; with permission.)

magnetic field manipulation allows the operator a great deal of flexibility in intracardiac catheter manipulation.

This magnetic navigation system is now integrated with one of the electroanatomic mapping system (CARTO RMT, Biosense Webster, Inc). The mapping system can precisely localize the catheter tip in space to a sub-millimeter resolution (Fig. 2A). Through precisely tracking the catheter location, this combination of mapping and navigation systems allows for a novel capability: automated chamber mapping. Briefly, the operator remotely manipulates the catheter within the left atrium to a few defined anatomic locations (eg, the ostia of the various PVs, the mitral valve annulus) and, based on these parameters, the system automatically manipulates the catheter throughout the chamber to facilitate the creation of an electroanatomic map. Future iterations of the software are planned to allow the system to automatically manipulate the catheter tip to create linear ablation lesions with the chamber as per the operator's wishes. However, the efficiency and accuracy of these automatic software solutions remain to be determined. The other significant advance is the ability to incorporate preacquired three-dimensional MRI or CT images into the system to allow mapping on a realistic model of the heart.

With the current generation software, some clinical data are available on its efficacy for AF ablation. In a consecutive series of 40 patients, Pappone and colleagues [9] used the mapping and navigation systems in tandem to

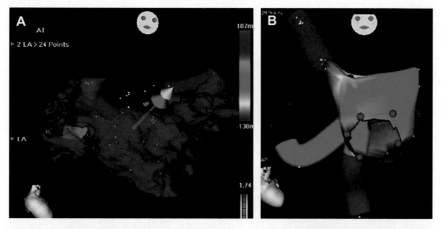

Fig. 2. (*A*) The magnetic navigation system is integrated with an electroanatomic mapping system that also permits integration of three-dimensional CT or MRI models. Once integrated, the magnetic field can be directly controlled with the computer mouse to the desired direction. The yellow arrow represents the current direction of magnetic field and the green arrow represents the desired direction of the field. Note that the catheter is oriented in the same direction as the field. (*B*) Magnetically enabled irrigated ablation catheters are not currently available for clinical use. However, as shown in this anterior view of the left atrial anatomic map, this catheter has been used in experimental protocols to show the ability to map the porcine left atrium and pulmonary veins.

determine the feasibility of circumferential PV ablation in patients undergoing catheter ablation of AF. Using a 4-mm–tip ablation catheter (with the requisite embedded magnets), they showed that the left atrium and PVs could be successfully mapped in 38 of 40 patients. Ablation lesions were placed in a circumferential fashion for a maximum of 15 seconds at any endocardial ablation site. They reported that procedure times decreased significantly with increased operator experience. Although this study clearly showed the feasibility of remote mapping of the left atrium and PVs, the procedural end point was not electrical PV isolation in the standard electrophysiologic sense. Instead, the end point was ">90% reduction in the bipolar electrogram amplitude, and/or peak-to-peak bipolar electrogram amplitude <0.1 mV inside the line" [9]. The significance of this end point is unclear.

To address some of these uncertainties, DiBiase and colleagues [10] examined the efficacy of PV isolation using this remote navigation system in a series of 45 patients using a stepwise approach. First, the ability to remotely map the chamber was again confirmed in this study. Second, these investigators performed circumferential ablation using the same 4-mm–tip radiofrequency ablation catheter as described in the initial paper by Pappone and colleagues. However, when a circular mapping catheter was deployed into the PVs to more precisely assess for vein isolation, no veins in any patient were shown to be electrically isolated. The operators then used the circular mapping catheter to remotely guide the ablation catheter to isolate the vein antra, but electrical disconnection was attained in only four veins in four different patients (8%). In the remaining 41 patients (92%), no evidence was found of disconnection in any of the veins. However, when the operators then targeted a portion of the veins using a standard manual radiofrequency ablation catheter (ie, not using the remote navigation system), they were able to achieve electrical isolation in all attempted veins.

Despite the sharply improved procedural outcome with manual catheter manipulation, concluding that PV isolation is not possible using the magnetic navigation system is inappropriate. Unlike with remote navigation, manual ablation in this study was performed using an irrigated radiofrequency ablation catheter. Unlike with standard radiofrequency ablation, irrigated ablation allows the operator to safely deliver more energy into the tissue, thereby achieving deeper ablation lesions. Significant charring on the ablation catheter tip was seen in 15 of 45 procedures (33%) when using the standard remote 4-mm–tip ablation catheter. The critical information that remains to be determined is whether remote PV isolation can be reproducibly achieved using an irrigated ablation catheter. An irrigated ablation catheter with the requisite embedded magnets to permit remote navigation exists but, at the time of this writing, has not been used clinically. However, in the experimental animal setting, the author has shown that this catheter can be remotely manipulated to map all chambers of the porcine heart (Fig. 2B), and can deliver ablation lesions of similar quality to those seen using a manual irrigated ablation catheter (Vivek Y. Reddy, unpublished data, 2006). How this finding translates during clinical use of this remote irrigated catheter will not be known until late 2007.

Remote robotic navigation

The remote navigation capability of the robotic system (Sensei, Hansen Medical, Inc.) is based on multiple pullwires that control the deflection capability of two steerable sheaths [11,12]. Briefly, this is a "master–slave" electromechanical system that controls an internal steerable guide sheath and an external steerable sheath (Fig. 3). The internal sheath contains 4 pullwires located at each quadrant; the range of motion includes deflection in 360° and the ability to insert/withdraw. The external sheath has a single pullwire to permit deflection, and can rotate and insert/withdraw. This combination of movements allows for a broad range of motion in virtually any direction. Unlike the magnetic navigation system, most standard ablation catheters can be used with this system, because the inner steerable sheath can accommodate any catheter up to 8.3-French diameter. By fixing the mapping/ablation catheter so that it is just protruding beyond the tip of the inner system, remotely driving these steerable sheaths translates to remote navigation of the catheter tip. The steerable sheaths are attached to the remote robotic arm unit, which can be mounted to any standard

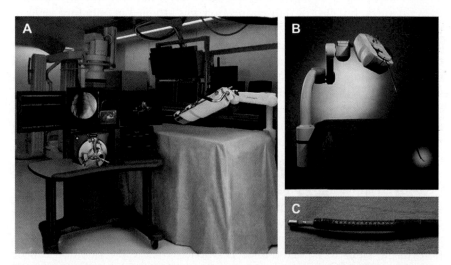

Fig. 3. The primary components of the robotic navigation system are shown (*A*), including the workstation and the robotic arm (*B*), which can be mounted at the foot of any standard fluoroscopy table. The two-piece sheath system extends from this robotic arm and is inserted through the femoral venous puncture site. Any standard ablation catheter can be manipulated within the heart by simply placing the catheter within the sheath system so that the tip of the catheter is protruding just beyond the tip of the inner sheath (*C*). (*Courtesy of* Hansen Medical, Inc., Mountain View, California; with permission.)

radiography procedure table. Using a software interface, a three-dimensional joystick allows the operator to remotely drive the catheter tip. Movements of the joystick are translated into a complex series of manipulations by the pullwires governing sheath motion.

The author examined the feasibility of synchronizing this robotic navigation system with electroanatomic mapping and three-dimensional CT imaging to perform view-synchronized left atrial ablation (Fig. 4) [13]. The mapping catheter was remotely manipulated with the robotic navigation system within the registered three-dimensional CT image of the left atrial PVs. The initial porcine experimental phase (N = 9) validated the ability of view-synchronized robotic navigation to guide atrial mapping and ablation. An irrigated radiofrequency ablation catheter was able to be remotely navigate into all of the PVs, the left atrial appendage, and circumferentially along the mitral valve annulus. In addition, circumferential radiofrequency ablation lesions were applied periosteally to ablate 11 porcine PVs. The consequent clinical phase (N = 9 patients who had AF) established that this paradigm could be successfully applied for all of the major aspects of catheter ablation of paroxysmal or chronic AF: electrical PV isolation in an extraostial fashion, isolation of the superior vena cava, and linear atrial ablation of typical and atypical atrial flutters. The electrophysiological end point of electrical PV isolation, as verified using a circular mapping catheter, was achieved in all patients. This study showed the safety and feasibility of

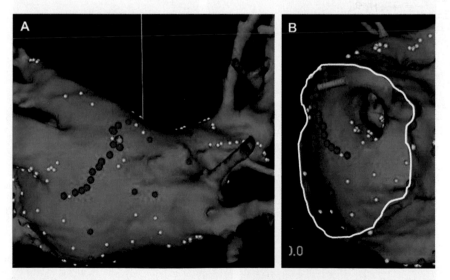

Fig. 4. View-synchronized robotic ablation was performed to treat atrial fibrillation. In this paradigm, the mapping system provided the location of the catheter tip, the CT scan identified where the catheter should be positioned, and the robotic navigation system was used to manipulate the catheter to each location. Shown are an external posterior view (A) and a left-sided endoluminal view showing the left PVs (B).

an emerging paradigm for AF ablation involving the confluence of three technologies: three-dimensional imaging, electroanatomic mapping, and remote navigation. However, this study involved a minimal number of patients treated by a single center. The long-term safety and efficacy of PV isolation performed by multiple operators in a larger patient cohort using this robotic navigation system remains to be established.

Image guidance

Three-dimensional imaging is playing an increasingly important role in guiding ablation procedures. It is now standard to integrate patient-specific preacquired three-dimensional models of the left atrium and PVs (generated using either contrast-enhanced CT or MRI) with mapping systems to better guide the ablation procedure (Fig. 5) [14–19]. However, this approach is somewhat limited by the variable chamber geometry and size that can occur as a result of various physiologic factors, such as heart rate, rhythm, and volume state. Accordingly, a significant amount of effort is being devoted

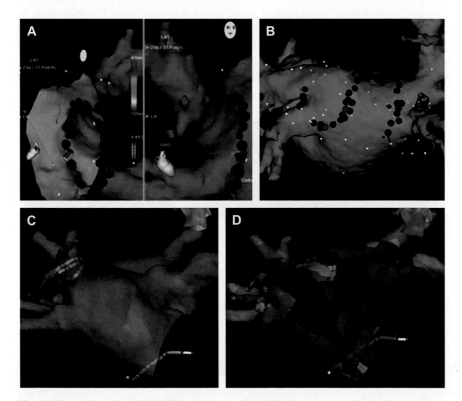

Fig. 5. Three-dimensional CT/MR image integration with electroanatomic mapping systems is now a standard procedure. Once the three-dimensional image is integrated, the ablation catheter can be manipulated to encircle the PVs with ablation lesions. Shown is integration with either the CARTO RMT (*A*, *B*) or NavX (*C*, *D*) systems.

to real-time or near–real-time imaging of the three-dimensional chamber anatomy during the ablation procedure. The modalities being explored include ultrasound imaging, three-dimensional rotational angiography, and MRI. Although three-dimensional surface transducers are already available for ultrasound imaging, obtaining accurate images of the left atrium and pulmonary veins through surface thoracic imaging can be difficult. Three-dimensional intracardiac ultrasound (ICE) imaging probes do not currently exist; however, localized three-dimensional ICE probes exist and can be used to generate three-dimensional images. Briefly, this consists of an ICE catheter with a localization sensor that precisely provides the location and direction of the catheter. Accordingly, a series of high-resolution two-dimensional images can be "stitched" together to generate a near–real-time three-dimensional image.

Rotational angiography consists of the injection of contrast followed by rotation of the x-ray fluoroscopy head around the patient to generate a three-dimensional image [20,21]. For example, the contrast can be injected directly into the pulmonary artery, and imaging can be performed during the levo-phase after the contrast traverses the pulmonary vascular bed and flows back through the PVs into the left atrium. As shown in Fig. 6, a volumetric three-dimensional image of the left atrium and PVs can be generated through properly timing the rotation of the x-ray fluoroscopy unit. The quality of these three-dimensional rotational angiography images was compared with the gold-standard, preacquired, three-dimensional CT or MR images in a consecutive series of 42 patients undergoing AF ablation procedures [21]. In this series, most of the three-dimensional rotational angiography acquisitions (71%) were qualitatively sufficient in delineating the left atrial and PV anatomy. A blinded quantitative comparison of PV ostial diameters resulted in an absolute difference of only 2.7 ± 2.3 mm, 2.2 ± 1.8 mm, 2.4 ± 2.2 mm, and 2.2 ± 2.3 mm for the left-superior, left-inferior, right-superior, and right-inferior PVs, respectively. In addition, the feasibility for registering the three-dimensional rotational angiography image with real-time electroanatomic mapping was also shown. More recent reconstruction algorithms that can resolve soft-tissue structures are likely to further increase the capability of three-dimensional rotational angiography through improving the image quality of data obtained with the current strategy (of intracardiac contrast injection) and potentially allowing for CT-like imaging of the left atrium and PVs using a peripheral intravenous injection of contrast.

Real-time interventional MRI involves the concept of performing the entire procedure in the MRI environment [22]. In this paradigm, various MRI-compatible catheters would be continuously imaged as they are positioned within the patient anatomy. MRI has the advantage of using nonionizing radiation, the ability to resolve soft-tissue with high resolution, and the potential for physiologic imaging; for example, during liver tumor ablation, MRI-based thermal imaging has been used to directly image

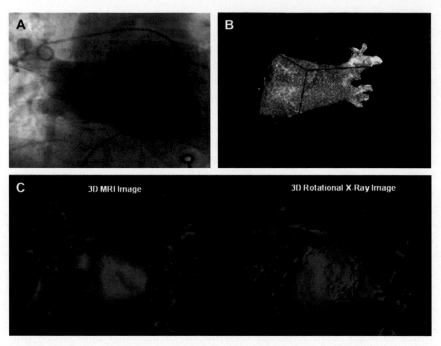

Fig. 6. Rotational angiography imaging can be used to generate volumetric images of the left atrium and PVs. Contrast is injected from a pigtail catheter positioned in the pulmonary artery, and rotational imaging is performed during the levo phase as the contrast courses back into the left atrium from the PVs (*A*) to generate a volumetric image of this anatomy (*B*). These intra-procedural rotational images are of comparable quality to preacquired three-dimensional MRI or CT images (*C*).

ablation lesion formation. Although this modality is in some respects the most powerful, it is also the one furthest away from clinical practice. A significant amount of research and development is required in the MR scanning equipment/protocols and MRI-compatible equipment (eg, catheters, patient monitoring equipment). Each of these three-dimensional imaging modalities will likely show a tremendous amount of progress.

Balloon ablation catheters

A significant effort has been put into developing balloon ablation catheter designs to quickly, easily, and effectively isolate the PVs. The first device tested clinically was an ultrasound balloon ablation catheter that delivered energy in a radial fashion at the level of the diameter of the balloon, hence necessitating that the balloon catheter be placed within the PV when delivering energy [23]. This balloon design was suboptimal because the level of electrical isolation typically excluded the proximal portions of the vein, and therefore pulmonary vein triggers of AF located at this region would not be included in the ablation lesion [24]. From a safety perspective, the intravenous location of the energy delivery resulted in PV stenosis. Since this first-generation device, balloon ablation catheters have evolved considerably. Four major balloon-based ablation devices are now used at various stages of clinical evaluation: (1) cryoballoon ablation, (2) endoscopic laser ablation, (3) high-intensity focused ultrasound (HIFU), and (4) balloon-based radiofrequency ablation (Fig. 7). Each of these devices was fashioned to be placed at the pulmonary vein ostia to theoretically isolate the veins outside their tubular portion.

Balloon cryoablation

The cryoballoon system is a deflectable catheter (manufactured by Cryocath Technologies Inc.) with a balloon-within-a-balloon design wherein the cryo refrigerant (N_2O) is delivered within the inner balloon. A constant vacuum is applied between the inner and outer balloons to ensure the absence of refrigerant leakage into the systemic circulation in the event of a breach in the integrity of the inner balloon. The cryoballoon catheter is manufactured in two sizes: 23 mm and 28 mm in diameter. After transseptal puncture, the deflated balloon catheter is deployed through a 12-French deflectable sheath. Once within the left atrium, the inflated balloon is positioned at each respective PV ostium to temporarily occlude blood flow from the targeted vein. Each balloon-based cryoablation lesion lasts 4 minutes. Because the cyrorefrigerant is delivered to the whole face of the balloon, any tissue in contact with the balloon is ablated. This function can be safely performed because the experimental results have shown that cryothermal ablation is associated with a minimal risk of PV stenosis [25,26]. Similarly, no evidence of stenosis has been seen in the clinical experience, perhaps because at the temperatures achieved with this system, the cryoablative energy is selective towards the cellular elements of the tissue and leaves the connective tissue matrix intact. Accordingly, cryothermy as an energy

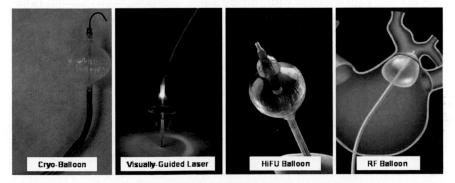

Fig. 7. Four major balloon ablation catheter technologies are currently in clinical trials to assess their safety and efficacy in treating patients who have paroxysmal AF.

source seems to have a good safety profile. However, the long-term efficacy of achieving permanent PV isolation has not been established.

Balloon-based visually guided laser ablation

The most unique aspect of this system is the capability for endoscopic visualization using a 2-French endoscope positioned at a proximal location in the balloon. This 12-French laser ablation catheter system (manufactured by CardioFocus, Inc.) is delivered using a deflectable sheath. Once in the left atrium, a 20-mm–, 25-mm– or 30-mm–diameter balloon is inflated and positioned at the PV ostia. The endoscope allows the operator to visualize the internal face of the balloon and identify areas of balloon–tissue contact (blanched white) versus blood (red) [27]. An optical fiber that projects a 90° to 150° arc is advanced and rotated to the desired location for energy delivery. Once the proper location is identified, a diode laser is used to deliver laser energy at 980 nm to electrically isolate the pulmonary vein. This endoscopic laser balloon catheter provides greater flexibility to the location of energy deposition and the total amount of energy applied to each site. For example, a greater amount/duration of energy may be applied anteriorly along the ridge between the left-sided PVs and left atrial appendage than that applied along the thinner posterior wall near the course of the esophagus.

Balloon-based high-intensity focused ultrasound ablation

The HIFU catheter (manufactured by ProRhythm, Inc.) is a 14-French system that, once inflated, consists of a fluid-filled balloon in front of a smaller carbon dioxide–filled balloon [28]. The ultrasound transducer delivers energy in a radially directed fashion; this energy reflects off the air–fluid interface to project forward and deposit and concentrate just beyond the face of the balloon. Because of the minimal chance of clot formation when sonicating through blood, contact with the atrial tissue is not necessary for ablation with this catheter. This deflectable catheter is delivered using a non-deflectable 14-French sheath. Lesions are delivered using either a 20-mm– or 25-mm–diameter balloon catheter for 40 to 60 seconds per lesion. To use this technology to ablate the PVs, a series of partially encircling ablation lesions sometimes must be stitched together as the balloon is precessed about the orifice of each vein.

Balloon-based radiofrequency ablation

This elastic balloon ablation catheter (Toray Industries, Inc.) is made of a heat-resistant, antithrombotic resin. Inside the fluid-filled balloon are a coil electrode for the delivery of radiofrequency energy and a thermocouple to monitor the electrode temperature [29]. The radiofrequency generator delivers a high-frequency current (13.56 MHz) to induce capacitive-type heating of the tissue in contact with the balloon. The energy output is modulated to maintain the temperature in the balloon at 60° to 75°C. During each application of energy, the venous blood is continuously suctioned through the central lumen of the catheter to protect the PV blood from excessive heating, thus preventing thrombus formation beyond the face of the balloon.

Clinical overview of balloon-based pulmonary vein isolation

Analysis of three-dimensional left atrial–PV surface reconstructions from MRI datasets on patients who had paroxysmal AF showed a marked intra- and interpatient variability in pulmonary vein ostial size and geometry [30]. The challenge to each of the balloon ablation catheters is to negotiate this venous anatomy so that the lesions are proximal enough to include all of the potentially arrhythmogenic periostial tissue and minimize the risk for PV stenosis. The energy source used also has important implications on the ablation strategy. For example, cryothermal ablation is believed to portend minimal risk for PV stenosis. Therefore, a balloon cryoablation catheter may be used safely even deep within large common PVs (ie, within the common truck to separately isolate the individual superior and inferior PVs). However, the adjustable lasing element of the endoscopic balloon catheter allows the operator to vary the circumference and location of the ablative beam. This catheter design may be considerably useful in patients who have veins with marked variability in size and shape. Alternatively, because HIFU energy can be delivered through blood with minimal risk, this energy modality might be efficacious in isolating large PV ostial or antral regions through delivering a series of sequential lesions as it is precessed about the long axis of the targeted vein.

Although the clinical experience is still very early, the results from nonrandomized feasibility studies suggest that most patients who have paroxysmal AF can be treated successfully with these balloon devices. Several balloon ablation catheters have received regulatory approval for clinical use in Europe, but none have been approved for general clinical use in the United States. Most of these devices are being studied in a randomized fashion versus antiarrhythmic medications in the United States. These investigations should determine conclusively whether all or any of these catheters will be able to provide facile, safe, and reproducibly effective PV isolation.

Catheter ablation of nonparoxysmal atrial fibrillation

Unlike catheter ablation of paroxysmal AF, considerably less consensus exists as to the proper approach to catheter ablation of chronic AF. There is a growing understanding is that as the pathophysiology of AF progresses from the paroxysmal to the persistent and eventual permanent state, significant electrophysiological and structural changes occur. These changes in ion channel physiology and increased extracellular fibrosis are believed to potentiate atrial myocardial substrate-driven reentry. Thus, when progressing on the continuum from paroxysmal to permanent AF, the pathophysiologic importance of focal triggers diminishes and the importance of substrate-driven reentry increases. Furthermore, because the latter perpetuating sources of AF are typically located outside the PVs in the atrial tissue itself, the efficacy of PV isolation alone is believed to decline in nonparoxysmal AF. However, this hypothesis has never been addressed conclusively because of the clinical difficulty in achieving permanent PV isolation. That is, because permanent vein isolation is difficult to reproducibly achieve, whether the cause of clinical arrhythmia recurrence is resumption of PV conduction or from the extravenous perpetuators of AF cannot be determined. If one or more of the balloon ablation catheters can consistently achieve permanent PV isolation, this cause can be determined. However, because of the limitations of current technology, a PV isolation–alone strategy is ineffective in many patients who have nonparoxysmal AF.

Intraoperative mapping studies of AF suggested the role of perpetuators of AF. These studies showed that complex fractionated atrial electrograms (CFAEs) were observed mostly in areas of slow conduction or at pivot points where the wavelets turn around at the end of the arcs of functional blocks (Fig. 8) [31]. These areas of fractionated electrograms during AF represent either continuous reentry of the fibrillation waves into the same area, or overlap of different wavelets entering the same area at different times. This complex electrical activity was characterized by a short cycle length and heterogeneous temporal and spatial distribution in humans. This observation led Nademanee and colleagues [32] to hypothesize that, if the areas of CFAEs could be identified through catheter mapping during AF, locating the areas where the wavelets reenter would be possible. They showed that they could terminate AF in 95% of patients, and reported that most patients were free of arrhythmia symptoms after these CFAE sites were ablated. These investigators concluded from this experience that CFAE sites represent the electrophysiologic substrate for AF and can be effectively targeted for ablation to achieve normal sinus rhythm.

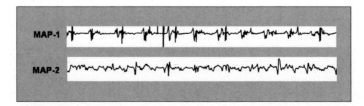

Fig. 8. Shown are two electrograms during AF. MAP-1 is a site with the usual degree of complexity (likely a passive site that would not be targeted or ablation), whereas MAP-2 is a site of complex fractionated activity (this site would be targeted for ablation). Note the continuous nature of electrogram activity in the latter.

Despite these encouraging clinical results, one of the difficulties other investigators have encountered in attempting to reproduce these results is the relative subjectivity inherent in defining whether a particular electrogram is complex enough to warrant ablation. In an effort to standardize the definition of a CFAE site, signal processing software to analyze atrial electrograms during AF is being developed. Several mapping systems now contain signal processing software to quantify the degree of electrogram complexity. However, further clinical work is necessary to determine whether catheter ablation of the sites identified by these software algorithms can truly convert AF into sinus rhythm.

Given the current clinical data, catheter ablation of chronic AF has evolved into an approach that incorporates strategies to address the AF triggers and perpetuators; that is, electrical isolation of the PVs to isolate the former, and ablation within the atria to eliminate the latter. Specifically, this stepwise approach initially involves electrical PV isolation and then targeting of CFAE sites within the left atrium, particularly the interatrial septum; the base of the left atrial appendage; and the inferior left atrium along the coronary sinus [33]. During this progressive ablation strategy, the rhythm often converts from AF to organized macro- or microreentrant atrial tachycardias (ATs). These organized ATs are then targeted for ablation to terminate the rhythm to sinus. Although feasible, this approach is limited by the long procedural duration and the extremely high rate of AT recurrence mandating second, and even third, ablation procedures [34].

Further technical and scientific advances are required to refine the ablation approach to overcome these limitations. One promising approach to these reentrant ATs is to use multielectrode mapping catheters in conjunction with advanced mapping systems to rapidly map these complex tachycardias (Fig. 9). In conclusion, although many questions are unanswered regarding ablation of nonparoxysmal AF, many patients at this end of the disease spectrum clearly require a more extensive procedure that is still being defined.

The safety of atrial fibrillation ablation

When performed by experienced operators, catheter ablation of AF is not a very high-risk procedure. However, as with all procedures, several potential complications are associated with ablation. Accordingly, improving the safety of the procedure has been and continues to be an important area of investigation. Several complications are associated with AF ablation, but the most important are PV stenosis, thromboembolism/stroke, perforation with cardiac tamponade, phrenic nerve injury, and atrioesophageal fistula.

It is now well established that if too much radiofrequency energy is applied within a PV, stenosis can occur [35,36]. Although this complication was common early in the ablation experience, symptomatic PV stenosis is now uncommon, with a frequency of approximately 1%. This decreased

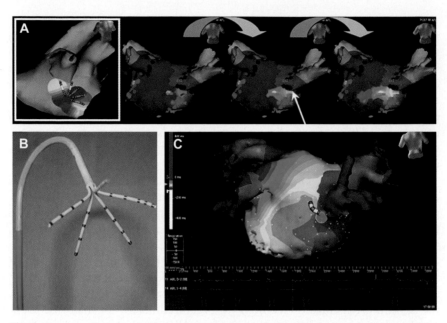

Fig. 9. One paradigm for rapid mapping of an atypical atrial flutter seen during an ablation procedure for nonparoxysmal AF (*A*). After isolating the PVs and placing additional lesions at sites of CFAEs, the rhythm had organized to the atypical flutter. Using a penta-array catheter (*B*) in conjunction with an electroanatomic mapping system (NavX), the atrium was rapidly mapped. Activation mapping showed an area of percolation of activity (*A, white arrow*) between the previously placed ablation lesions isolating the RIPV and the inferior left atrium region below the right inferior pulmonary vein. Entrainment of the flutter from this site showed a post-pacing interval–tachycardia cycle length. As shown on the activation map projected onto a three-dimensional CT image, an ablation lesion placed at this location terminated and eliminated the flutter (*C*).

incidence is partly a result of the more careful use of various imaging modalities (eg, intracardiac ultrasound, three-dimensional CT/MRI) to prevent inadvertent ablation deep within a PV (Fig. 10). Future developments include continued refinements in real-time imaging, such as three-dimensional ultrasound imaging or direct visual guidance (eg, endoscopic visualization using the laser balloon catheter), and the use of alternative energy modalities such as cryothermal energy that seem to have minimal risk for PV stenosis [37].

During radiofrequency energy delivery, the temperature of the catheter tip increases when in contact with the tissue being ablated. However, when this temperature exceeds approximately 50°C, coagulum can accumulate and embolize to cause a stroke. The simple solution has been to irrigate the tip of the ablation catheter with saline to prevent overheating. Future approaches include the use of other ablation technologies that either work by generating more volumetric heating (eg, focused ultrasound, laser energy) or have an inherently low thrombogenic potential (eg, cryothermal energy).

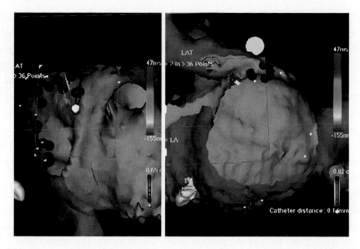

Fig. 10. Using a properly registered CT image, the ablation catheter is precisely positioned at the ridge, separating the left PVs and left atrial appendage. In avoiding placing the catheter deep inside the PV, the risk for PV stenosis can be minimized. An endoluminal image of the left PVs (*left*) and a posterior view with the posterior atrial wall clipped away to show the relative incursion of the ablation catheter into the PV (*right*).

When too much radiofrequency energy is delivered into the tissue, steam formation can rapidly occur, culminating in a "pop." Although some of these pops are clinically insignificant, others can result in cardiac perforation and pericardial effusion with tamponade physiology. However, the amount of power that qualifies as too much varies significantly according to the catheter tip–tissue contact force. That is, mild contact may require 35 Watts of energy to generate an adequate lesion, but forceful contact with the tissue may require only 15 Watts, with 35 Watts causing a pop. Thus, one of the important areas of active investigation is the development of a force-sensing mechanism on the catheter tip to optimize energy delivery.

The right phrenic nerve is typically located just lateral to the superior vena cava in proximity to the right superior PV but several centimeters distal to the vein ostium. Therefore, phrenic nerve injury can occur if radiofrequency energy is delivered at this location [38]. From a practical perspective, this complication is now uncommon during radiofrequency ablation, because ablation is now typically delivered at the vein ostium and not within the vein. However, because of the typical funnel-shaped morphology of the right superior PV, balloon ablation catheters tend to lodge further inside the vein. Accordingly, phrenic nerve injury has been a more common issue associated with these devices. One of the important goals in the further development of these balloon catheters is to either minimize the impact of this complication or avoid this complication altogether.

Although certainly one of the most infrequent complications associated with AF ablation (estimated at less than 1:10,000), atrioesophageal fistula formation remains the most feared because of its high mortality. This complication occurs from inadvertent damage to the esophagus as ablation energy is applied to the posterior left atrium [39–41]. Although the exact pathophysiology of atrioesophageal fistula formation is unknown, the outcome is dismal [42]. Recent experience suggests that early recognition and treatment may prevent a fatal outcome. With an esophageal ulcer, mild interventions may be required, such as treatment with proton pump inhibiting medications and not giving patients anything by mouth. However, esophageal stent placement has been used successfully in a patient who had a transmural esophageal ulcer, without a frank fistula to the atrium [43]. Furthermore, with prompt recognition that an atrioesophageal fistula has already formed, cardiac surgery can correct the defect.

Although the best strategy is prevention, further work is needed to best define the most appropriate means to avoid esophageal injury. The strategies that are currently being used include minimizing the overall amount of energy delivered to the posterior wall, visualizing the real-time position of the esophagus during catheter ablation with either intracardiac ultrasound or fluoroscopy, and esophageal temperature monitoring to help titrate the magnitude and duration of energy delivery. Two other concepts being explored are the use of a cooling balloon catheter placed inside the esophagus to counteract the thermal effect of the ablation energy, and deflecting an endoscope positioned within the esophagus to deviate it away from the ablation catheter [44,45]. Further work is required to fully determine the usefulness of these various maneuvers. This investigation is particularly important as the ablation energy sources become progressively more powerful (eg, balloon ablation catheters).

Stroke prophylaxis in patients who have atrial fibrillation

Little doubt exists that Warfarin treatment should be instituted in patients who have AF and additional risk factors (eg, advanced age, hypertension, congestive heart failure, diabetes, prior personal history of thromboembolism). However, less well-understood is whether successful catheter ablation can substantially and favorably modify this risk to obviate the need for oral anticoagulation treatment. Some data suggest that catheter ablation can favorably modify the risk to a level safe without Warfarin [46]. However, one very important observation from the AFFIRM study was that patients who were believed to be treated successfully with antiarrhythmic medications still developed strokes as a result of asymptomatic AF [47]. Thus, although catheter ablation can treat symptoms of AF, further studies are required to fully assess the effect of ablation on the long-term risk for thromboembolism and stroke.

Several other oral anticoagulant medications are being investigated as alternatives to Warfarin (see the article by Waldo, found elsewhere in this issue), but none has gained clinical approval. However, one nonpharmacologic approach is currently being investigated as an alternative to

Warfarin: the Watchman device. This device consists of a nitinol spline and is covered by a 120-μm pore filter made of polytetrafluoroethylene. When delivered through a long transseptal sheath, it can be placed at the ostium of the left atrial appendage to cause permanent occlusion (Fig. 11). After undergoing significant evolution in a preliminary safety study, the device is now being studied in the pivotal phase in the United States [48]. In this U.S. Food and Drug Administration study, patients who have AF and at least one other risk factor for stroke are randomized to treatment with either the Watchman device or continued usual therapy (Warfarin), with stroke as the primary end point [49]. This noninferiority study is designed to determine whether the Watchman device can replace Warfarin for treating patients who have AF. In addition to assessing the safety of the Watchman device, this study will directly assess the true import of the left atrial appendage in the pathogenesis of stroke in patients who have AF. If positive, the Watchman device may be relevant in managing patients who have asymptomatic AF who do not want to take Warfarin and those who undergo catheter ablation (as concomitant therapy).

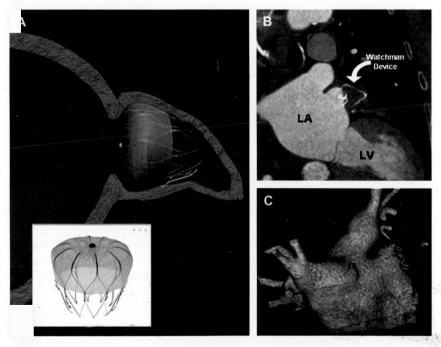

Fig. 11. The Watchman device (*A, inset*) is designed to occlude the left atrial appendage at its ostium. In a patient treated with this device, two-dimensional (*B*) and three-dimensional (*C*) CT images of the left atrium were obtained 1 year after implantation. Note the location of the Watchman device and the absence of contrast in the left atrial appendage, indicating its successful exclusion from the systemic circulation. (Part A *courtesy of* Atritech, Inc., Plymouth, Minnesota; with permission.)

Summary

Considerable progress has been made in understanding the pathogenesis of and approaches to the treatment of AF. However, more unanswered questions than answered questions remain, including: What is the best approach to achieve permanent PV isolation? Which patients who have nonparoxysmal AF can be treated with PV isolation alone? What is the proper follow-up for patients who have undergone AF ablation? How much ablation should be performed during catheter-based substrate modification of nonparoxysmal AF? Which energy sources are the best for achieving long-term safety while maintaining an acceptable level of efficacy? What are the precise electrogram characteristics during AF that best identify an active source of AF as opposed to irrelevant areas of passive activation? In which patients can Warfarin treatment be stopped after catheter ablation? Further studies are required to answer these questions.

References

[1] Haissaguerre M, Jais P, Shah DC, et al. Spontaneous initiation of atrial fibrillation by ectopic beats originating in the pulmonary veins. N Engl J Med 1998;339:659–66.
[2] Chen SA, Hsie MH, Tai CT, et al. Initiation of atrial fibrillation by ectopic beats originating from the pulmonary veins: electrophysiological characteristics, pharmacological responses, and effects of radiofrequency ablation. Circulation 1999;100:1879–86.
[3] Jais P, Weerasooriya R, Shah DC, et al. Ablation therapy for atrial fibrillation (AF): past, present and future. Cardiovasc Res 2002;54:337–46.
[4] Marrouche NF, Dresing T, Cole C, et al. Circular mapping and ablation of the pulmonary vein for treatment of atrial fibrillation: impact of different catheter technologies. J Am Coll Cardiol 2002;40:464–74.
[5] Oral H, Scharf C, Chugh A, et al. Catheter ablation for paroxysmal atrial fibrillation: segmental pulmonary vein ostial ablation versus left atrial ablation. Circulation 2003;108:2355–60.
[6] Ouyang F, Bansch D, Ernst S, et al. Complete isolation of left atrium surrounding the pulmonary veins: new insights from the double-lasso technique in paroxysmal atrial fibrillation. Circulation 2004;110:2090–6.
[7] Callans DJ, Gerstenfeld EP, Dixit S, et al. Efficacy of repeat pulmonary vein isolation procedures in patients with recurrent atrial fibrillation. J Cardiovasc Electrophysiol 2004; 15:1050–6.
[8] Faddis MN, Chen J, Osborn J, et al. Magnetic guidance system for cardiac electrophysiology: a prospective trial of safety and efficacy in humans. J Am Coll Cardiol 2003;42:1952–8.
[9] Pappone C, Vicedomini G, Manguso F, et al. Robotic magnetic navigation for atrial fibrillation ablation. J Am Coll Cardiol 2006;47:1390–400.
[10] DiBiase L, Tahmy TS, Patel D, et al. Remote magnetic navigation: human experience in pulmonary vein ablation. J Am Coll Cardiol 2007;50:868–74.
[11] Al-Ahmad A, Grossman JD, Wang PJ. Early experience with a computerized robotically controlled catheter system. J Interv Card Electrophysiol 2005;12:199–202.
[12] Saliba W, Cummings JE, Oh S, et al. Novel robotic catheter remote control system: feasibility and safety of transseptal puncture and endocardial catheter navigation. J Cardiovasc Electrophysiol 2006;17:1–4.
[13] Reddy VY, Neuzil P, Malchano ZJ, et al. View-synchronized robotic image-guided therapy for atrial fibrillation ablation: experimental validation and clinical feasibility. Circulation 2007;115:2705–14.

[14] Mikaelian BJ, Malchano ZJ, Neuzil P, et al. Integration of 3-dimensional cardiac computed tomography images with real-time electroanatomic mapping to guide catheter ablation of atrial fibrillation. Circulation 2005;112:E35–6.

[15] Noseworthy PA, Malchano ZJ, Ahmed J, et al. The impact of respiration on left atrial and pulmonary venous anatomy: implications for image-guided intervention. Heart Rhythm 2005;2:1173–8.

[16] Tops LF, Bax JJ, Zeppenfeld K, et al. Fusion of multislice computed tomography imaging with three-dimensional electroanatomic mapping to guide radiofrequency catheter ablation procedures. Heart Rhythm 2005;7:1076–81.

[17] Kistler PM, Eaerley MJ, Harris S, et al. Validation of three-dimensional cardiac image integration: use of integrated CT image into electroanatomic mapping system to perform catheter ablation of atrial fibrillation. J Cardiovasc Electrophysiol 2006;17:341–8.

[18] Dong J, Dickfeld T, Dalal D, et al. Initial experience in the use of integrated electroanatomical mapping with three-dimensional MR/CT images to guide catheter ablation of atrial fibrillation. J Cardiovasc Electrophysiol 2006;17:459–66.

[19] Malchano ZJ, Neuzil P, Cury R, et al. Integration of cardiac CT/MR imaging with 3-dimensional electroanatomical mapping to guide catheter manipulation in the left atrium: implications for catheter ablation of atrial fibrillation. J Cardiovasc Electrophysiol 2006; 17:251–5.

[20] Orlov MV, Hoffmeister P, Chaudhry GM, et al. Three-dimensional rotational angiography of the left atrium and esophagus—a virtual computed tomography scan in the electrophysiology lab? Heart Rhythm 2007;4:37–43.

[21] Thiagalingam A, Manzke R, d'Avila A, et al. Intra-procedural volume imaging of the left atrium and pulmonary veins with rotational x-ray angiography. J Cardiovasc Electrophysiol, in press.

[22] Thiagalingam A, D'Avila A, Schmidt EJ, et al. Feasibility of MRI-guided mapping and pulmonary vein ablation in a swine model. Heart Rhythm 4(5S):S13.

[23] Natale A, Pisano E, Shewchik J, et al. First human experience with pulmonary vein isolation using a through-the-balloon circumferential ultrasound ablation system for recurrent atrial fibrillation. Circulation 2000;102:1879–82.

[24] Saliba W, Wilber D, Packer D, et al. Circumferential ultrasound ablation for pulmonary vein isolation: analysis of acute and chronic failures. J Cardiovasc Electrophysiol 2002;13: 957–61.

[25] Sarabanda AV, Bunch TJ, Johnson SB. Efficacy and safety of circumferential pulmonary vein isolation using a novel cryothermal balloon ablation system. J Am Coll Cardiol 2005; 46:1902–12.

[26] Reddy VY, Neuzil P, Pitschner HF, et al. Clinical experience with a balloon cryoablation catheter for pulmonary vein isolation in patients with atrial fibrillation: one-year results. Circulation 2005;112:II491–2.

[27] Reddy VY, Neuzil P, Themisotoclakis S, et al. Long-term single-procedure clinical results with an endoscopic balloon ablation catheter for pulmonary vein isolation in patients with atrial fibrillation. Circulation 2006;114:II747.

[28] Nakagawa H, Antz M, Wong T, et al. Initial experience using a forward directed, high-intensity focused ultrasound balloon catheter for pulmonary vein antrum isolation in patients with atrial fibrillation. J Cardiovasc Electrophysiol 2007;18:1–9.

[29] Satake S, Tanaka K, Saito S, et al. Usefulness of a new radiofrequency thermal balloon catheter for pulmonary vein isolation: a new device for treatment of atrial fibrillation. J Cardiovasc Electrophysiol 2003;14:609–15.

[30] Ahmed J, Sohal S, Malchano ZJ, et al. Three-dimensional analysis of pulmonary venous ostial and antral anatomy: implications for balloon catheter-based pulmonary vein isolation. J Cardiovasc Electrophysiol 2006;17:251–5.

[31] Konings KT, Smeets JL, Penn OC, et al. Configuration of unipolar atrial electrograms during electrically induced atrial fibrillation in humans. Circulation 1997;95:1231–41.

[32] Nademanee K, McKenzie J, Kosar E, et al. A new approach for catheter ablation of atrial fibrillation: mapping of the electrophysiologic substrate. J Am Coll Cardiol 2004;43: 2044–53.

[33] Haïssaguerre M, Sanders P, Hocini M, et al. Catheter ablation of long-lasting persistent atrial fibrillation: critical structures for termination. J Cardiovasc Electrophysiol 2005;16: 1125–37.

[34] Haïssaguerre M, Hocini M, Sanders P, et al. Catheter ablation of long-lasting persistent atrial fibrillation: clinical outcome and mechanisms of subsequent arrhythmias. J Cardiovasc Electrophysiol 2005;16:1138–47.

[35] Robbins IM, Colvin EV, Doyle TP, et al. Pulmonary vein stenosis after catheter ablation of atrial fibrillation. Circulation 1998;98:1769–75.

[36] Packer DL, Keelan P, Munger TM, et al. Clinical presentation, investigation, and management of pulmonary vein stenosis complicating ablation for atrial fibrillation. Circulation 2005;111:546–54.

[37] Tse HF, Reek S, Timmermans C, et al. Pulmonary vein isolation using transvenous catheter cryoablation for treatment of atrial fibrillation without risk of pulmonary vein stenosis. J Am Coll Cardiol 2003;42:752–8.

[38] Bai R, Patel D, Biase LD, et al. Phrenic nerve injury after catheter ablation: should we worry about this complication? J Cardiovasc Electrophysiol 2006;17:944–8.

[39] Doll N, Borger MA, Fabricius A, et al. Esophageal perforation during left atrial radiofrequency ablation: is the risk too high? J Thorac Cardiovasc Surg 2003;125:836–42.

[40] Sosa E, Scanavacca M. Left atrial-esophageal fistula complicating radiofrequency catheter ablation of atrial fibrillation. J Cardiovasc Electrophysiol 2005;16:249–50.

[41] Pappone C, Oral H, Santinelli V, et al. Atrio-esophageal fistula as a complication of percutaneous transcatheter ablation of atrial fibrillation. Circulation 2004;109:2724–6.

[42] Cummings JE, Schweikert RA, Saliba WI, et al. Brief communication: atrial-esophageal fistulas after radiofrequency ablation. Ann Intern Med 2006;144:572–4.

[43] Bunch TJ, Nelson J, Foley T, et al. Temporary esophageal stenting allows healing of esophageal perforations following atrial fibrillation ablation procedures. J Cardiovasc Electrophysiol 2006;17:435–9.

[44] Tsuchiya T, Ashikaga K, Nakagawa S, et al. Atrial fibrillation ablation with esophageal cooling with a cooled water-irrigated intraesophageal balloon: a pilot study. J Cardiovasc Electrophysiol 2007;18:145–50.

[45] Yokoyama K, Nakagawa H, Reddy VY, et al. Esophageal cooling balloon prevents esophageal injury during pulmonary vein ablation in a canine model. Heart Rhythm 4(5S): S12–S13.

[46] Oral H, Chugh A, Ozaydin M, et al. Risk of thromboembolic events after percutaneous left atrial radiofrequency ablation of atrial fibrillation. Circulation 2006;114:759–65.

[47] The Atrial Fibrillation Follow-up Investigation of Rhythm Management (AFFIRM) Investigators. A comparison of rate control and rhythm control in patients with atrial fibrillation. N Engl J Med 2002;347:1825–33.

[48] Sick PB, Schuler G, Hauptmann KE, et al. Initial worldwide experience with the WATCHMAN left atrial appendage system for stroke prevention in atrial fibrillation. J Am Coll Cardiol 2007;49:1490–5.

[49] Fountain RB, Holmes DR, Chandrasekaran K, et al. The PROTECT AF (WATCHMAN Left Atrial Appendage System for Embolic PROTECTion in Patients with Atrial Fibrillation) trial. Am Heart J 2006;151:956–61.

ELSEVIER
SAUNDERS

Med Clin N Am 92 (2008) 259–264

THE MEDICAL
CLINICS
OF NORTH AMERICA

Index

Note: Page numbers of article titles are in **boldface** type.